Praise for the Growing G.R.E.E.N. InterActions Program®

From a teacher:

The Growing G.R.E.E.N. InterActions program provides students with the opportunity to develop perspective-taking skills and to practice prosocial responses through role-play activities. The students in my class really enjoy the feeling of acting on stage. There are roles for everyone, including being the director, scene writers, movie characters, and audience members. The role-play activities provide students with the opportunity to practice new coping skills in a safe environment. There is nothing more enjoyable than to hear a student learn to use a response during the Growing G.R.E.E.N. InterActions program and generalize it to a situation.

Rosanne Lewton, Special Education Teacher

From a cotreating occupational therapist:

It has truly been a pleasure to have a collaborative relationship with Herb as he developed the G.R.E.E.N. approach. It has been enjoyable to watch the children learn and implement an approach that allows for proper expression of complex relation building ideas. The concepts and tools developed created a common language for all children and adults that opened successful positive communication where once there was an environment of closed and negative thoughts.

Mark Wilson, OTR, Occupational Therapist

From a cotreating counselor:

Working with Herb on Growing G.R.E.E.N. InterActions in the classroom was a fun and interactive way to teach our students about social skills and social communication. His approach to social communication is very helpful for all students regardless of primary diagnosis (i.e., ASD, ADHD, PTSD, Mood Disorder, ODD, etc.). Growing G.R.E.E.N. InterActions approaches communication using a framework from Cognitive Behavioral Therapy. It helps the student understand the processes behind specific interactions and the reasons why talking about the feelings of yourself and the feelings of others is important. It teaches kids how our behaviors do impact and affect the feelings, thoughts, and actions of those around us. Herb's approach is to help the students understand that everyone works as a team and how we affect one another. I think this is a much-needed aspect of social skills training. I highly recommend that SLPs, counselors, social workers, OTs, teachers and therapists use his curriculum in any school across the world.

Arielle Lugn, MA, PPS

Growing GREEN InterActions—*InterActive Lesson Book*

A Social Literacy Program to Be Our Better Selves in a Better World

Herb Hein, MMSc, CCC-SLP

Hein SLP, Inc. San Diego, California

Growing G.R.E.E.N. InterActions—*InterActive Lesson Book*

A Social Literacy Program to Be Our Better Selves in a Better World

Published by Hein SLP, Inc. San Diego, California

www.HeinSLPinc.com

Permissions, requests, and correspondence should be directed to the publisher.

ISBN-13: 978-0-9659878-1-3

This first edition printed in the United States of America.

Contents

1 Introduction

1.1 What Is the Growing G.R.E.E.N. InterActions Program? 1
1.2 Read and Discuss: What Does It Mean to Act G.R.E.E.N.? 2
1.3 Wise Action Tools Help You Act G.R.E.E.N. 5
1.4 Acting Civilized and G.R.E.E.N. during G.R.E.E.N. Team Lessons 5
1.5 Why Are Some Words in This Book in Different Colors? 7
1.6 What Does It Mean to Survey the Scene? 7
1.7 Survey the Scene: How Are These People Acting G.R.E.E.N.? 8

2 What Makes Our Civilization Work?

2.1 Read and Discuss: A Great Civilization Grows from People Working Together 11
2.2 Draw People Working Together in Our Civilization 12
2.3 Read and Discuss: Building Great Civilizations in Ancient Times 15
2.4 Draw Something Beautiful and Useful for Our Civilization 16
2.5 Read and Discuss: Civilization Goes Backward in the Dark Ages 17
2.6 Questions about Being Civil 19
2.7 Survey the Scene: Civilized Action or Not? 21

3 Growing Your Team Power

3.1 Read and Discuss: Who Is on Your Team? 23
3.2 Actions That Are Good for Everyone Help Everyone Win 25
3.3 Draw a Scene of Team Members Helping Each Other 26
3.4 Read and Discuss: What Is Your Potential to Have Team Power? 27

4 Helping Everyone Reach Common Team Goals

4.1 What Are Common Team Goals? 29

4.2 Typical Common Team Goals 29

5 Tracking Your G.R.E.E.N. Actions for the Team

5.1 Why Act G.R.E.E.N. with Your Teams? 33

5.2 Start Tracking G.R.E.E.N. Action—What's Your Baseline? 34

5.3 Self-Evaluation: How G.R.E.E.N. Am I Acting Today? 35

5.4 Getting Feedback from Others: How G.R.E.E.N. Do You Think I Am Acting Today? 35

5.5 Using G.R.E.E.N. Action Reports 37

5.6 What Are Personal and Team G.R.E.E.N. Action Trackers? 39

6 The Importance of Team Rules

6.1 Read and Discuss: Keeping the Civil in Civilization Requires Rules 45

6.2 Each Team Has Its Own Rules to Follow 46

7 Being Your Best Self with Personal Goals

7.1 Read and Discuss: Being Your Best Self in Your Best Life 53

7.2 Setting Personal Goals for Your Own Best Life 58

7.3 How to Choose a Goal Area to Improve Your Life! 59

7.4 Read and Discuss: Being Honest and Realistic to Achieve Your Goals 60

7.5 Reviewing and Choosing Personal Goals 61

7.6 Some Great Personal Goals for School Scenes 61

7.7 Some Great Personal Goals for Home Scenes 62

7.8 Some Great Personal Goals for Friendship Scenes 63

7.9 Examples of Goals That People Set for Themselves 64

7.10 Take Positive Action to Take the Next Step Forward! 68

7.11 Survey the Scene: Positive or Negative Action in the School Scene 69

7.12 Survey the Scene: Positive or Negative Action in the Home Scene 70

8 Achieving Personal Goals and Common Team Goals

8.1 Achieving Your Personal Goals and Common Team Goals! 71
8.2 Survey the Scene: Basketball Practice at Home—Which Action Choices Let John Achieve Both Goals at Home? 72
8.3 Survey the Scene: Asking Questions—Which Action Choice Lets Trent Achieve Both Goals in Class? 74

9 Getting Power from Guiding G.R.E.E.N. Thoughts®

9.1 What Is a Guiding G.R.E.E.N. Thought®? 77
9.2 Reaching Up for a Guiding G.R.E.E.N. Thought 77
9.3 Guiding G.R.E.E.N. Thoughts for G.R.E.E.N. Action 79
9.4 Practice Makes Perfect 80
9.5 Strategy: Challenge Your Memory for Guiding G.R.E.E.N. Thoughts 84

10 Examples of Guiding G.R.E.E.N. Thoughts® to Use

GRATEFUL 87
RESPECTFUL 88
EMPATHETIC 89
EASYGOING 90
NAVIGATING 91

11 Thinking First to Make the Best Choices

11.1 Read and Discuss: You Have the Power to Make Your Team Great 93
11.2 Positive and Negative Consequences of Your Actions 95
11.3 Survey the Scene: Will These Actions Lead to Positive or Negative Consequences? 96
11.4 Read and Discuss: What Is a R.E.D. Interaction? 98
11.5 Survey the Scene: Is This Action G.R.E.E.N. or R.E.D.? 100
11.6 Read and Discuss: Drivers Learn to Take G.R.E.E.N. Actions on the Road 103
11.7 Read and Discuss: Red Lights and G.R.E.E.N. Lights Are in Your Brain! 104
11.8 You Can Think First with Your Powerful Brain! 107

11.9 Do You Think First or Do You Act Impulsively? ... 108
11.10 Survey the Scene: Is This Action Thoughtful or Impulsive? ... 108
11.11 Using the Civilized Choice Checker to Make the Best Choices for the Team 109
11.12 Making Choices That Are Logical, Safe, and Good for Everyone ... 111
11.13 Logical or Illogical? ... 112
11.14 Survey the Scene! Are These Actions Logical or Illogical? ... 113
11.15 Survey the Scene: Are the Actions in These Scenes Good for Everyone? ... 115
11.16 Guiding G.R.E.E.N. Thoughts for Actions That Are Logical, Safe, and Good for Everyone ... 117

12 Getting Ready for G.R.E.E.N. Scene Action
12.1 Why Are We Acting in G.R.E.E.N. Scenes? ... 119
12.2 Making the Best G.R.E.E.N. Scenes ... 120
12.3 Rules for Acting in G.R.E.E.N. Scenes ... 122
12.4 Using the G.R.E.E.N. Scene Review Form ... 122
12.5 G.R.E.E.N. Scene Warm-Ups ... 123
12.6 Start with Quick G.R.E.E.N. Scenes ... 126
12.7 Directions for Quick G.R.E.E.N. Scenes ... 126
12.8 Quick G.R.E.E.N. Scene Score Sheet—Basic G.R.E.E.N. Skills ... 127
12.9 Basic G.R.E.E.N. Skills Score Sheet: ... 128
12.10 Quick Grateful G.R.E.E.N. Scene ... 128
12.11 Quick Respectful G.R.E.E.N. Scene ... 130
12.12 Quick Empathetic G.R.E.E.N. Scene ... 131
12.13 Quick Easygoing G.R.E.E.N. Scene ... 132
12.14 Quick Navigating G.R.E.E.N. Scene ... 133

13 Self-Calming Strategies
13.1 Learning How to Get Calm ... 135
13.2 Check Yourself! Are You Calm Enough to Think First? ... 136
13.3 Guiding G.R.E.E.N. Thought: I Use Feedback to Get Calm ... 137
13.4 Powerful Self-Calming Strategies ... 138

13.5 You Can Think First after Your Calming Break! ... 142
13.6 Picture a Peaceful Scene to Help Yourself Stay Calm ... 143
13.7 G.R.E.E.N. Scene #1 ... 147

14 Flipping the Switch for Self-Control

14.1 Read and Discuss: Powerful Humans Have Self-Control to Act Safely ... 151
14.2 Step on the Brake and Flip the Switch! ... 153
14.3 Survey the Scene: Who Needs Their Switch Flipped for Self-Control? ... 154
14.4 Guiding G.R.E.E.N. Thought: I Control My Own Body So No One Else Is Bothered ... 155
14.5 Bothering Someone or Not! What Are the Consequences? ... 156
14.6 Things to Do before G.R.E.E.N. Scene #2 ... 158
14.7 Guiding G.R.E.E.N. Thought Choices for G.R.E.E.N. Scene #2 ... 160
14.8 Things to Do before G.R.E.E.N. Scene #3: ... 162

15 Making Powerful Transformations

15.1 Guiding G.R.E.E.N. Thought: I Make Transformations to Improve the Scene 167
15.2 Transform Yourself to Reconnect with Others ... 169
15.3 A Transformation Story: A Solitary R.E.D. Brain Is Transformed ... 172
15.4 When to Use the Thought Transformation Scene Changer ... 174
15.5 How to Use the Thought Transformation Scene Changer ... 175
15.6 Survey the Scene: What Changes Are Needed for G.R.E.E.N. Scene #4? .. 177
15.7 Change the Scene to Make It G.R.E.E.N.: Help Travis Make a Transformation ... 178
15.8 Help Travis Choose Guiding G.R.E.E.N. Thoughts for His Transformation ... 179
15.9 G.R.E.E.N. Scene #4: I Can Follow Your Plan ... 180
15.10 A Word Problem for Travis to Use in G.R.E.E.N. Scene #4 ... 182

16 T.O.P. Ideas Help You Make Transformations

16.1 T.O.P. Ideas: Think First, Be Open-Minded, and Be Positive ... 183
16.2 G.R.E.E.N. Scene #5: Thirsty but Still Thinking First (Remember Team Rules before You Act) ... 184

16.3 G.R.E.E.N. Scene #5: Thirsty but Still Thinking First! ... 185
16.4 Choosing Guiding G.R.E.E.N. Thoughts for G.R.E.E.N. Scene #5 ... 186
16.5 Be Open-Minded to New Ideas ... 187
16.6 G.R.E.E.N. Scene #6: Open-Minded Like Oscar! ... 188
16.7 Choosing Guiding G.R.E.E.N. Thoughts for G.R.E.E.N. Scene #6 ... 189
16.8 Be Positive; Things Will Get Better! ... 190
16.9 G.R.E.E.N. Scene #7: Acting Positive Makes It Better ... 190
16.10 G.R.E.E.N. Scene #7: Acting Positive Makes It Better ... 191
16.11 Choosing G.R.E.E.N. Thoughts for G.R.E.E.N. Scene #7 ... 192

17 Being Grateful

17.1 Acting in a Grateful Way ... 193
17.2 Guiding G.R.E.E.N. Thoughts for Acting Grateful ... 195
17.3 Telling What We Are Grateful for Is Powerful ... 195
17.4 Survey the Scene: Using Grateful Words and Actions for Getting Help with Math ... 197
17.5 Survey the Scene: Using Grateful Words and Actions to Get Help during a Sad Time ... 198
17.6 Survey the Scene: Using Grateful Words and Actions for Getting Help Playing Basketball ... 199
17.7 Change the Scene to Make It G.R.E.E.N.: Help Lily Get Help ... 200
17.8 G.R.E.E.N. Scene #8: Help Lily Say, "I Am Grateful for Your Help!" ... 201
17.9 Change the Scene to Make It G.R.E.E.N.: Greedy or Grateful for Ice Cream? ... 202
17.10 Change the Scene to Make It G.R.E.E.N.: Is One Enough? ... 206
17.11 G.R.E.E.N. Scene #9: Thank You! One Is Enough for Me ... 207

18 Learning to Respectfully Respond to Others

18.1 Add Respect to Your Interactions! ... 209
18.2 What Does It Mean to Be Respectful? ... 209
18.3 Guiding G.R.E.E.N. Thoughts for Being Respectful ... 210

18.4 Ways to Act Respectfully 211
18.5 Survey the Scene: Choose to Act Respectfully.... 212
18.6 Quick G.R.E.E.N. Scenes for Eye Contact and Quick Responses.... 214
18.7 Change the Scene to Make It G.R.E.E.N.!: Help Matthew Respectfully Answer.... 215
18.8 Change the Scene to Make It G.R.E.E.N. at School: Please Answer My Question 217
18.9 Change the Scene to Make It G.R.E.E.N. at School: Tell Me You Need More Time 219
18.10 Change the Scene to Make It G.R.E.E.N. at School: Please Tell Me You Didn't Hear Me....222
18.11 Change the Scene to Make It G.R.E.E.N. at School: Ask Me to Help You Understand 224

19 Respectfully Choosing Topic, Volume, and Tone of Voice

19.1 Being Respectful by Staying On-Topic....227
19.2 Using the On-Topic Tracker for a Respectful Conversation 228
19.3 Change the Scene to Make It G.R.E.E.N.!: Help Julia Be On-Topic 230
19.4 Being Respectful by Talking about Someone Else's Preferred Topic.... 231
19.5 Why Choose the Best Voice Volume for Each Scene?....236
19.6 Survey the Scene: What Is the Best Voice Volume for This Situation? 237
19.7 Guiding G.R.E.E.N. Thoughts for a Respectful Tone of Voice....238
19.8 Telling the Truth Leads to Positive Consequences 240
19.9 Change the Scene to Make It G.R.E.E.N.: Help Charlie Ask Politely Instead of Demand 241
19.10 Survey the Scene: Can You Tell the Difference Between Politely Asking and Demanding? 243
19.11 Should I Be Serious or Funny in This Conversation? 244
19.12 Read and Discuss: Sincere and Serious, or Sarcastic?....245
19.13 Change the Scene: What Can Be Said Instead of Sarcastic Words? 246
19.17 Read and Discuss: Hein Conversational Rating Scale....256

19.18 Change the Scene and Make It G.R.E.E.N.: Help Mark Be Respectful and Responsible 257

19.19 Survey the Scene: How Is Samantha Acting with Her School Team? 261

19.20 Change the Scene: Help Samantha Be a More Respectful Team Member 262

19.21 Quick G.R.E.E.N. Scenes: Showing Samantha How to Be Respectful in Class 263

20 Learning How to Be More Empathetic

20.1 What Does It Mean to Be Empathetic? 265

20.2 How to Be Empathetic 266

20.3 Why Act Empathetically? 267

20.5 Underline Red or Green: Which Actions Show Empathy for Others? 270

21 Survey the Scene: Infer How Others Feel

21.1 Making Inferences by Surveying the Scene 271

21.2 With Practice, You Can Notice How People Feel 272

21.3 How to Survey the Scene to Match Your Words with Their Feelings 273

21.4 Survey the Scene and Choose Empathetic Words at Home 274

21.5 Survey the Scene and Choose Empathetic Words at School 278

21.6 Survey the Scene and Choose Empathetic Words with Friends 281

21.7 Steps for Being Empathetic in Quick G.R.E.E.N. Scenes 284

21.8 Directions for Quick Empathetic G.R.E.E.N. Scenes 285

21.9 Quick G.R.E.E.N. Scene Challenge: Making Supportive Comments with My Teams 286

21.10 Acting Empathetic at Home 286

21.11 Acting Empathetic at School 288

21.12 Acting Empathetic with Your Friend 289

21.13 Quick G.R.E.E.N. Scene Tracking Sheet: How Well Did I Support My Teammates with Supportive Comments? 290

22 Expanding Empathy and Support with Peers

22.1 Expanding Your Vocabulary of Feelings 291
22.2 Survey the Scene and Choose Your Feeling Words: Situations 1–5 292
22.3 Survey the Scene and Choose Your Feeling Words: Situations 6–10 294
22.4 Using Different Supportive Words to Match the Situation 298
22.5 Survey the Scene and Choose the Best Words for Each Situation................ 299
22.6 Directions for Quick G.R.E.E.N. Scenes for Supporting Peers...................... 300
22.7 Quick G.R.E.E.N. Scenes: Showing Support for Peers!................................ 301
22.8 Keeping Track: How Supportive Was I with My Peers? 302
22.9 Choosing a Supportive Scene for Eddie 302
22.10 G.R.E.E.N. Scene #10: Write a Supportive Scene for Eddie 304
22.11 Read and Discuss: Really Winning by Showing Good Sportsmanship 305
22.12 Survey the Scene: What to Say after the Game.. 307
22.13 Showing Empathy by Making Comments and Asking Questions 308
22.14 Building a Bridge to a Related Topic in an Empathetic Conversation........... 309
22.15 Take These Steps for an Empathetic Conversation: 310
22.16 Fill in the Blanks: Steps to Take in an Empathetic Conversation 311
22.17 G.R.E.E.N. Scene #11: Write It and Act It Out: No One to Play With 312
22.18 G.R.E.E.N. Scene #12: Write It and Act It Out: Help! I Lost the Key! 313
22.19 G.R.E.E.N. Scene #13: Write It and Act It Out: Help Me Carry the Load! .. 314
22.20 G.R.E.E.N. Scene #14: Write It and Act It Out: Please Help Me Remember 315
22.21 G.R.E.E.N. Scene #15: Write It and Act It Out: Please Help Me Play Better 316

23 Being Easygoing

23.1 What Is Easygoing? 317
23.2 Guiding G.R.E.E.N. Thoughts: Ways to Be Easygoing 318
23.3 Change the Scene to Make It G.R.E.E.N.: Please Help Steve Cooperate!.... 320
23.4 G.R.E.E.N. Scene #16: I Cooperate with a Positive Attitude 322
23.5 Change the Scene to Make It G.R.E.E.N.: Please Help Marco Share!.......... 323
23.6 Scene #17: I Share the Ball with My Team... 325

24 Take Steps to Make Connections with Teams

24.1 Thinking of Being on Friendship Teams 327
24.2 Read and Discuss: Why Do Humans Have Friends? 328
24.3 What Common Team Goals Can You Share with Your Friends? 329
24.4 Survey the Scene: Are They Connecting to Friendship Teams or Disconnecting from Them? 331
24.5 Using the Connection Direction Tracker: Am I Moving Forward or Backward with My Team? 333
24.6 Quick G.R.E.E.N. Scenes: Connecting on a Home Team 336
24.7 Quick G.R.E.E.N. Scenes: Connecting on a Classroom Team 338
24.8 Quick G.R.E.E.N. Scenes: Connecting on Friendship Teams 340
24.9 Survey the Scene at Dinnertime—Scene #1: Who Is Connecting on the Home Team? 343
24.10 Survey the Scene at Dinnertime—Scene #2: Who Is Disconnecting from the Home Team? 345

25 Being Easygoing When You Have Mixed Feelings

25.1 Read and Discuss: Having Mixed Feelings 347
25.2 Using Wise Action Tools to Take Positive Outside Action 349
25.3 Drawing Your Choices to Help Show Positive Outside Action Control! 350
25.4 Show Positive Outside Action Control to Act Generous, Not Jealous 352
25.5 Guiding G.R.E.E.N. Thoughts about Sharing While Controlling Selfish, Jealous Feelings 354
25.6 G.R.E.E.N. Scene #17: I Act Friendly with My Friend's Other Friend 355

26 Sharing Points of View

26.1 Read and Discuss: Different People Have Different Points of View 357
26.2 Survey the Scene: Different Points of View about Waiting in Line 358
26.3 Survey the Scene: Different Points of View about Setting the Table 360
26.4 The Necessary Ingredients for a Cooperative Conversation 362
26.5 Survey the Scene: Is This a Cooperative Conversation? 364

26.6 Survey the Scene: Can Everyone Get Their Needs Met When Justin Gets Home? 367

26.7 Survey the Scene: Birthday Plans Need to Change 369

26.8 G.R.E.E.N. Scene #18: Write Your Own Cooperative Conversation Scene about Changing Birthday Plans 370

26.9 Read and Discuss: Being Easygoing When Receiving Feedback 371

26.10 Survey the Scene: Seeing Point of View about Following Advice 373

26.11 Accepting Advice or Not: Help Alan Make the Wisest Choice 375

26.12 G.R.E.E.N. Scene #19: Write Your Own Script to Accept Advice 378

26.13 Change the Scene to Make It G.R.E.E.N.!: Accepting Advice to Go to Bed Earlier 379

26.14 Change the Scene to Make It G.R.E.E.N.: Please Set the Table, Tommy! 380

26.15 G.R.E.E.N. Scene #20: Write a Better Scene with Tommy Asking to Quickly Save His Work before Doing a Chore 382

27 Is It Time for a Compromise?

27.1 Read and Discuss: What Does It Mean to Make a Compromise? 383

27.2 Survey the Scene: Is this a Time for a Compromise? Late for School 385

27.3 Survey the Scene: Is this a Time for a Compromise? Setting the Table 386

27.4 Survey the Scene: Is this a Time for a Compromise? While Watching a Show 387

27.5 Guiding G.R.E.E.N. Thoughts for Compromising 388

27.6 Survey the Scene: Help Roger and Carlos Make a Compromise 390

27.7 Drawing the Steps of the Compromise Plan: Please Wait to Tell Me after Class 390

28 What Does It Mean to Be Navigating?

28.1 Guiding G.R.E.E.N. Thoughts to Help You Navigate Successfully 394

29 Wait for the Best Time to Act

29.1 It Helps to Know Why You Must Wait 396

29.2 I Can Think of Why I Must Wait 397

29.3 G.R.E.E.N. Scene #21: I Wait for the Best Time to Act 398

29.4 The Scene: I Wait for the Best Time to Act! ... 398
29.5 Guiding G.R.E.E.N. Thought Choices for G.R.E.E.N. Scene #21 ... 399

30 Ask for Help When You Need It

30.1 Asking for Help Can Be Helpful! ... 401
30.2 Being Open-Minded to Ask for Help ... 402
30.3 How Much Help Do You Need? ... 403
30.4 Change the Scene to Make It G.R.E.E.N.: Tommy Doesn't Understand the Directions! ... 407
30.5 G.R.E.E.N. Scene #22: I Get Calm and Ask for Help ... 409

31 Accepting When Someone Tells Me "No"

31.1 You Can Accept When Someone Tells You "No" When You Know Why ... 413
31.2 Thinking of Reasons Why People Say "No" ... 414
31.3 G.R.E.E.N. Scene #23: Why Did Kevin's Parents Say "No"? ... 415
31.4 G.R.E.E.N. Scene #24: Let's Navigate Past the Word "No" ... 418
31.5 The Scene: Let's Navigate Past the Word "No" ... 419
31.6 The Writing Assignment That Needs to Be Finished ... 421
31.7 Write Guiding G.R.E.E.N. Thoughts You Think Carl Chose to Make a Transformation ... 422

32 Adjusting to Changes

32.1 Adjusting to Changes by Being Open-Minded ... 425
32.2 Survey the Scene: Helping Nathan Adjust to Changes at School ... 426
32.3 Guiding G.R.E.E.N. Thoughts for Nathan to Choose ... 427
32.4 Thought Transformation Scene Changer for Nathan ... 429
32.5 Stating What Is Being Learned ... 430
32.6 Positive Reinforcement for Acting G.R.E.E.N. ... 430

Glossary ... 435

Musical Transcriptions ... 447

SONGS

Keep the Civil in Civilization 20
Wake Up 57
Guiding G.R.E.E.N. Thought Song 83
What's Best for the Team? 97
Brake to Take a 5 Break 141
Don't Listen to the Moon 171
Transformation Song 173
I Appreciate 196
I Don't Ignore You 213
It's Not All about Me 268
Cooperation's in the Air 319
You Are a Friend of Mine 330

Wise Action Tools

G.R.E.E.N. Token Tracker 6

Who Is on a Team with You? 24

Our Common Team Goals 31

G.R.E.E.N. Actions Evaluation Chart 36

G.R.E.E.N. Action Report 38

My Personal G.R.E.E.N. Action Tracker 40

Classroom Team G.R.E.E.N. Action Tracker 41

Home Team G.R.E.E.N. Action Tracker 42

Work Team G.R.E.E.N. Action Tracker 43

Our Classroom Team Rules 49

Our Home Team Rules 50

Our Friendship Team Rules 51

Our Work Team Rules 52

Self-Check: Are You Making Your Best Life Story? 54

Picture Your Own Best Life! 56

My Personal Goal Worksheet 66

Noting Progress on My Personal Goals 67

Ready, Set, Goal! My Goal for Right Now 81

I Draw Myself Using a Guiding G.R.E.E.N. Thought 82

Guiding G.R.E.E.N. Thought Memory Challenge 85

Civilized Choice Checker 110

Surveying the Scene before Taking Action 121

G.R.E.E.N. Scene Review Form 125

Brake to Take a 5 Break 139
Peaceful Scenes to Help Me Stay Calm 144
Creating My Own Self-Calming Scene 145
This Is How I Look after I Use a Self-Calming Strategy 146
Self-Calming by Quietly Squeezing a Fidget 157
Writing Your Own Guiding G.R.E.E.N. Thought for Self-Control 161
My Own Guiding G.R.E.E.N. Thought for Having Self-Control to Stop Harmful Action 165
Thought Transformation Scene Changer 176
Appreciation Box 194
Please Tell Me Something Right Away When I Ask you a Question! 216
On-Topic Tracker 229
Take the Conversation Power Challenge! 232
Building My Conversation Power by Paying Attention, Asking Questions & Taking Notes ... 233
Topics for Caring Conversations 234
Voice Volume Chart 235
Hein Conversational Rating Scale 255
Connection Direction Tracker 334
Name Mixed Feelings and Think of Action Consequences 348
Show Positive Outside Action Control! 351
Cooperative Conversation Ingredients Checklist 363
I Accept Constructive Feedback in These Areas 372
Worksheet for Making a G.R.E.E.N. Team Compromise 389
Charting How Much Help I Need Today 406
Lesson Log for What I Am Learning 431
Growing G.R.E.E.N. Certificate 432

1 Introduction

1.1 What Is the Growing G.R.E.E.N. InterActions Program?

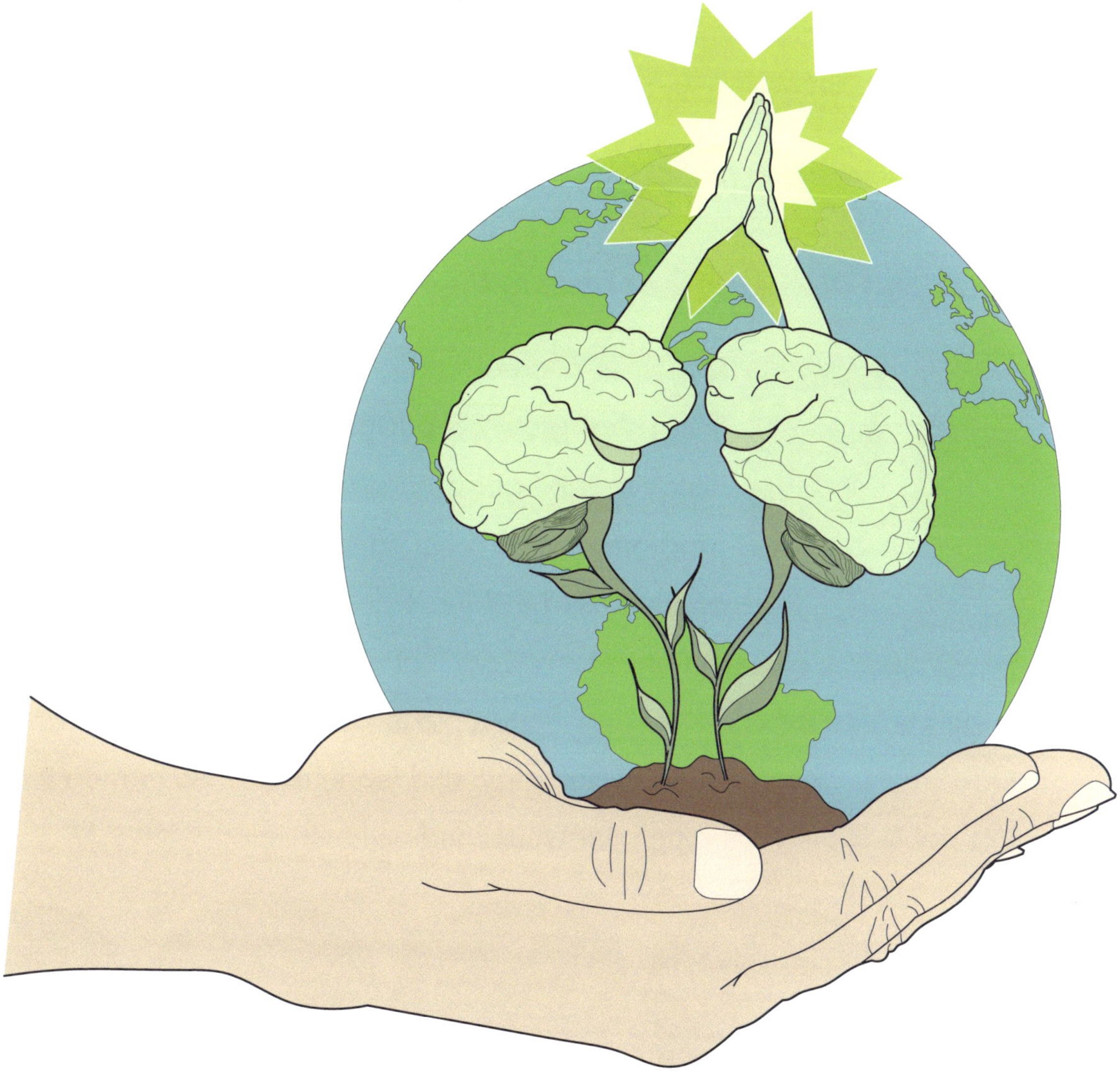

Growing G.R.E.E.N. InterActions is a program designed to help you become a **positive** member of your world.

By paying attention to the lessons and participating in the activities of the **Growing G.R.E.E.N. InterActions** Program, you will find yourself growing. This program does not focus on growth in height or weight—its **goal** is for you to grow in using your **powerful** brain to think about people around you being on a Team with you. You will learn to be **thoughtful** instead of impulsive. You will grow in your ability to make choices to say and do things that make any situation **better** for you and others on your Teams. You will have the chance to analyze and act out scenes to practice your skills. You will learn the skills and strategies needed to be **G.R.E.E.N.**: **Grateful**, **Respectful**, **Empathetic**, **Easygoing**, and **Navigating**. Get ready to be **open-minded** so you can help yourself, your Team, and our civilization grow in the best possible ways.

Thank you for being part of this program!

1.2 Read and Discuss: What Does It Mean to Act G.R.E.E.N.?

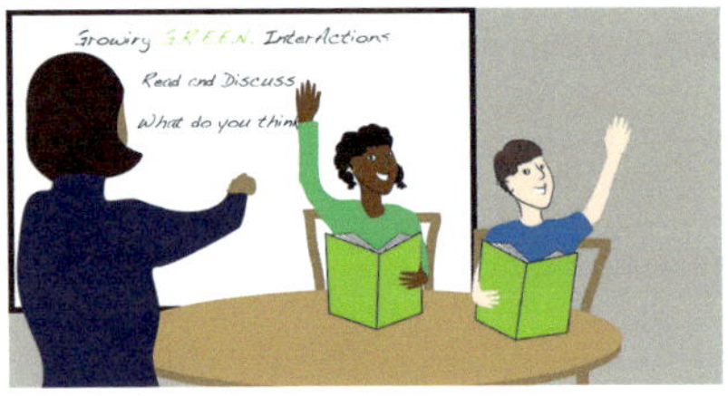

Green is a great color. It is the color of many wonderful things that grow on our planet. Being green means we do things to take good care of our home, planet Earth. In this program, **G.R.E.E.N.** stands for acting to take care of one another. **G.R.E.E.N.** is an acronym, meaning that each letter—**G**, **R**, **E**, **E**, and **N**—stands for a word that reminds us how to act when we want to do our best for ourselves and the people in our lives. We can learn to act more **G.R.E.E.N.** where we live, learn, play, and work; really, we can do it anywhere. We act **G.R.E.E.N.** through our words and actions:

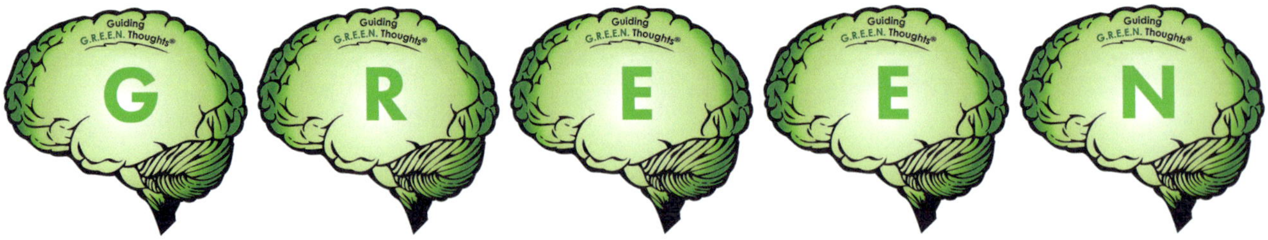

Grateful **Respectful** **Empathetic** **Easygoing** **Navigating**

Grateful means appreciating what we have. You interact **gratefully** when you say and do things that show you are **thankful** for what you have. You **appreciate** what you have and the people with you. When you and the people around you act **grateful**, you let one another know with your words and actions that you are glad to be in one another's lives.

Respectful means choosing our words carefully. You interact **respectfully** when you **treat people politely** and recognize their right to be just as safe as you are and to work on their **Personal Goals**. When you are **respectful**, you listen when people talk so they know that you have heard them. When you and the people around you **respect** one another, you take the time to hear their words.

Empathetic means caring about how others feel. Interacting **empathetically** shows that you care about the feelings of the people you are with. You take time to understand their feelings and do your best to think about their feelings when you interact with them.

Easygoing means working together toward **common goals**. When you are **easy-going**, you are **cooperative**. You do your best to work easily and peacefully with others, acknowledging that they are on your Team and working with you to meet **Common Team Goals**. You learn to **take turns** and **share** with others.

Navigating means using our **powerful** brains to choose the best things to say and do when challenges cross our path as we try to move **forward**. You are **navigating** when you find ways to manage any challenges and keep moving forward without getting upset. You use strategies to control yourself. You think about self-guiding thoughts and use words that help you move through challenging life scenes successfully.

Matching G.R.E.E.N. to the Meaning of G.R.E.E.N.

Use a green pencil to help each person connect their G.R.E.E.N. brains with the meaning of being G.R.E.E.N.

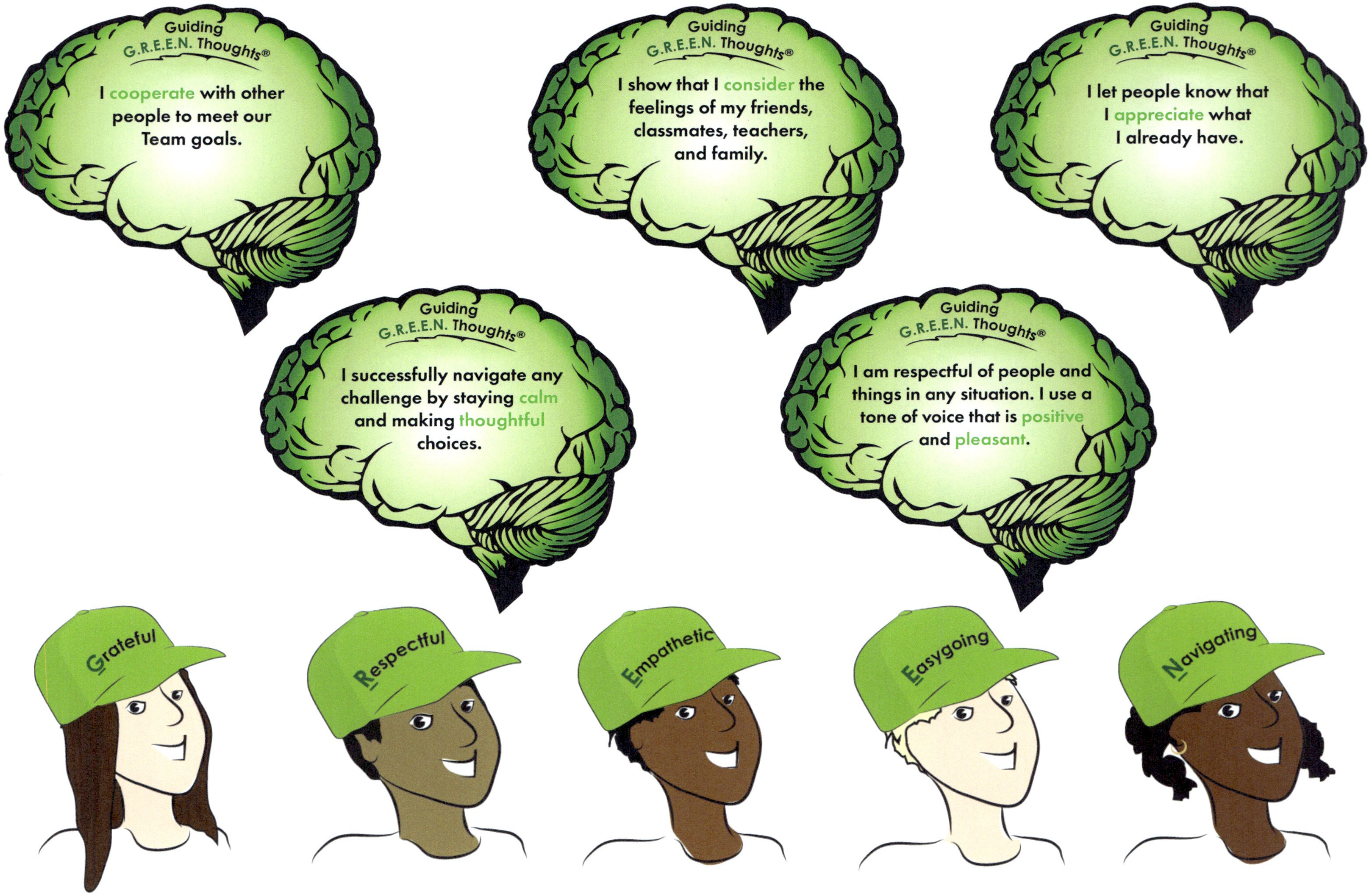

1.3 Wise Action Tools Help You Act G.R.E.E.N.

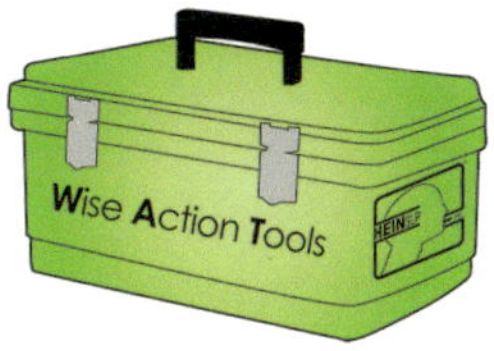

Wise Action Tools are pages that you can view, think about, write on, and draw on to help you take the best actions when you are with people. The **Growing G.R.E.E.N. InterActions** Program has many Wise Action Tools, which your guide will help you use in future lessons.

The first Wise Action Tool is the **G.R.E.E.N.** Token Tracker! This Wise Action Tool helps you and your guide track how **G.R.E.E.N.** you are acting during lessons. Keep focused and act **G.R.E.E.N.** to fill all the circles with **green** tokens.

1.4 Acting Civilized and G.R.E.E.N. during G.R.E.E.N. Team Lessons

It is easy to learn to act more **G.R.E.E.N.** with others. When you act civilized and **G.R.E.E.N.**, your teaching guide can give you **green** tokens to let you know that you have been successful. In each lesson, your **goal** will be to collect at least five **green** tokens on the Token Tracker by showing that you can be civilized and **G.R.E.E.N.** Getting **green** tokens is easy when you listen to your guide and follow their directions.

When you get a token, put it right on top of a circle on the Token Tracker. You will be challenged to practice your **self-control** by leaving the tokens on the circles. If the circles fall on the floor, they won't count! When you get a token on each of the five **G.R.E.E.N.** words, you can be proud of yourself. Your teaching guide will reward you for making choices to act **civilized** and **G.R.E.E.N.** as you work together with your Team.

It is up to you to work on getting all five tokens during a lesson. Your teaching guide will notice how you act during the lesson. If you don't get all five tokens, you will have a chance to think about what you can do better to get all five tokens during the next lesson.

For more advanced lessons, you may need to fill your card two or three times before you get a reward. Your guide will tell you the number of tokens you will need for each lesson.

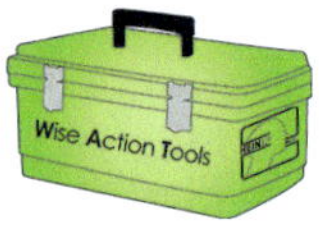

G.R.E.E.N. Token Tracker

I AM CIVILIZED & G.R.E.E.N.

G rateful — **Grateful**—I appreciate what I have

R espectful — **Respectful**—I am polite and well mannered

E mpathetic — **Empathetic**—I care about the feelings of others

E asygoing — **Easygoing**—I am cooperative

N avigating — **Navigating**—I use strategies to cope with challenges

1.5 Why Are Some Words in This Book in Different Colors?

To help you see signals while you read this book, words related to **helpful, positive G.R.E.E.N.** actions are in **green,** whereas those related to negative, **R.E.D.** actions are in red.

Words related to **self-control** are in **purple** to indicate that you are using your **power** to control how you act. **Purple** also is found whenever your **powerful** human brain is mentioned. You use your **powerful** human brain to **flip the switch** to make **transformations** and **change** your actions to make better choices.

Having **self-control** when deciding on and making important **changes** and **transformations** helps you achieve **goals**, which are in **gold**.

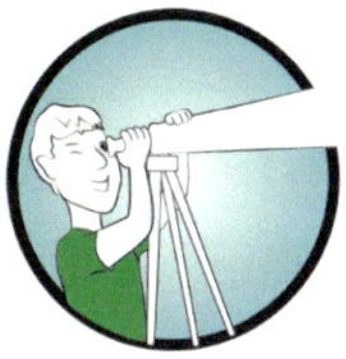

By **surveying the scene** around you, you will become aware of what is happening within you. You will be able to make the best action choices. When you are asked to **survey the scene**, the color will be **blue.**

The colored signals in these lessons help make it easier for you to learn to act G.R.E.E.N. with your Teams as we work together to make a great civilization.

1.6 What Does It Mean to Survey the Scene?

In the **Growing G.R.E.E.N. InterActions** Program, you will learn to do your best job of **surveying the scene**. What does it mean to **survey the scene**?

Before a civilization can build something great, a person called a surveyor must check out the land to determine whether buildings and roads can be built logically and safely. The surveyor makes sure that whatever is built can last a long time. This makes buildings and roads better.

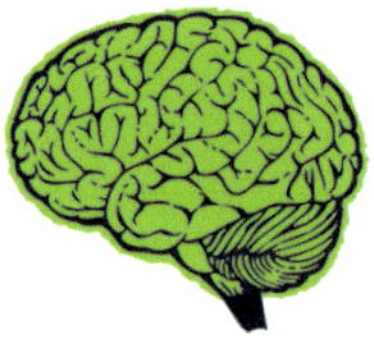

Because you have a human brain, you have the **power** to **survey the scene** before taking any action. But you don't use surveying equipment like that used by a surveyor. Instead, you **use your eyes to see** and **your ears to listen to what is happening around you**. You can see who else is on your Team and what everyone is trying to do in the scene. You then make your best guess about what others want and need. By **surveying the scene**, you can take your best action and work together with your Team to make the best possible scene!

In the **Growing G.R.E.E.N. InterActions** Program, you will be asked to find clues about how other people feel. You will learn to find the words in sentences, scenarios, and G.R.E.E.N. Scenes that will help you understand how people are acting. This allows you to tell how they and the people around them might feel.

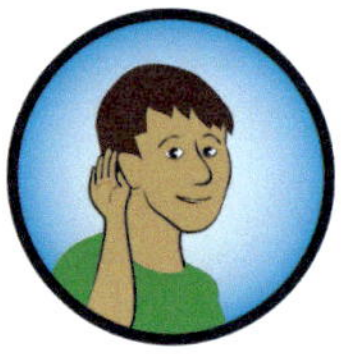

1.7 Survey the Scene: How Are These People Acting G.R.E.E.N.?

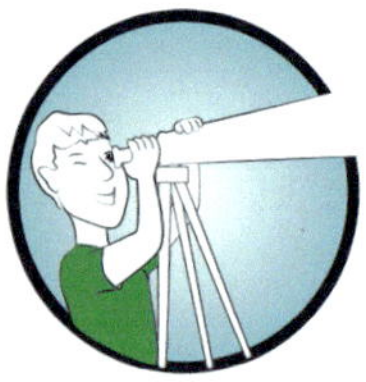

Survey the scene below and see if you can tell how these people are acting and feeling. As you learn more in this program, you can return to this activity to see what else you have learned about acting G.R.E.E.N., and how G.R.E.E.N. actions affect others.

Directions: Can you recognize different kinds of G.R.E.E.N. action? Underline G.R.E.E.N. actions with a green pencil. Then circle the G.R.E.E.N. behavior that tells how the people were acting. You may circle more than one G.R.E.E.N. behavior for these questions:

1. Josh thanked his brother for the gift.

   A. How was Josh acting?

   Grateful **Respectful** **Empathetic** **Easygoing** **Navigating**

   B. How did Josh's words make his brother feel? ______________________________

   ____

2. Katrina listened while her grandfather told her about something that happened to him a long time ago.

   A. How was Katrina acting?

   Grateful **Respectful** **Empathetic** **Easygoing** **Navigating**

   B. How did Katrina's actions make her grandfather feel? ____________________

   ____

3. Carl took turns using the magnifying glass with his brother.

   A. How was Carl acting?

   Grateful **Respectful** **Empathetic** **Easygoing** **Navigating**

   B. How did Carl's actions make his brother feel? ____________________

   ____

4. Paul congratulated his classmate for winning the "Student of the Week" award, even though he thought he was going to win it himself.

   A. How was Paul acting?

   Grateful **Respectful** **Empathetic** **Easygoing** **Navigating**

   B. How did Paul's actions make his classmate feel? ____________________

   ____

5. Sarah told Audrey that she couldn't be her partner in the dance competition because she had sprained her ankle. Audrey told Sarah that she hoped she felt better soon and told her not to worry about it because there was enough time to find a replacement partner to practice with.

   A. How was Audrey acting?

   Grateful Respectful Empathetic Easygoing Navigating

   B. How did Audrey's words make Sarah feel? ______________________________

   ____

6. When Mark arrived late to a rock-climbing party, John let him go in front of him so that he could have the next turn climbing the wall.

   A. How was John acting?

   Grateful Respectful Empathetic Easygoing Navigating

   B. How did John's actions make Mark feel? ______________________________

   ____

2 What Makes Our Civilization Work?

2.1 Read and Discuss: A Great Civilization Grows from People Working Together

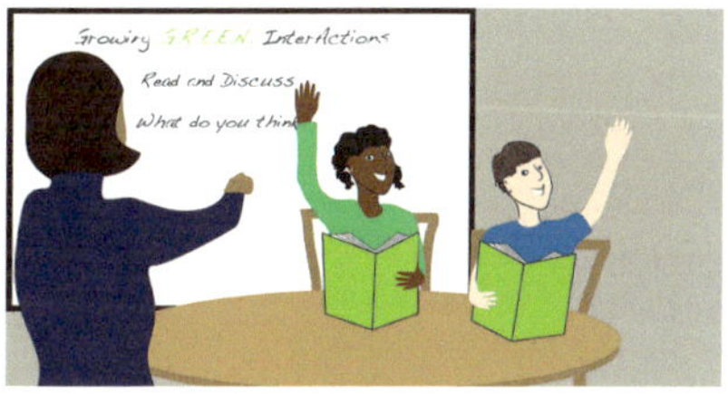

We are human beings.

We don't live by ourselves.

We don't live on our own separate islands.

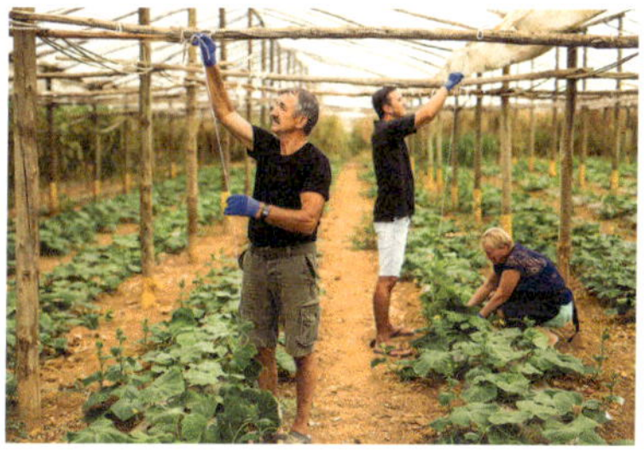

We live and work with other people.

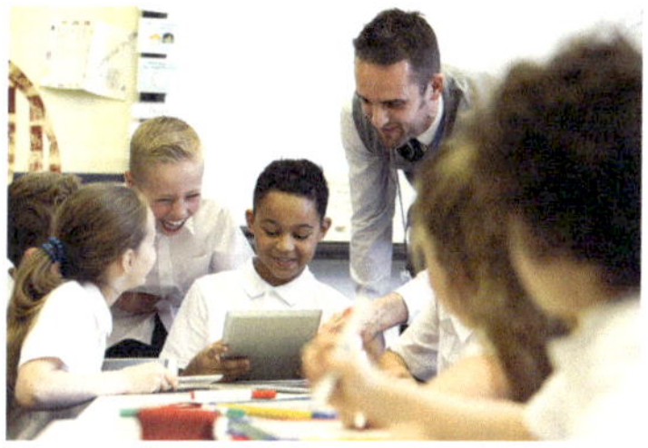

We learn things from other people, and they learn things from us.

When many people live and work together, each person is a part of a civilization.

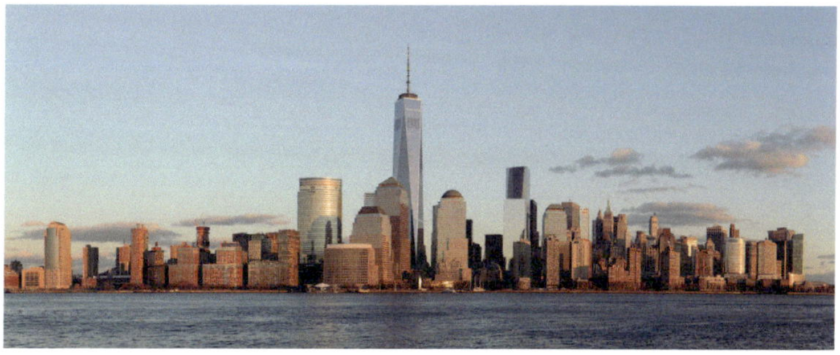

When we are part of a civilization, we can make life better for everyone.

2.2 Draw People Working Together in Our Civilization

What is the name of your city or town? ______________________________

____

Your city or town is an important part of our civilization. It is the place where you get to see how our civilization works.

People in our civilization must learn how to live together so our civilization will keep getting **better**.

For our civilization to work well, people must do things that make their lives **better**. Each person's actions can make things better for the other people in their city or town.

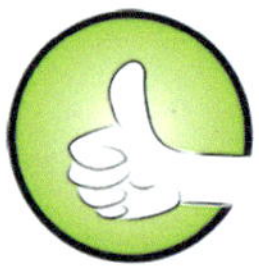

Think about the people who live in your city, town, or neighborhood. What jobs do they have? Draw a picture that shows some ways that people work together and help each other.

When you choose actions that help our civilization move **forward** in a **helpful** direction, you are acting **civil**. This means you are **respectful**, **cooperative**, and **positive**. You have the **power** to choose to be **civil** in our civilization!

You can learn to use your **power** with this **Growing G.R.E.E.N. InterActions** Program. This book will teach you how to make choices that help you work with others to make your civilization **better**.

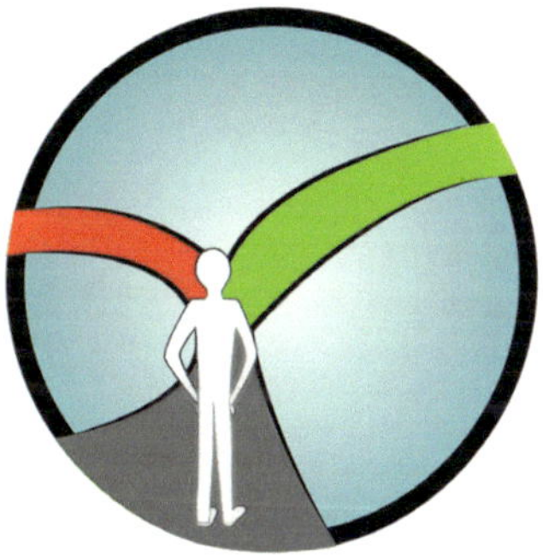

Words are **powerful**! When you think about making your civilization better, the words you choose will guide you to think in **positive** ways. You can then make **positive** choices for yourself and those you are with. You use words to make situations with other people the best they can be. Your **powerful** use of words can help our civilization move **forward**.

Thank you!

I would like to understand what you mean.

How Can I Help?

Let's figure this out together!

Interestingly, you and the people with you are on the same track and trying to move ahead.

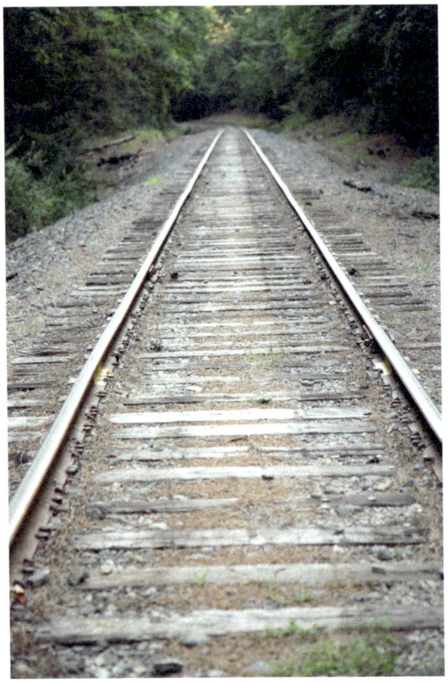

By making **positive** connections with other people, you are taking steps to move our civilization **forward** along the track.

Take a step forward to connect →

I took steps to *disconnect* from other people.	-4	-3	-2	-1	0	+1	+2	+3	+4	I took steps to make positive civilized connections with other people.

← Take a step backward to disconnect

2.3 Read and Discuss: Building Great Civilizations in Ancient Times

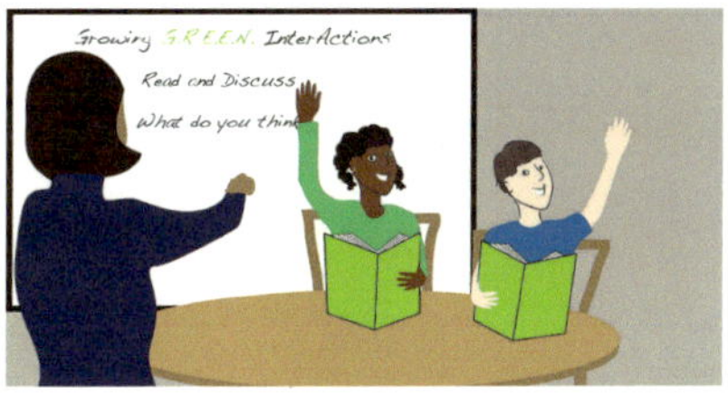

Let's learn about the great things that human beings have done throughout history when they have worked together well.

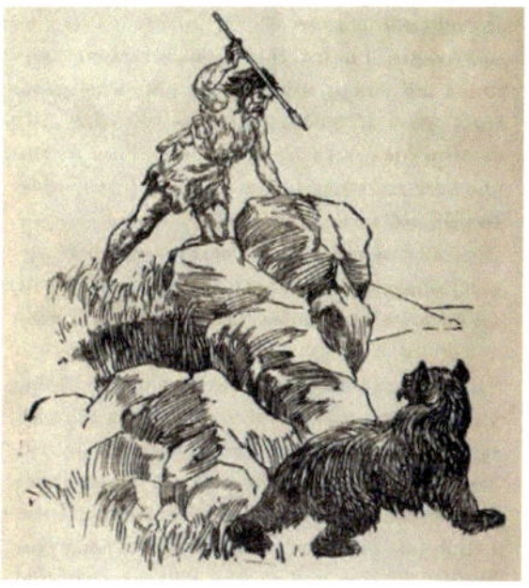

A long time ago, humans were hunters and gatherers. This means they had to move from place to place to hunt and collect food.

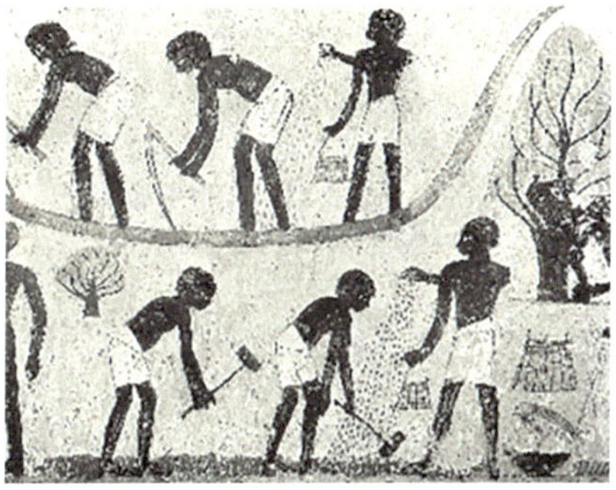

Then they learned to do things in new ways, which led to a **transformation** in how they lived. One big **change** was learning how to plant and take care of crops in one place. Humans no longer had to move around to find food. They began to live together in one place.

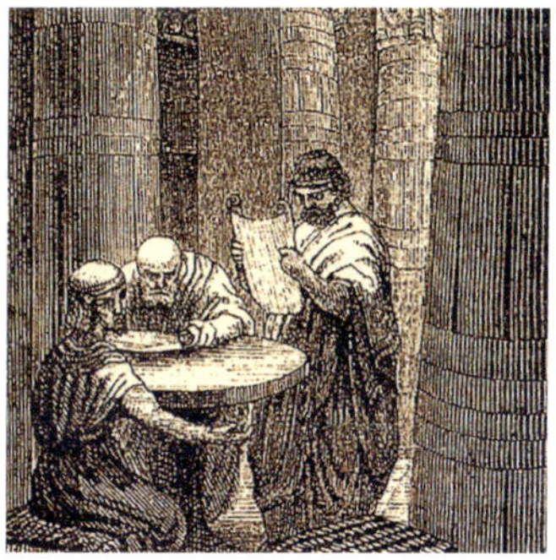

Because people no longer had to move from place to place, they learned to work together to build towns and cities. The people of these civilizations made beautiful buildings and gardens. They learned to live together and **cooperate** with each other. They **shared** interesting thoughts through music, poetry, and books. Schools, libraries, and workshops were built so that people could learn together.

Discuss: What would you like to learn from people so that you can help make your civilization great? ______________________________

____

____

2.4 Draw Something Beautiful and Useful for Our Civilization

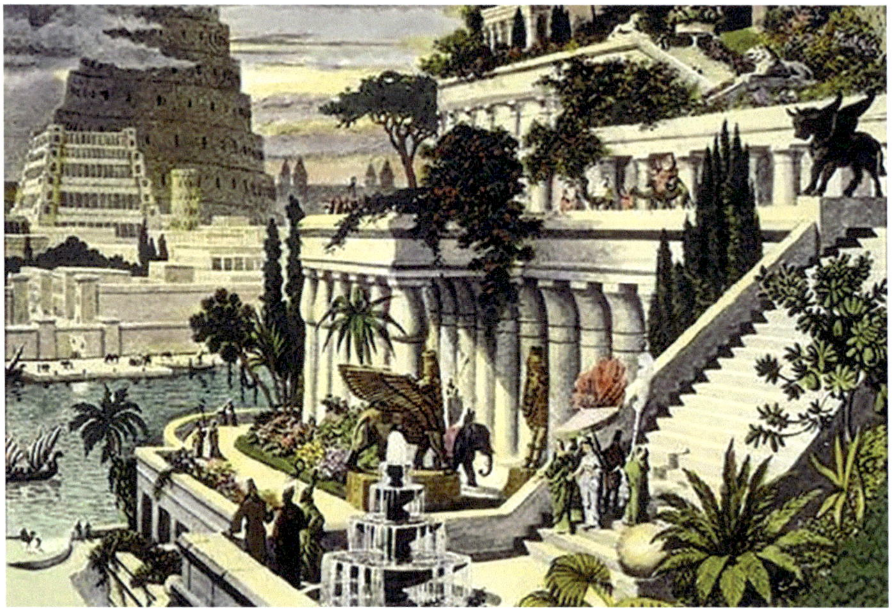

If you could work together with other humans to build something beautiful and useful, what would it be? You can use the box below to plan and draw what you would like to build for our civilization.

2.5 Read and Discuss: Civilization Goes Backward in the Dark Ages

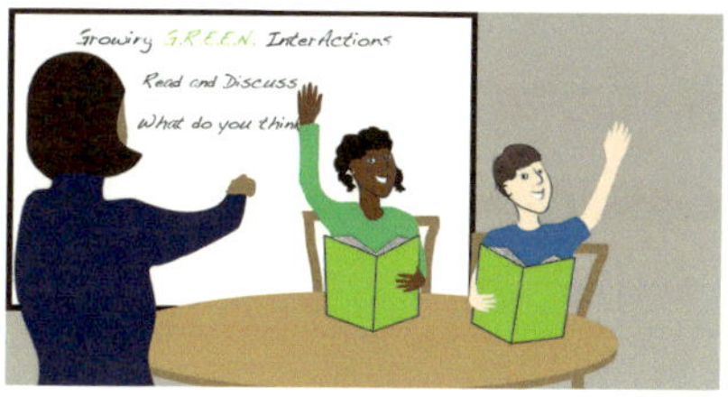

Unfortunately, some people in the past did not get along well with their neighbors. They were more interested in destroying things than **creating** and **building** them. Sadly, such people did not make **positive** choices to move civilization **forward**. For this reason, many human civilizations were completely destroyed.

It is hard to believe that human civilization could go backward and get worse. But at some points in our human history, that is what happened!

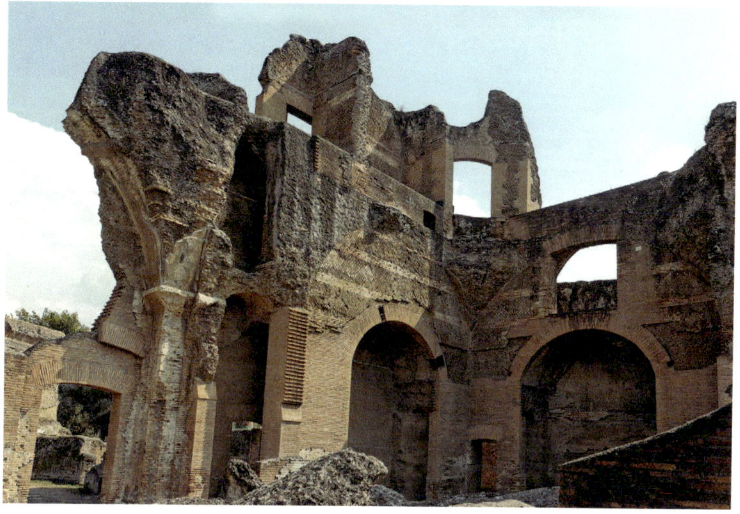

Take a step forward to connect →

I took steps to *disconnect* from other people.	-4	-3	-2	-1	0	+1	+2	+3	+4	I took steps to make positive civilized connections with other people.

← Take a step backward to disconnect

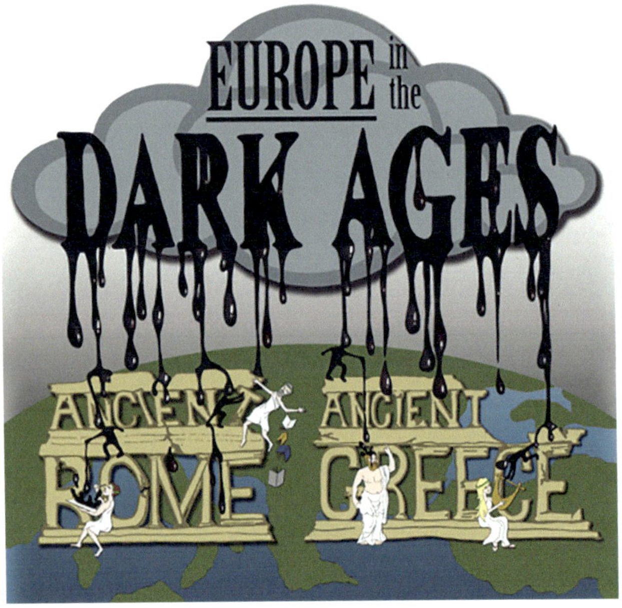

The Greek and Roman Empires had wonderful music, art, and architecture (buildings), as well as great writers and poets. Many people learned to read, write, and create things. Because learning was considered important, teachers were highly respected. But when the great civilizations of ancient Europe were destroyed, civilization went backward! The next period became known as the **Dark Ages**.

The Dark Ages lasted for hundreds of years. People stopped learning how to create amazing things because there were no more schools and libraries. Most people even stopped learning to read and write! People forgot how to share ideas and build things together as the great civilizations of Ancient Greece and Ancient Rome had. Civilization had stopped moving **forward** and had gone backward instead.

When people no longer cared about building human civilizations, they stopped working together. They fought and destroyed the property of others. People in the Dark Ages did not know how to act **politely** and **respectfully** toward one another. They forgot how to be **civil**, so they did not continue to have great civilizations.

Unfortunately, this still happens in our world today. What happened in the Dark Ages reminds us that our civilization and everything in it can be destroyed if we do not work together to maintain it. Instead, we must use our **power** to make good choices for ourselves and the people in our lives. Then our civilization can move **forward** and get even **better**.

Many people today play games in which they pretend to destroy things for fun. We must remember that acting like that in our real lives is a bad choice. We need to make sure we keep our real civilization alive. We want to keep the **civil** in civilization! We don't want the Dark Ages to come back!

2.6 Questions about Being Civil

1. Have humans always acted **thoughtful**, **helpful**, **kind**, and **civil** with one another?

   yes no

2. What was life like in the Dark Ages when people stopped acting **civil** with one another?____

   ____

3. Can a human civilization be destroyed if people forget how to learn and live together?

   yes no

4. What does it mean to be "**civil**" (see Section 2.2)? ____________________

   ____

5. Do you think you can do your part to act **civil** so that our civilization can continue to be great?

   yes no

6. Does it matter whether we treat each other in thoughtful, helpful, and kind ways?

   yes no

7. What thought do you think we can all have in our brains to help our civilization be great? ____

   ____

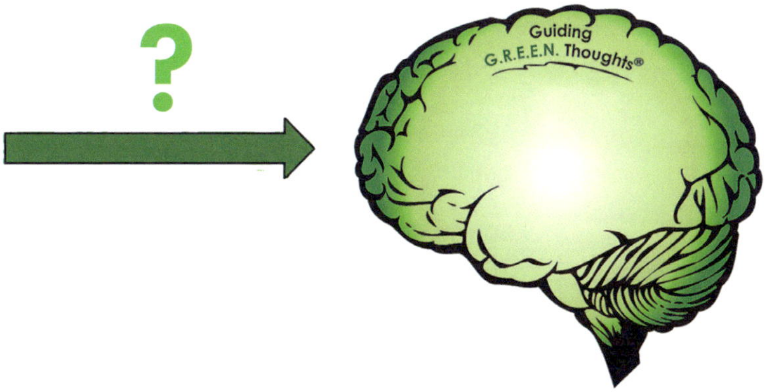

KEEP THE CIVIL IN CIVILIZATION

A Song for **Guiding G.R.E.E.N. Thoughts**®

by Herb Hein

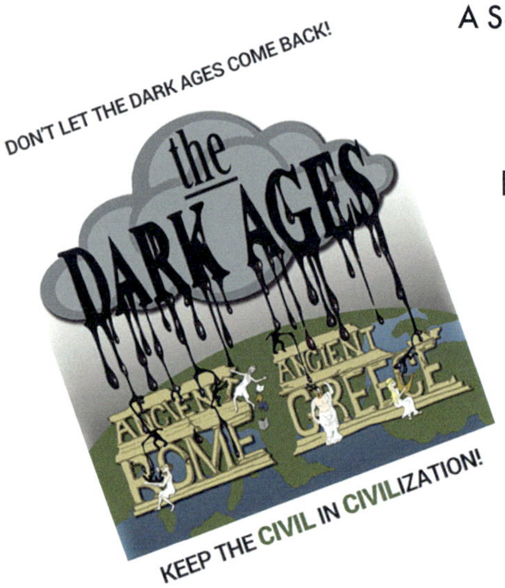

Don't let the Dark Ages come back,
Don't make us fall off the track,
Keep the civil in civilization.
Act up to high expectations
That we can learn to live together
In any kind of weather.
Yes, we can learn to act together
To make a better world.
And move forward, ever forward,
Let's move forward, let's move ahead.
And move forward, ever forward,
Let's move forward, let's move ahead.
Don't get us pulled off the stage,
Don't start to spin in a rage,
Keep the civil in civilization
And use our education
To help improve our relations
To make a better world.
And move forward, ever forward,
Let's move forward, let's move ahead.
And move forward, ever forward,
Let's move forward, let's move ahead,
Let's move ahead.
I said, "Let's move ahead!"
I said, "Let's move ahead!"
I said, "Let's move ahead!"
Let's move forward...Let's move forward...

2.7 Survey the Scene: Civilized Action or Not?

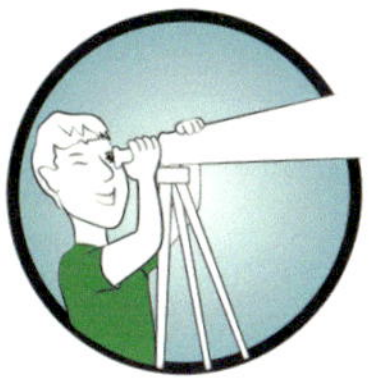

Directions: Pay attention to the action being described. Put a green check ✓ next to helpful, thoughtful, and civilized actions that move people forward in a positive direction. Put a red X by what you think are unhelpful, uncivilized actions:

__ 1. When Paul sees people get hurt, he tries to help them.

__ 2. When Paul sees people get hurt, he laughs.

__ 3. When people stand or walk near Harry, he moves carefully so he does not bump into them.

__ 4. When people stand or walk near Harry, he bumps into them on purpose.

__ 5. When Julia looks at things that belong to others, she is careful.

__ 6. When Julia looks at things that belong to others, she tries to break them.

__ 7. When his parent or teacher gives him directions, Robbie ignores them and makes noises instead.

__ 8. When his parent or teacher gives him directions, Robbie pays attention and listens so that he can follow them.

__ 9. When Carla sees that something is messy, she makes it messier.

__ 10. When Carla sees that something is messy, she takes time to help clean it up.

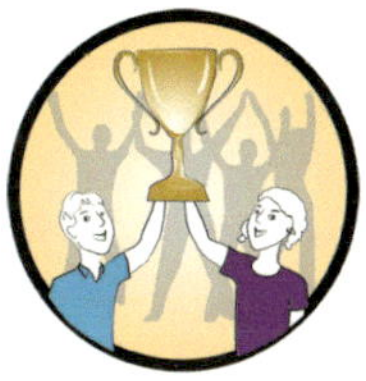

3 Growing Your Team Power

TEAM POWER

3.1 Read and Discuss: Who Is on Your Team?

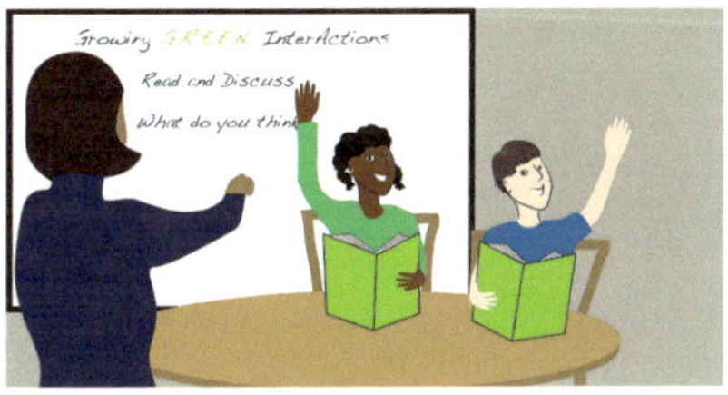

Throughout history, when people worked together to make civilizations great, they accomplished amazing things. By working together, they were on the same Team and **shared** similar thoughts about creating the best civilization. They **cooperated** with each other.

This may have been a **powerful** thought they all **shared**:

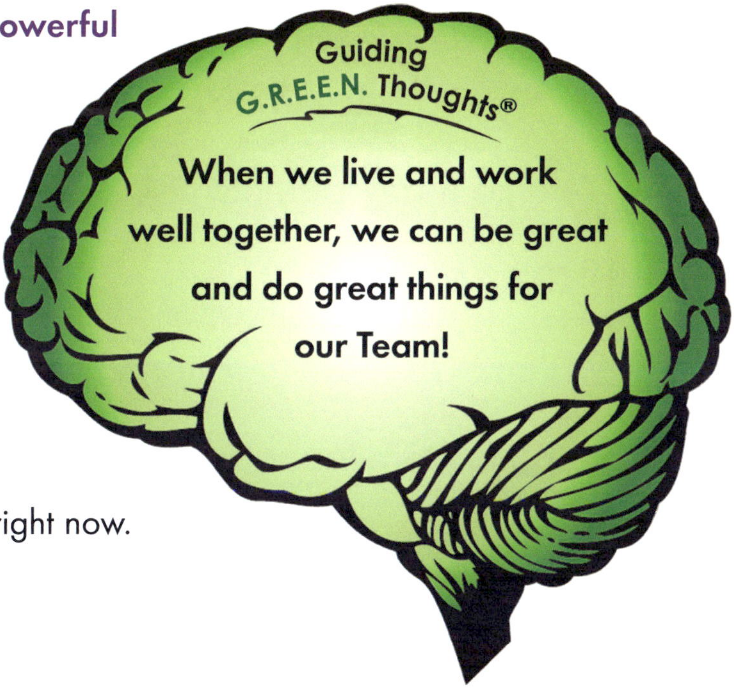

We can be inspired by the humans who came before us. We can follow their good examples in making our world **better**.

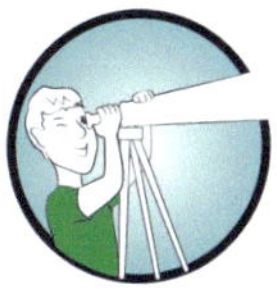

Survey the scene right now. Who is with you?

Who is on your Team?

____

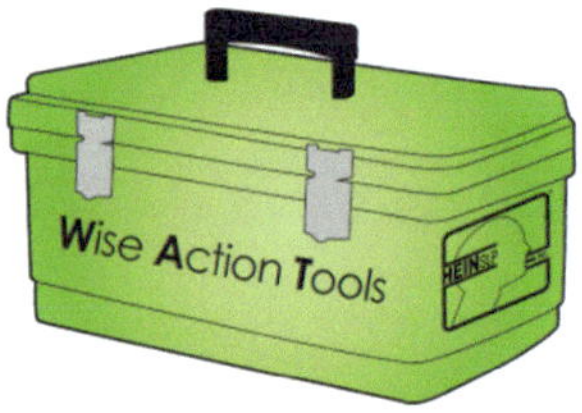

WHO IS ON A TEAM WITH YOU?

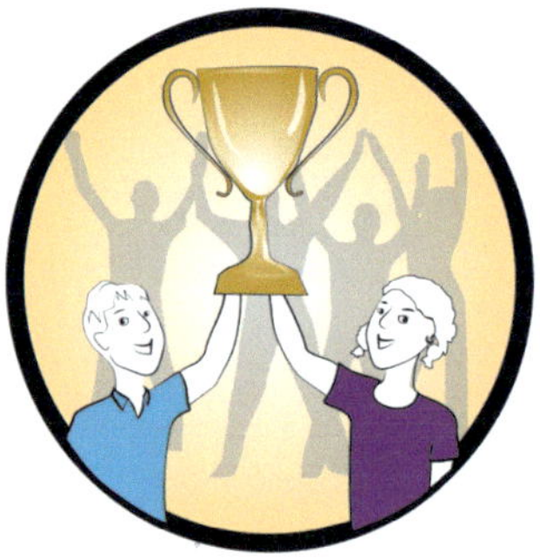

You make the world better when you think of other people. in addition to yourself. You can be more **civil** and help your part of civilization be more civilized! You have more **power** when you realize that you and the people around you are all on the same Team!

Who is on your Team? Who else should you be thinking about besides yourself?

What are your **powerful** Teams? If you are a member of a Team, check it off to show you are part of it. Add any other Teams that you might be on if they are not listed already:

______ Home Team (parents, siblings, children)

______ Classroom Team (teacher, aides, therapists, classmates, students)

______ Friendship Team (old friends, new friends, future friends)

______ Sports Team (coaches, teammates, umpires, referees)

______ Work Team (boss, coworkers)

______ ____

______ ____

3.2 Actions That Are Good for Everyone Help Everyone Win

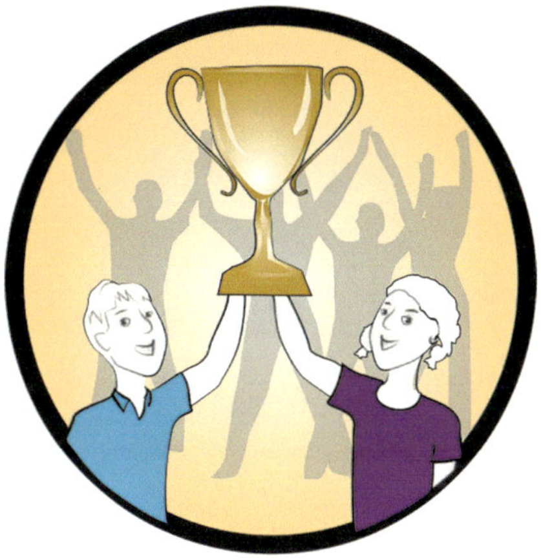

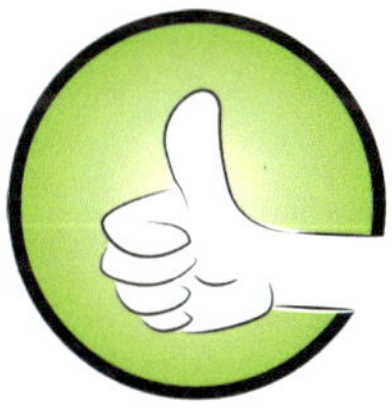

Do you and the other people on your Teams help each other by **connecting** with each other and **helping** to make things **better**, or do you block yourself from working together well with other people by disconnecting from them?

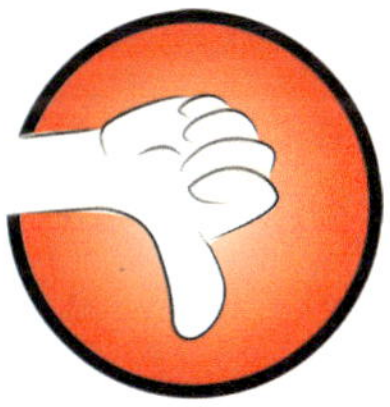

You may not always think about how important your actions are to the Teams you are on. But it is important to understand that you can make a difference to your civilization every single day.

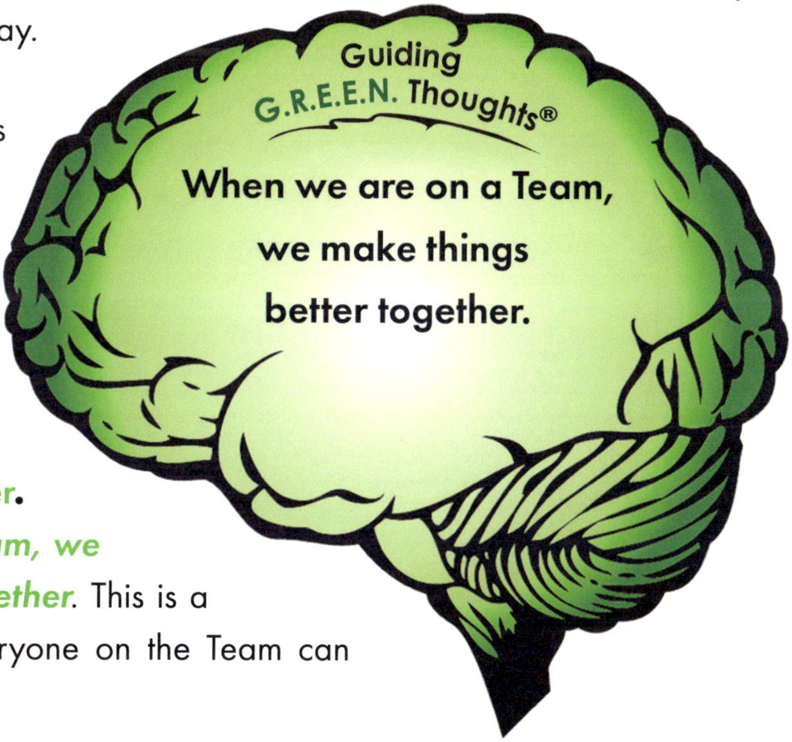

When everyone does their part to help the Team, then everyone can win! When everyone can live, play, and work well with all the other people on their Teams, things get **better**. ***When we are on a Team, we make things better together***. This is a guiding thought that everyone on the Team can have in their own minds.

3.3 Draw a Scene of Team Members Helping Each Other

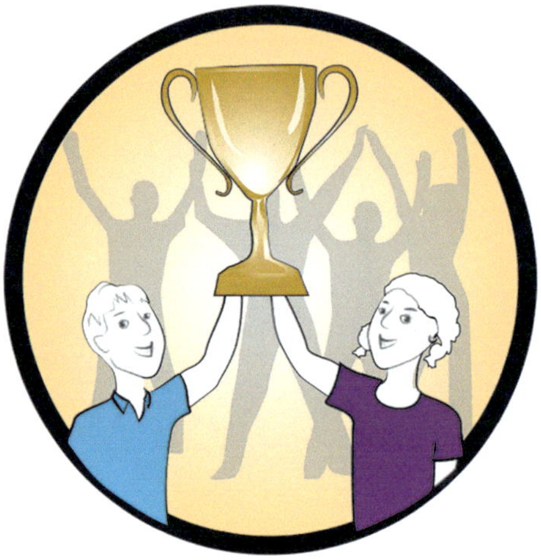

Draw a picture of yourself living, working, or playing well with others on one of your Teams. Show that you are helping each other with your actions.

3.4 Read and Discuss: What Is Your Potential to Have Team Power?

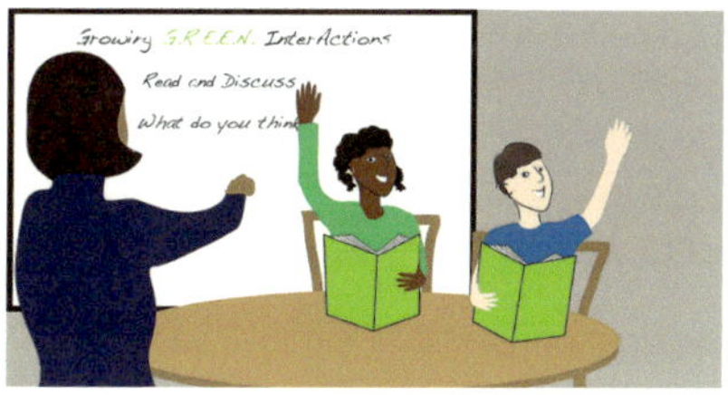

The word **potential** means something that has not happened yet but could possibly happen. It is related to the word **power**.

You might not ever have thought about how you are on the same Team with the people in your family or in your classroom. But once you start to think of yourselves as a Team and act together as a Team, you can start to see the **power** of **cooperating** with each other. You can have the same **positive, helpful** thought in common to make choices to act as a Team to make things **better** for the Team.

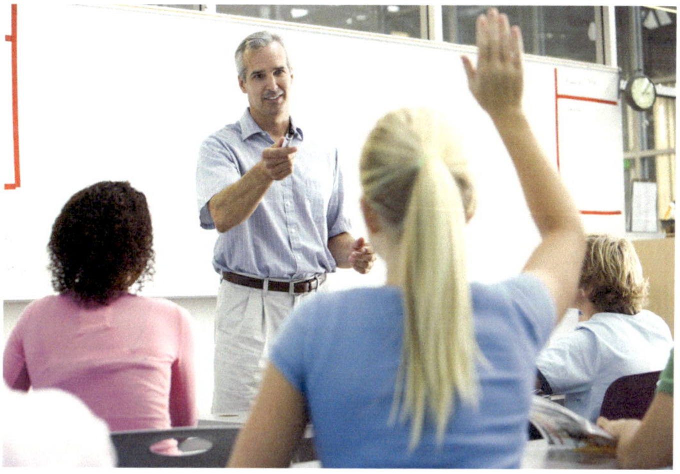

Think about the **potential** Teammates on your **potential**, **powerful** Teams.

Think about what you want to achieve together.

What do you want to achieve together with your Teams? ____________________

____

____

____

____

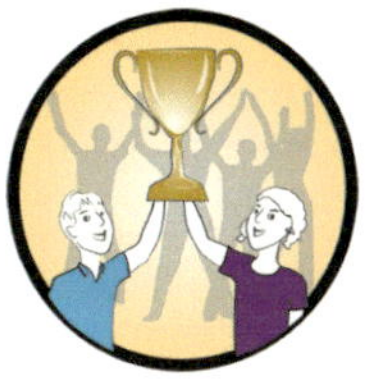

4 Helping Everyone Reach Common Team Goals

4.1 What Are Common Team Goals?

When you think about being on the same Team as the people around you, you can think about the **goals** the Team wants to accomplish. What are you trying to do together? These are the **goals** everyone on the Team has in common.

Once you have decided on **Common Team Goals**, you can work together as a Team each time you are together in the same life scene.

Think about some **Common Team Goals** each of your Teams might have. These are the **goals** that Team members have in common, which means they are the same for everyone.

Read the **Common Team Goals** listed for each Team and add any others you can think of.

4.2 Typical Common Team Goals

Common Team Goals for the Home Team

- We make a peaceful place to live.
- We show that we care about each other.
- We support each other so we can grow to be our best selves.
- Everyone can have a turn to share ideas.

Common Team Goals *for the Classroom Team*

- We make a place where we can all learn.
- We treat each other with respect.
- We learn from and help each other.

Common Team Goals *for the Friendship Team*

- We support each other to be our best.
- We show that we care about each other.
- We enjoy being with each other.
- We take turns talking and sharing ideas.

Common Team Goals *for the Sports Team*

- We follow the rules of the game.
- We play fairly every time.
- We do our best to work together.
- We are good sports when we don't win.

Common Team Goals *for the Work Team*

- We follow the rules of the workplace.
- We try to do our best work every time.
- We do our best to work together.
- We try to learn from our mistakes so we can be more successful next time and move the Team forward.

Remember that once you have decided on **Common Team Goals**, you can work together as a Team each time you are together in the same life scene.

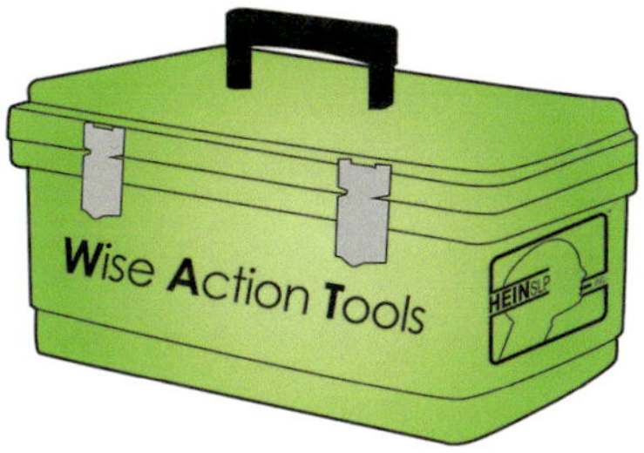

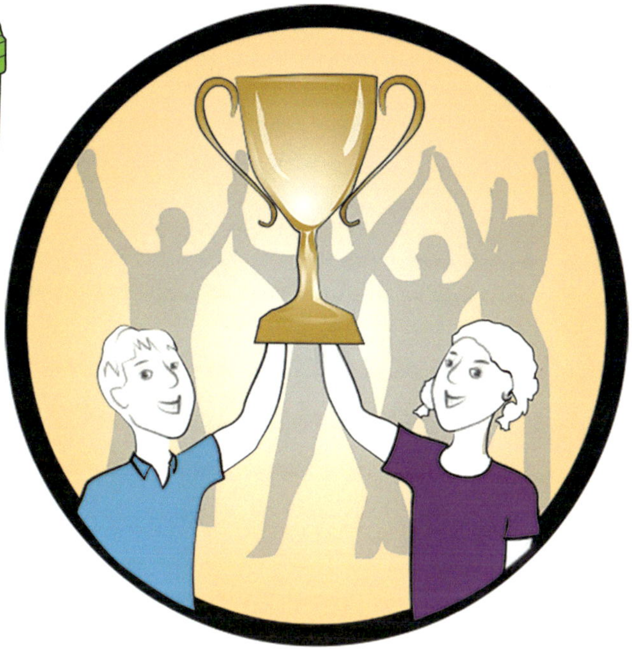

OUR TEAM NAME ______________________________

OUR COMMON TEAM GOALS

____

____

____

____

____

____

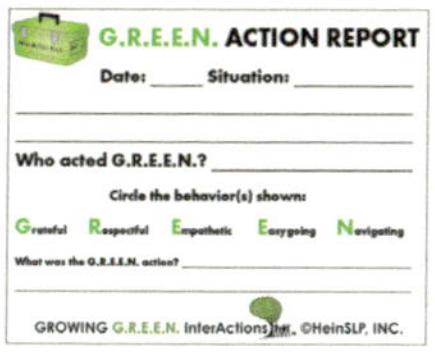
G.R.E.E.N. ACTION REPORT

Date: ____ Situation: ____

Who acted G.R.E.E.N.? ____

Circle the behavior(s) shown:

Grateful Respectful Empathetic Easygoing Navigating

What was the G.R.E.E.N. action? ____

GROWING G.R.E.E.N. InterActions Inc. ©HeinSLP, INC.

5 Tracking Your G.R.E.E.N. Actions for the Team

5.1 Why Act G.R.E.E.N. with Your Teams?

Any time you are with others, it is as if you are in the same scene. In any scene in your life, you can choose how you act. This includes following the rules so that everyone can do their best to act civilized in the scene.

When Team members act G.R.E.E.N. and expect others on your Team to act the same way, you can all expect the following:

- All of you will **survey the scene** so that everyone knows what is happening and can work together.
- You and other Team members will act **grateful**, appreciating what you have and the people around you.

You and other Team members will

- do your best to care about one another's feelings
- keep working on your **Personal Goals** and those that everyone shares—**Common Team Goals**
- **act safely** so that the scene can be as peaceful and successful as possible
- do your best to **act logically and with good judgment** so the scene can get even **better**
- **navigate** as well as you can using coping strategies to avoid upsetting yourselves and others

5.2 Start Tracking G.R.E.E.N. Action—What's Your Baseline?

The goal of the **Growing G.R.E.E.N. InterActions** Program is to teach you how to act more G.R.E.E.N. than you did before. So you need to know how G.R.E.E.N. you are acting at the start of this program. You can also find out how those on your Team think you are acting. This will be your **starting point**, also known as your **baseline**. You and your Teammates can honestly score how you are doing today and then rescore yourselves each month to see how much you have improved. You can be proud of yourself when you notice how your actions have become more civil. It will be exciting to "grade yourself" on how much you have improved the skills that are most important to you and your Team.

Using a self-checking chart to honestly determine your baseline is a wise strategy for self-improvement. When you evaluate yourself with these self-checking charts, you are using Wise Action Tools, which also can be used to track your Team's progress. In this way, everyone learns how to act more G.R.E.E.N. together.

If you have been acting G.R.E.E.N. all or most of the time, you can be proud of yourself and how you act with others. You can predict that you will continue to act G.R.E.E.N. with these people. If you honestly determine that you usually do not think about acting G.R.E.E.N. with others or rarely act G.R.E.E.N., you still have the potential to start doing it a little more each day. As you start taking steps toward acting more G.R.E.E.N., you can be proud of yourself and your choices.

5.3 Self-Evaluation: How G.R.E.E.N. Am I Acting Today?

This G.R.E.E.N. Actions Evaluation Chart can help you honestly describe your own starting point for your G.R.E.E.N. actions. Take time now to think about how G.R.E.E.N. you are acting today. How much of the time do you think you are

Grateful?

Respectful?

Empathetic?

Easygoing?

Navigating?

Fill out the chart as honestly as you can. Then get a total score to see what your baseline is. Then you will be able to compare your total score with the next time you fill out this evaluation chart.

5.4 Getting Feedback from Others: How G.R.E.E.N. Do You Think I Am Acting Today?

It is often difficult to listen to feedback from others around you. Sometimes, what others think about how you are acting does not completely match what you think about yourself. Be willing to let your teacher, therapist, coach, or parents evaluate how G.R.E.E.N. you are acting by filling out this chart too. You will find that you will benefit from their feedback. You will see if you are rating yourself too high or too low.

You and your other evaluators can fill out this form again in a month or at the end of every school quarter. You will be able to compare your G.R.E.E.N. baseline now with a future time as you learn to act more G.R.E.E.N. with your Teams.

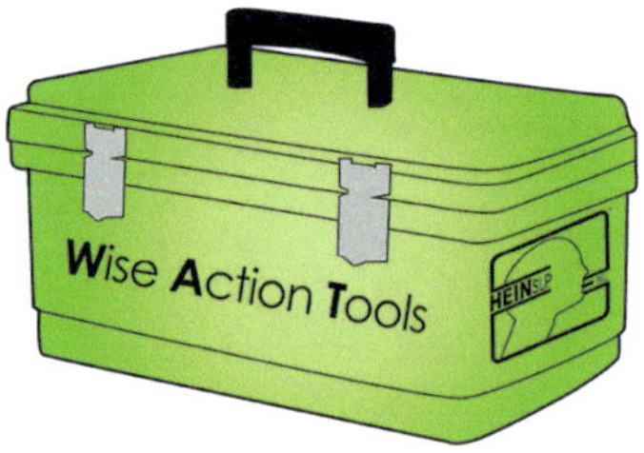

G.R.E.E.N. ACTIONS EVALUATION CHART

Team Member: ______________________________ Today's Date ____________________

Evaluation by:

- ☐ Self
- ☐ Teacher
- ☐ Parent
- ☐ Peer
- ☐ Other ________________

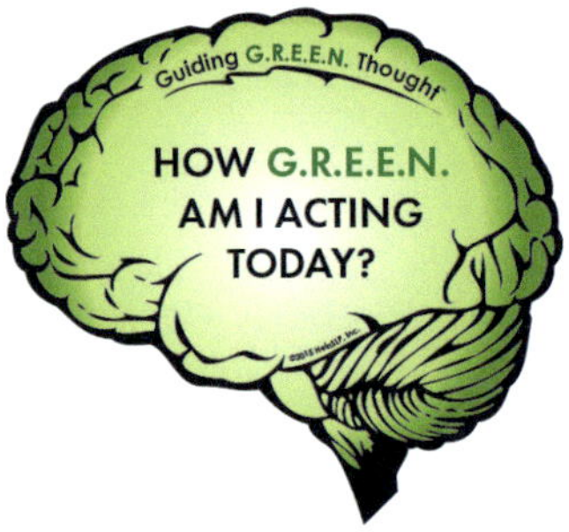

HONESTLY EVALUATE ACTIONS BY CHECKING THE BOX THAT IS TRUE TODAY

	NEVER 0	A LITTLE BIT 1	HALF THE TIME 2	MOST OF THE TIME 3	ALL THE TIME 4	TOTAL
GRATEFUL- I let people know that I appreciate what I have.						
RESPECTFUL- I am respectful of the people and things in every situation. I use a tone of voice that is positive and polite.						
EMPATHETIC- I show that I am considerate of the feelings of my friends, classmates, and family.						
EASYGOING- I am open-minded and cooperate with people to meet Team goals.						
NAVIGATING- I am flexible when I manage challenges because I stay calm and make wise choices.						
I take responsibility for my actions and accept consequences.						
				GRAND TOTAL		

5.5 Using G.R.E.E.N. Action Reports

We all have **Personal Goals** we are trying to achieve. Your **Personal Goals** might include acting more G.R.E.E.N. with the people on your Teams. You can use a G.R.E.E.N. Action Report to help you notice when you act G.R.E.E.N. You also can notice the G.R.E.E.N. actions of people on your Teams and fill out an Action Report for them, and they can write an Action Report when they notice you acting G.R.E.E.N. Your Team will get more G.R.E.E.N. because all of you are noticing the G.R.E.E.N. actions of others. Put the G.R.E.E.N. Action Reports in a special place and choose a time to share them at a weekly G.R.E.E.N. Action Celebration. G.R.E.E.N. actions can then be added to a Personal or Team G.R.E.E.N. Action Tracker.

To fill out a G.R.E.E.N. Action Report:

1. Write down the date of the action.

2. Write a summary of the situation.

3. Write down who acted G.R.E.E.N.

4. Circle one or more G.R.E.E.N. words that show the G.R.E.E.N. behavior you saw:

   Grateful **Respectful** **Empathetic** **Easygoing** **Navigating**

5. Write down the G.R.E.E.N. action.

Notice G.R.E.E.N. Action! Report it! Track it!

G.R.E.E.N. ACTION REPORT

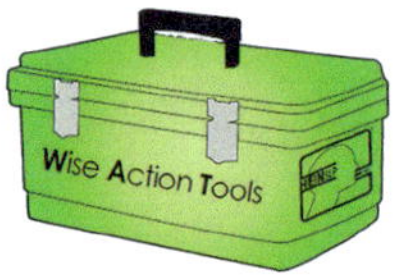

Date: ________________ Situation: ________________

____

____

Who acted G.R.E.E.N.? ________________________________

Circle the behavior(s) shown:

Grateful **R**espectful **E**mpathetic **E**asygoing **N**avigating

What was the G.R.E.E.N. action? ______________________________

____

____

5.6 What Are Personal and Team G.R.E.E.N. Action Trackers?

My Personal G.R.E.E.N. Action Tracker

This page helps you track G.R.E.E.N. actions in your real-life scenes. Add a check mark when someone on your Team notices you acting G.R.E.E.N.

Give yourself a check mark when you have written a G.R.E.E.N. Action Report about your action. Total the check marks you received during the week. Compare the total check marks with the number you received last week. See if you can increase your G.R.E.E.N. action each week!

Classroom Team G.R.E.E.N. Action Tracker

This page tracks how well everyone on the Classroom Team is working to act more G.R.E.E.N. and can be filled out when G.R.E.E.N. Action Reports are shared. Your Classroom Team could be the people in your classroom, on your Recess/Playground Team, or on any other Team you are with at school. Your teacher, therapist, or coach will be responsible for filling this in.

Home Team G.R.E.E.N. Action Tracker

This page tracks how well every person on the Home Team is working to act more G.R.E.E.N. with others. Home Team members can take turns filling out this form when the Home Team shares its G.R.E.E.N. Action Reports.

Work Team G.R.E.E.N. Action Tracker

This page tracks how well every person on the Work Team is working to act more G.R.E.E.N. with others. Work Team members can take turns filling out this form when the Work Team shares its G.R.E.E.N. Action Reports.

MY NAME ______________________________

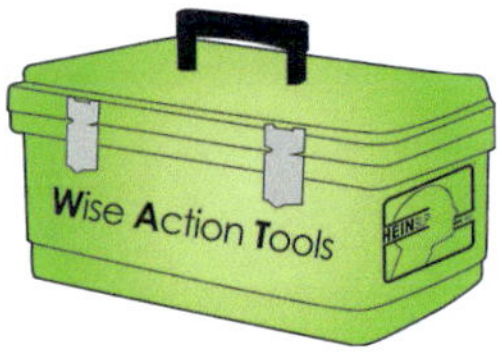

MY PERSONAL G.R.E.E.N. ACTION TRACKER

How many times can I act G.R.E.E.N. this week?

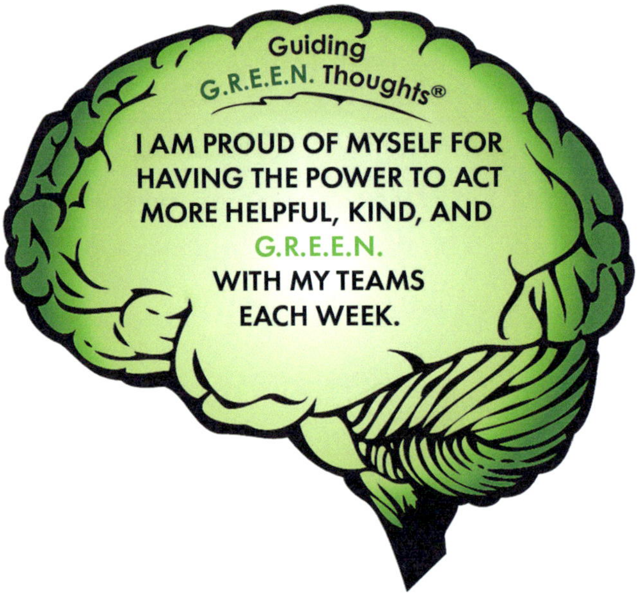

I am acting G.R.E.E.N. when I take action that others think is caring, civil, cooperative, considerate, easygoing, empathetic, grateful, helpful, kind, navigating, polite, positive, respectful, supportive, or thoughtful. When others on my Teams notice me acting G.R.E.E.N. and give me a G.R.E.E.N. **Action Report**, I put a check mark in the box for that day. I also can fill out a G.R.E.E.N. **Action Report** for myself when I notice that I have acted G.R.E.E.N.with someone, and I can then give myself a check mark in the box for that day.

I see how many times I can act G.R.E.E.N. this week.
Then I can see if I can act G.R.E.E.N. even more times next week!

Date	Date	Date	Date	Date	Date	Date

This week's G.R.E.E.N. Action Total: __________

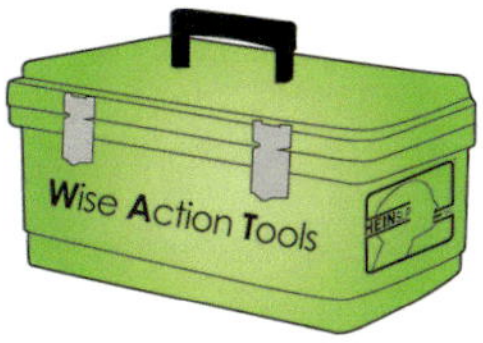

CLASSROOM TEAM G.R.E.E.N. ACTION TRACKER

Name of our Classroom Team: ______________________________

This is our Team Action Tracker for the week starting on ________________
(date)

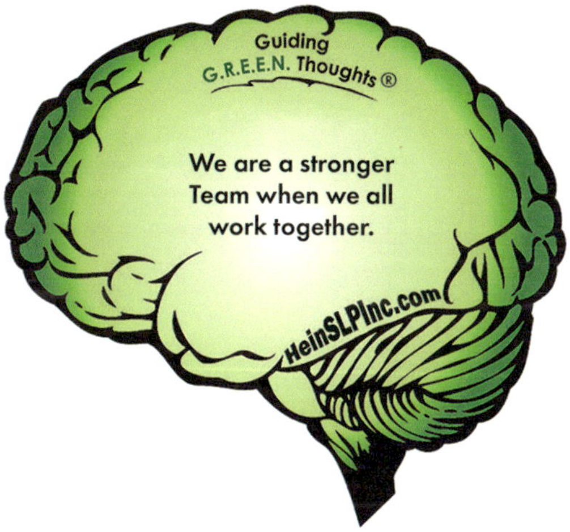

Fill in the names of everyone on the Team.

√ Check the box under the date each time a Classroom Team member acted G.R.E.E.N. or transfer the total from each Team member's **Personal G.R.E.E.N. Action Tracker.**

Classroom Teammates	Monday	Tuesday	Wednesday	Thursday	Friday	Individual Totals

This week's Team total: ____________

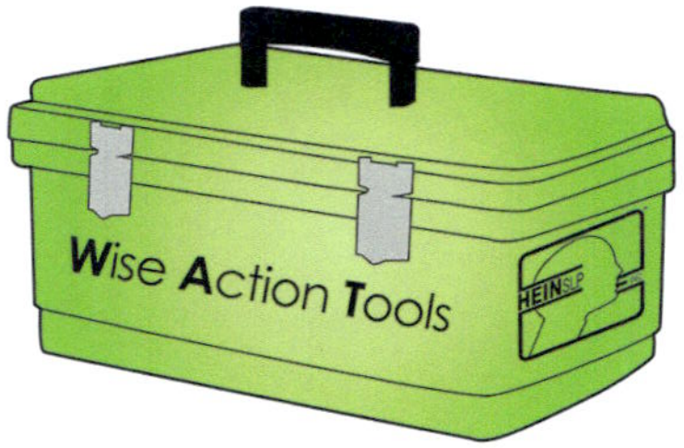

HOME TEAM G.R.E.E.N. ACTION TRACKER

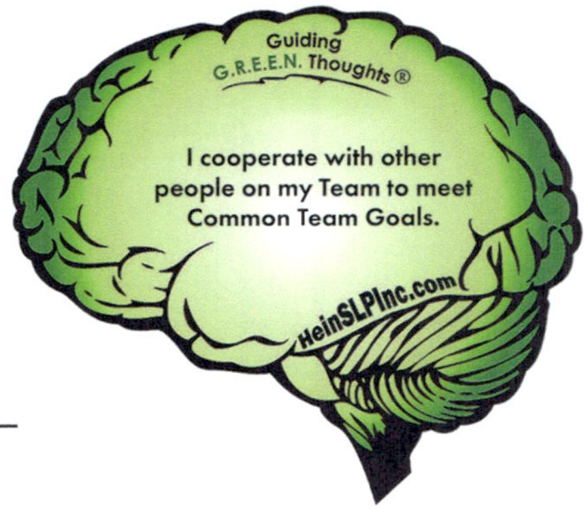

Name of our Home Team: ______________________________

This is our G.R.E.E.N. Action Tracker for the week starting on ______________
(date)

Fill in the names of all members of the Home Team. Fill out and then review the G.R.E.E.N. Action Reports. Put a check in a box to give a Home Team member credit on each date when he or she acted G.R.E.E.N.

Home Team Members	Mon	Tue	Wed	Thu	Fri	Sat	Sun	7-Day Total

This week's Home Team G.R.E.E.N. Action Total: ____________

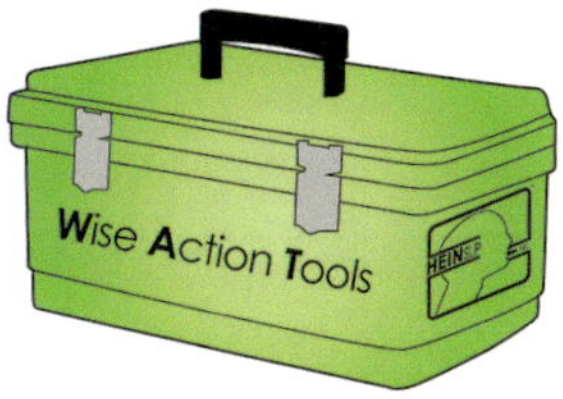

WORK TEAM G.R.E.E.N. ACTION TRACKER

Name of our Work Team: ______________________________

This is our Team Action Tracker for the week starting on ________________
(date)

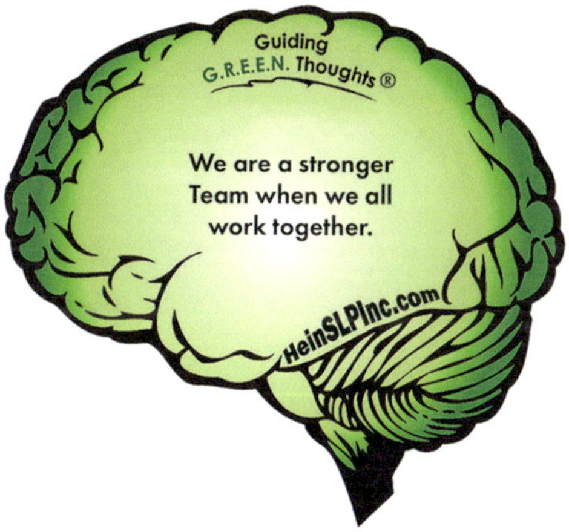

Fill in the names of everyone on the Team.

√ Check the box under the date each time a Work Team member acted G.R.E.E.N. or transfer the total from each Team member's **Personal G.R.E.E.N. Action Tracker.**

Work Teammates	Mon	Tue	Wed	Thu	Fri	Sat	Sun	Individual Totals

This week's Team total: ____________

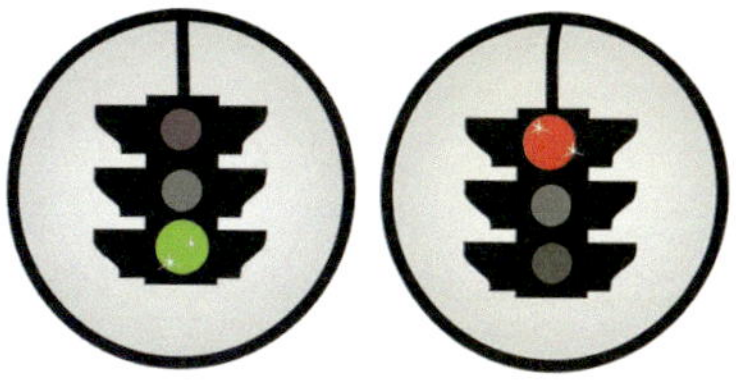

6 The Importance of Team Rules

6.1 Read and Discuss: Keeping the Civil in Civilization Requires Rules

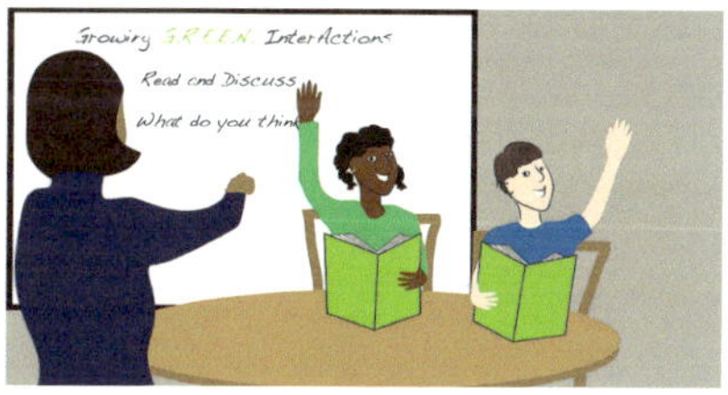

People living together in past civilizations created laws and rules to protect their food, their houses, and things that people made. When civilizations worked well, people learned to **respect** their rules. Citizens knew that the rules helped them know how to treat one another. The rules guided people to be **civil** toward each other. People learned that when they followed the rules, it was easier for everyone to get along. When people followed the rules, citizens could live their lives knowing that they were safe and their hard work respected.

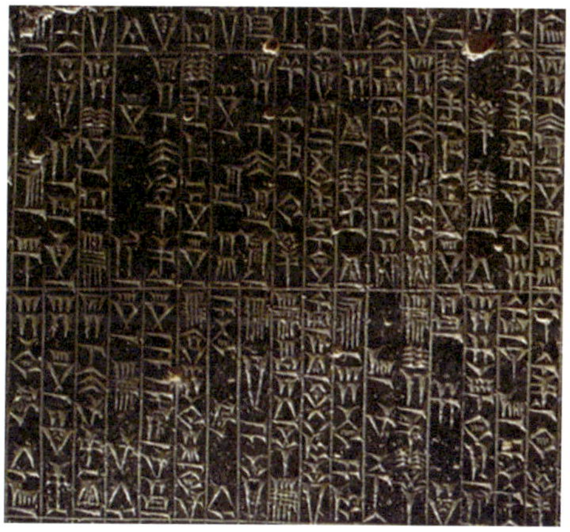

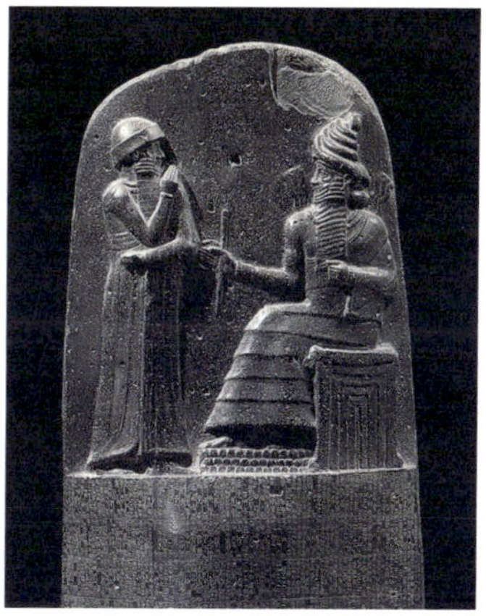

In today's civilization, we also live with laws and rules. We follow them so that people in our countries, states, and cities can all act in a **civil** manner.

Discuss: What do you think? What are some useful rules that help make our civilization a place where people can live, learn, and work peacefully, and make and do great things? ______________________________

____

____

6.2 Each Team Has Its Own Rules to Follow

Just as we must follow the laws and rules of our countries, states, and cities, we also must follow the rules of each Team. It is important to know each Team's rules and why it has them. It is a good idea to talk with your Team members to decide which rules help Team members know how to act. With Team rules in place, each Team can be at its best.

Reasons for Classroom Team Rules

You learn Classroom Team rules so everyone can get along well and be successful with their schoolwork. When everyone interacts well, it is easy to focus on learning. The teacher will do the best possible job teaching. Classroom Team members will move **forward** and **navigate** challenges together to meet Classroom **Common Team Goals**. Also, when Team members follow the Classroom Team rules, each student's **Personal Goals** can be met. If Classroom Team rules are not followed, the Team gets stuck and cannot move **forward**—it becomes disconnected. Students don't learn and the teacher is unable to teach. To help the Team be **powerful** and move **forward**, everyone must make the best choices and follow Classroom Team rules.

Discuss:

What Classroom Team rule do you think is important? ______________________________

____

How does this rule help the Team move **forward**? ______________________________

____

Reasons for Home Team Rules

Your Home Team develops rules so everyone in your home feels safe, respected, and appreciated. Everyone on the Home Team likes to feel that they can move **forward** and have their best lives doing the important things they want to do. When members of the Home Team **support** one another, they feel good about moving the Home Team **forward**. When you don't follow the Home Team rules, the Team gets stuck—people on the Team cannot move **forward**. They will not feel safe enough or respected enough to move in their best directions. The Team loses some **power** because it becomes disconnected and distracted. To help the Home Team stay **powerful** and move **forward**, everyone must make the best choices and follow Home Team rules.

Discuss:

What Home Team rule do you think is important? ______________________

____

How does this rule help the Team move **forward**? ______________________

____

Reasons for Friendship Team Rules

Your Friendship Team also has rules to follow, just as the Classroom and Home Teams do. There are rules about how friends should interact so that everyone feels safe and can trust (page 240) one another. If you don't follow the Friendship Team rules, you may not develop strong and lasting friendships, or you may even lose your friends. However, if you follow the Friendship Team rules, your friendships can grow **better** and stronger.

Discuss:

What Friendship Team rule do you think is important**?** ______________________

____

How does this rule help the Team move **forward?** ______________________

____

Reasons for Work Team Rules

Your Work Team also has rules to follow, just as the Classroom, Home, and Friendship Teams do. There are rules about how coworkers should communicate so that everyone feels safe and can trust one another. If you don't follow the Work Team rules, you may not develop strong and lasting work relationships, and you may have difficulty being successful in your job. However, if you follow the Work Team Rules, your work connections can grow **better** and stronger. When you can be trusted to follow the Work Team rules, you may be given more responsibility in getting things done and get rewarded for your hard work.

Discuss:

What Work Team rule do you think is important? ______________________

____

How does this rule help the Team move **forward**? ______________________

____

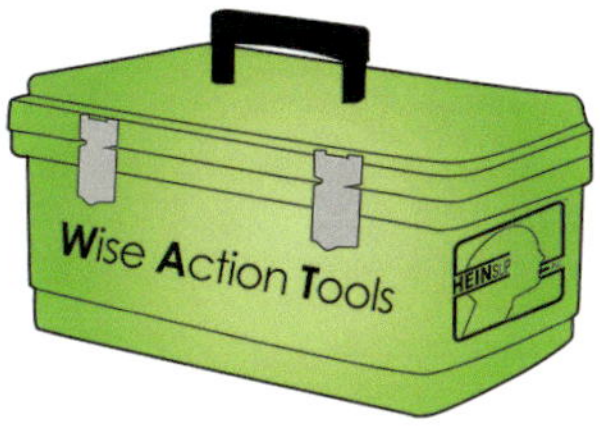

OUR CLASSROOM TEAM RULES

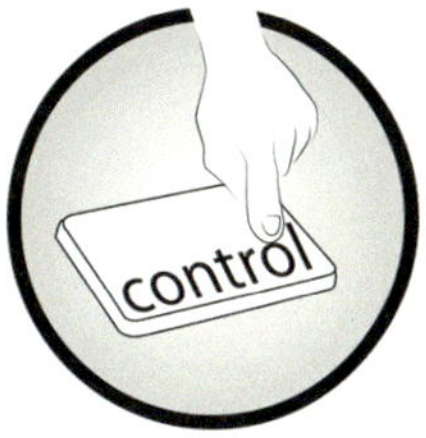

Everyone on our Classroom Team works to find the control to follow our Classroom Team rules.

These are the Classroom Team rules everyone on the Team follows so our Team can be great and powerful and keep moving forward!

1. ____

2. ____

3. ____

4. ____

5. ____

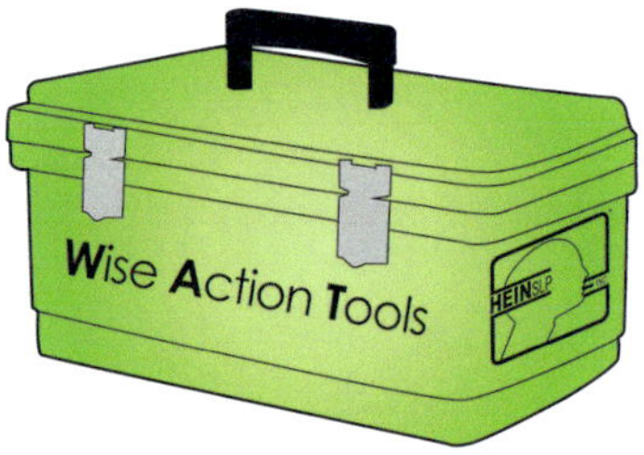

OUR HOME TEAM RULES

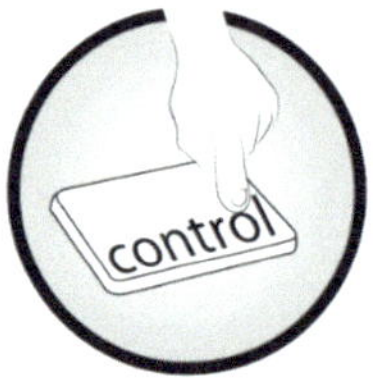

Everyone on our Home Team uses **self-control** and follows our Home Team Rules.

Here are our Home Team Rules.

Everyone on the Team follows these rules so our Team can be great and **powerful** and keep moving **forward**!

1. ____

____

2. ____

____

3. ____

____

4. ____

____

5. ____

____

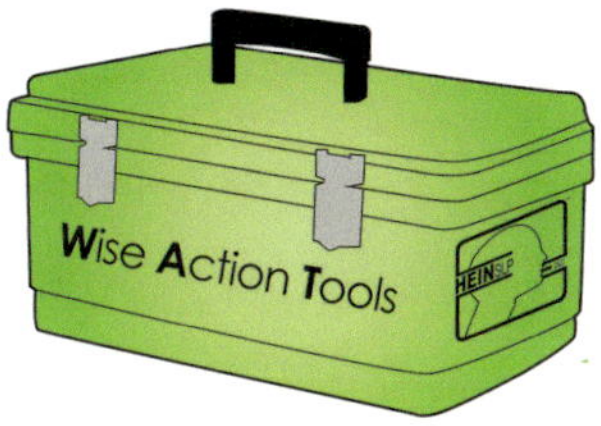

OUR FRIENDSHIP TEAM RULES

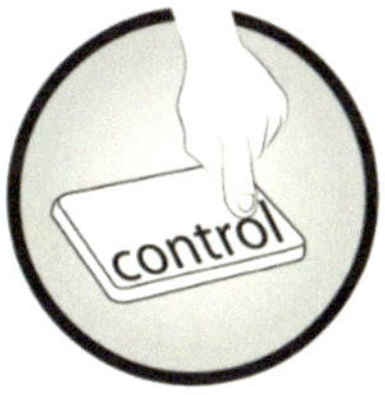

Everyone on our Friendship Team uses **self-control** and follows our Friendship Team Rules.

These are our Friendship Team Rules.

Everyone on the Team follows these rules so our Team can be great and **powerful** and keep moving **forward**!

1. ____

____

2. ____

____

3. ____

____

4. ____

____

5. ____

____

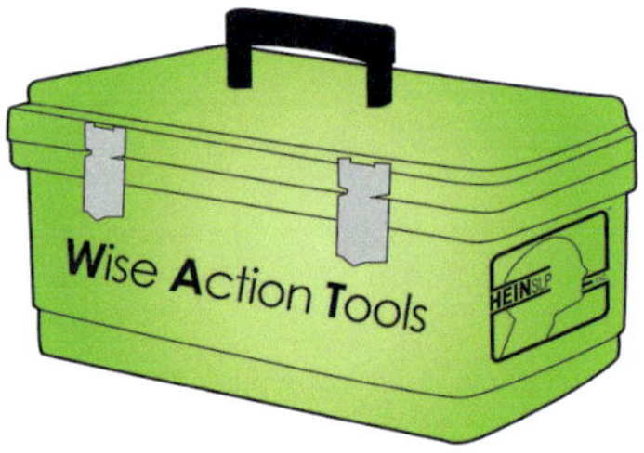

OUR WORK TEAM RULES

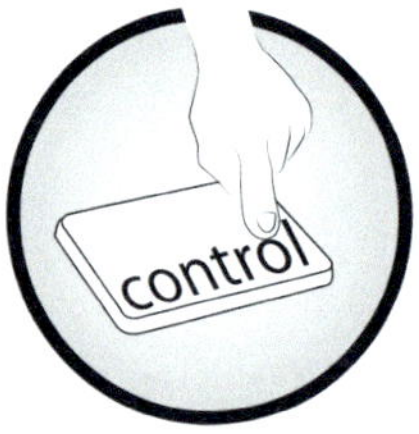

These are the Work Team Rules that everyone on our Team follows so our Team can be great and powerful and keep moving forward.

1. ____

____

2. ____

____

3. ____

____

4. ____

____

5. ____

____

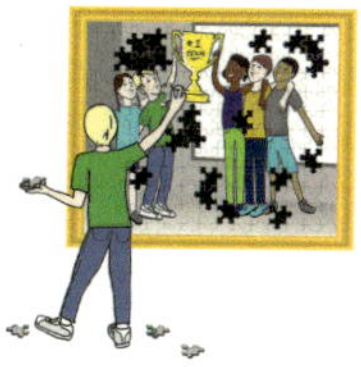

7 Being Your Best Self with Personal Goals

7.1 Read and Discuss: Being Your Best Self in Your Best Life

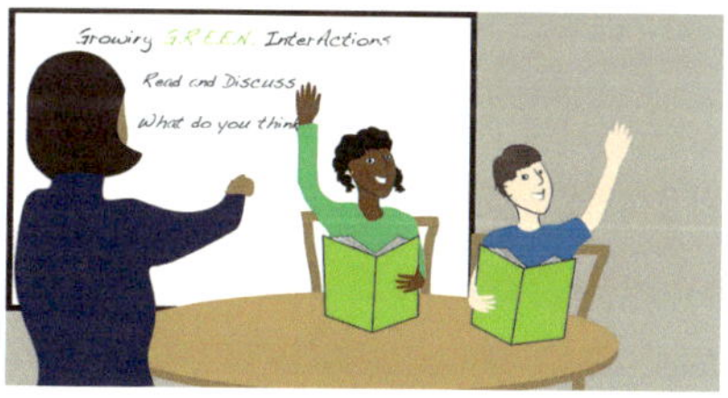

Have you ever thought of *yourself* as the main character in your own life story? Think about it. This is quite a **powerful** thought! It helps you consider how you act each day. Knowing that you are the main character can guide your choices. Every time you are with someone, you are in a new scene. You get to decide what to say and do with the people you are with so that the scene is the best it can be. You can take an active role and have more control over your life. You have the **power** to take action to be your **best self** in your own **best life** story. You can set **goals** to have your **best life**.

Who is the main character in your favorite story? ______________________________

____

Why do you like this character? ______________________________

____

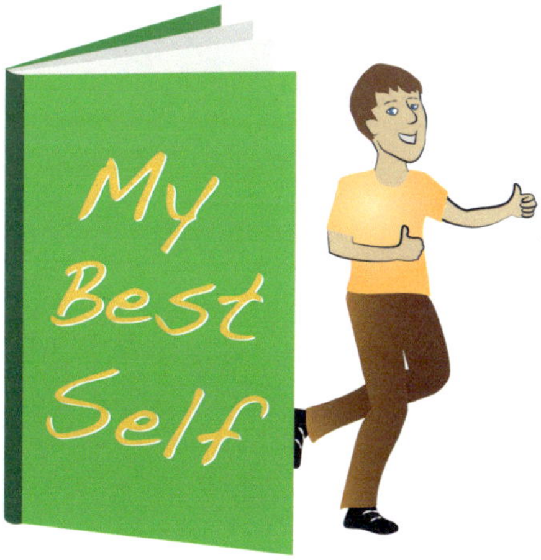

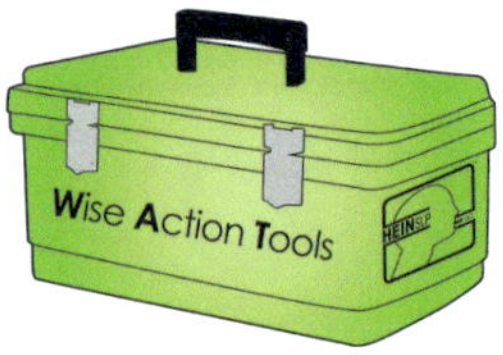

SELF-CHECK:
ARE YOU MAKING YOUR BEST LIFE STORY?

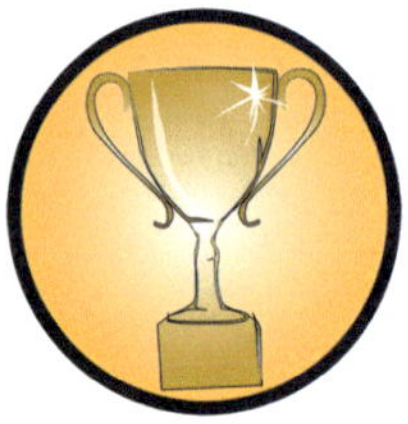

Answer these questions to help you think about whether you are making choices to help *your* life story be the best it can be:

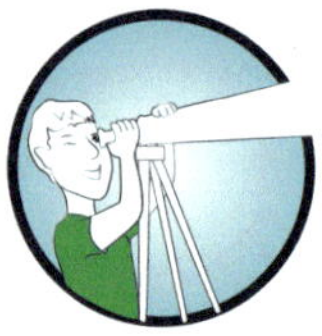

1. As the main character in your own life, are you alert and **paying attention to what's happening around you**?
   most of the time/ some of the time/ never

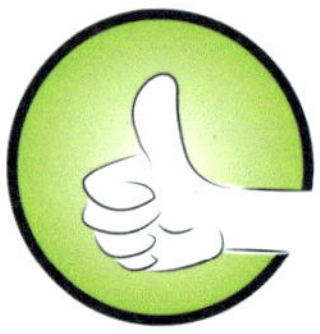

2. As the main character in your own life, are you making your best decisions so your life story gets **better**?
   most of the time/ some of the time/ never

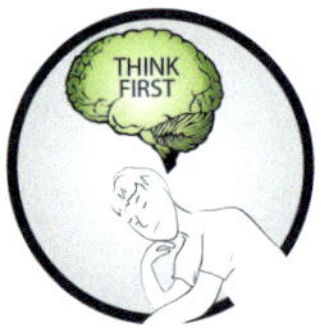

3. Do you think about acting **G.R.E.E.N.** in your own life story? Do you think about helping the other people in your life have **better** life stories too?
   most of the time/ some of the time/ never

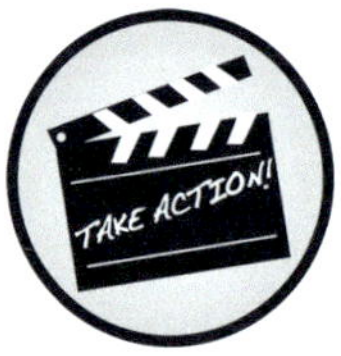

4. As the main character in your own life, do you take **positive** action when things need to be solved or fixed so each scene can be the best it can be?
   most of the time/ some of the time/ never

To be your **best self** in each scene in your own life story you can follow these steps. The more you practice these skills, the more you strengthen the pathways in your brain that guide you to take **positive** action.

IT IS NEVER TOO LATE TO START GUIDING YOURSELF TO BE THE BEST CHARACTER IN YOUR OWN BEST LIFE STORY!!! You have the **power** to choose the best action more often.

Think about making a **change** for the **better.** 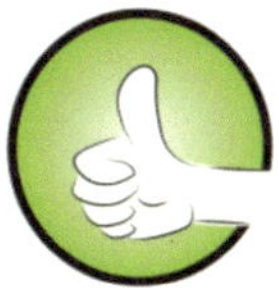 Every day you have the **power** to guide yourself to be the **best character** in your own **best life** story!!

Learn to make choices for your own **best life.** Act **G.R.E.E.N.** with others around you. It will change your attitude about what can happen each day. When you see **positive** things happening because of your actions, you will notice more **positive** energy growing inside of you. This will help you take the next steps toward the **best life** for yourself and people on your TEAMS.

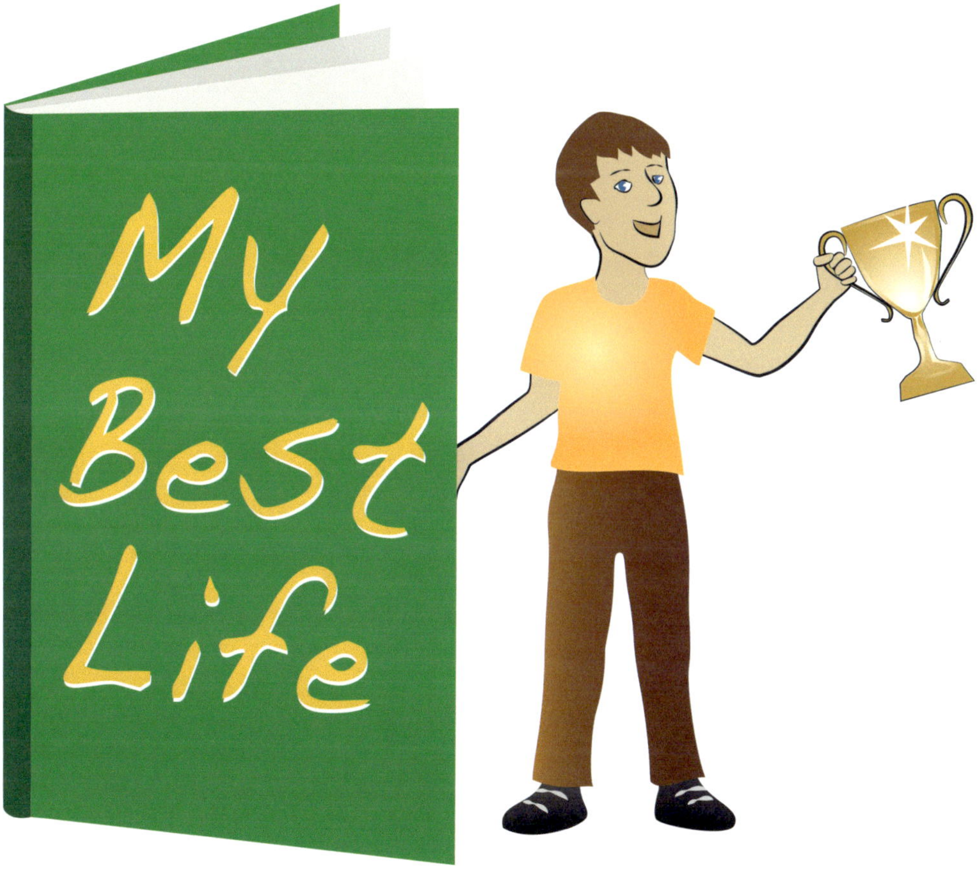

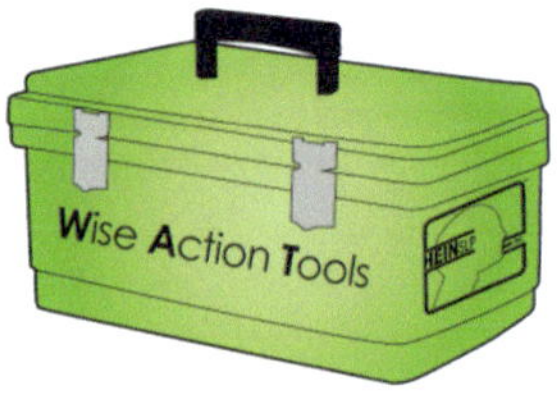

PICTURE YOUR OWN BEST LIFE!

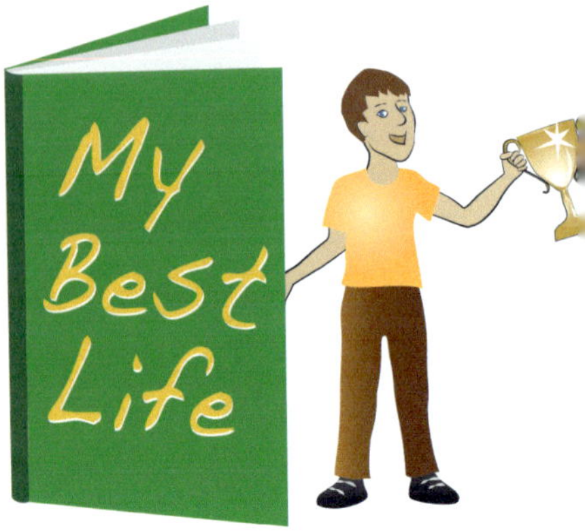

Now see if you can picture your own **best life**.

1. **Where** is your **best life** happening?
2. **Who** is with you in your own **best life**?
3. **What** are you doing in your life that makes it the best?
4. **When** is this **best life** of yours happening?

   tomorrow   next week   next month   next year   in five years

5. Draw your own **best life** in the box below or write in the words that describe the life you want to have. Start taking the road to your best life by taking your best steps in each and every one of your life scenes.

This is a picture of my own **best life**:

WAKE UP

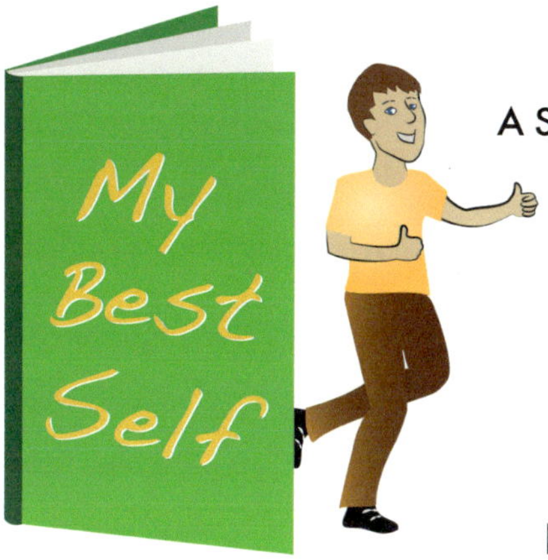

A Song for Guiding G.R.E.E.N. Thoughts®

by Herb Hein

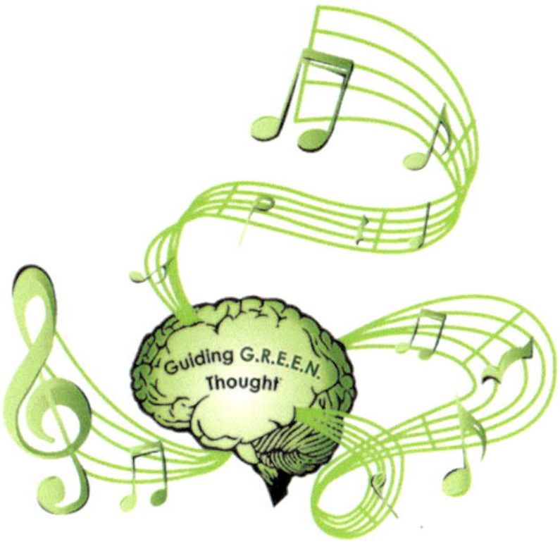

Hey you, the sun is shining,
Time to get up and do your thing.
No use in lying, dreaming,
New day is knockin' waitin' for you.
Come on baby, open your eyes.
Clock says it's time to rise.
Give a kiss and step on the floor,
Grab your clothes and out the door.
Pick up that feeling, moving ahead.
Let it surround you.
You'll be glad you moved beyond your bed.
Start to feel the wheels a-hummin'.
Time to hear the rhythm strummin'.
Learn your lessons from yesterday,
Give them meaning as you go on your way.
Don't be worried if you make a mistake;
It's only natural when you're awake.
Try again and you'll get it right.
You'll deserve your sleep tonight.
Pick up that feeling, moving ahead.
Let it surround you,
You'll be glad you moved beyond your bed.
Pick up that feeling, moving ahead.
Let it surround you,
You'll be glad you moved beyond your bed.

7.2 Setting Personal Goals for Your Own Best Life

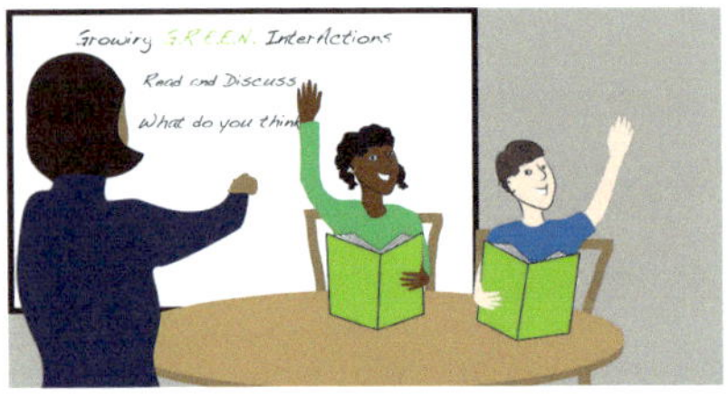

After you evaluate yourself and get feedback from others, you will want to decide on a **Personal Goal** that will increase the number of **G.R.E.E.N.** actions you take. This **goal** can guide you to do even **better** for your next evaluation. **Personal Goals** are those you want to accomplish so your life gets even **better**. You set **goals** to help you take steps **forward** toward your **best life**.

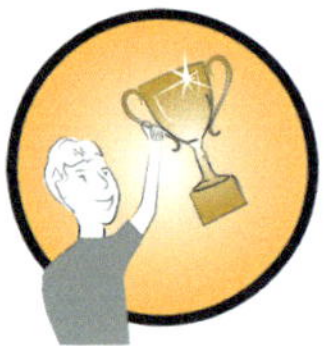

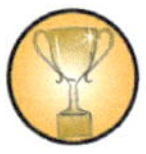

You can have smaller **goals** to reach *today* or *this week*.

Discuss: What goal can you accomplish today or this week? ____________________

____

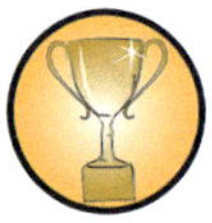

You can have bigger **goals** to accomplish *this month* or *this year*.

Discuss: What goal do you want to accomplish this month or this year? ________

____

Setting small **goals** and achieving them helps you take the steps toward bigger future **goals**. Where would you like to be? Who would you like to have with you? What would you like to be doing in one year? Five years? Ten years? What smaller steps do you need to take today to fulfill that future **best-life goal**?

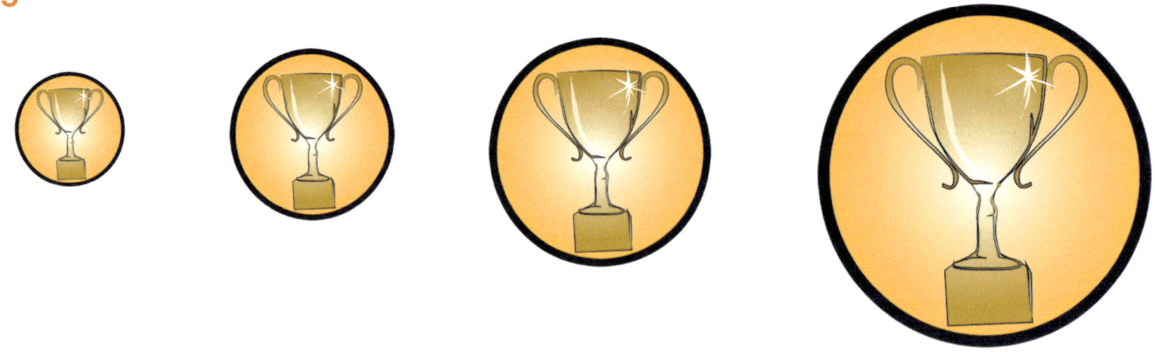

7.3 How to Choose a Goal Area to Improve Your Life!

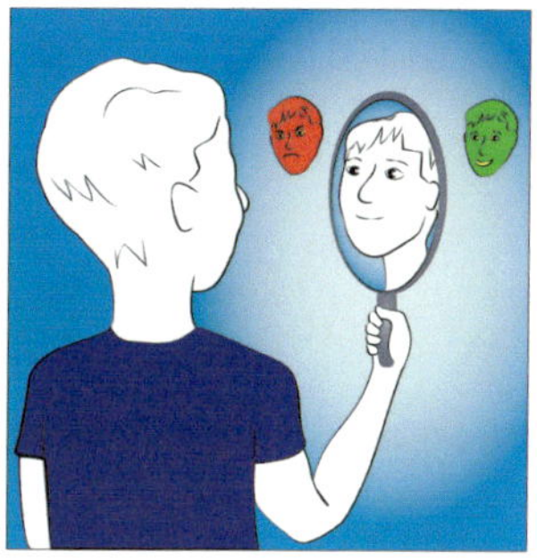

Look at yourself and imagine looking in the mirror to see how you really act. How do you behave? As you **pay attention and survey your actions**, what things are you doing that make your life **better**? What things are you doing that make your life worse? Is there a behavior or action you can do more often that will make your life **better**? Make it a **goal** to do this behavior or action more often. You can choose something you already do sometimes and decide to do it more frequently. Honestly think about how often you perform this behavior now. Consider this your starting point or *baseline*.

You can mark your starting point on the **goal** baseline chart.

A. Your Baseline: You will circle how often you do the action at your starting point.

never sometimes half the time most of the time almost always

0 5 10 15 20 25 30 35 40 45 50 55 60 65 70 75 80 85 90 95 **100**

Next, think realistically about how much progress you can make. Circle those words and that number on the **goal** setting chart. That will be your **goal** for you to achieve!

B. Your Goal: You will circle the number that shows how often you will be able to do the action that will be in your goal.

(You circle how far you will be able to *realistically* move to the right.)

never sometimes half the time most of the time almost always

0 5 10 15 20 25 30 35 40 45 50 55 60 65 70 75 80 85 90 95 **100**

7.4 Read and Discuss: Being Honest and Realistic to Achieve Your Goals

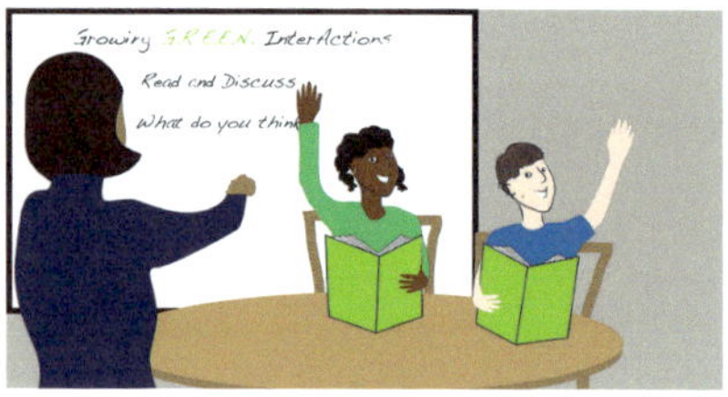

It often requires real effort to take the steps needed to reach and achieve **goals**. That is why it is important to set **goals** that you can achieve. When you are **realistic**, you are honest with yourself about what you can actually accomplish. Will it take just one day or one week to reach the **goal**, or will it take a month or longer? If you are **realistic** about setting your **goals**, you will find that you are more likely to achieve them in a **realistic** amount of time. The most important thing is to start taking steps toward achieving the **goal** you set for yourself. Then keep taking more steps. After you take the first step, you can watch yourself improve a little bit at a time. As you start to achieve your **goals**, you will learn how much you can realistically achieve in a week, a month, or longer.

It may not be realistic to improve yourself so much that you act **better** all the time. This is especially true if you are trying to reach a **goal** in just a week or month. However, you can start to act **better** more often.

Let's look at **goals** people have set for themselves and decide whether they are **realistic** about achieving their **goals**.

Discuss which goals you think are more realistic because the person could *really* achieve the goal.

Choosing a Realistic Personal Goal for the Week

So far this school year, Beth has been receiving 60% on her math quizzes. What is a realistic **goal** for Beth's next quiz if she studies?

A. I will study and get 100% on my next quiz. I will be perfect at math.

B. I will study and get 80% on my next quiz. I will become better at math.

Choosing a Realistic Personal Goal for the Month

So far, Jim has been getting the basketball into the basket two out of every ten shots. This means he is making baskets 20% of the time. What is a realistic **goal** for Jim for the next month if he practices?

A. I will make my shot 60% of the time.

B. I will make my shot 100% of the time.

7.5 Reviewing and Choosing Personal Goals

The next few pages will give you ideas about some **goals** you might choose at school, at home, or with friends. Choose one or more or think of your own and write them on the blank lines. In the future, you may want to add **goals** as you have new thoughts about what you want to achieve.

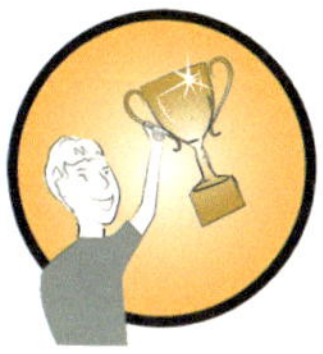

7.6 Some Great Personal Goals for School Scenes

If you go to school, think about your real-life school scene. Think about what you want to accomplish in the next *week* or *month* to make your school life **better**. You

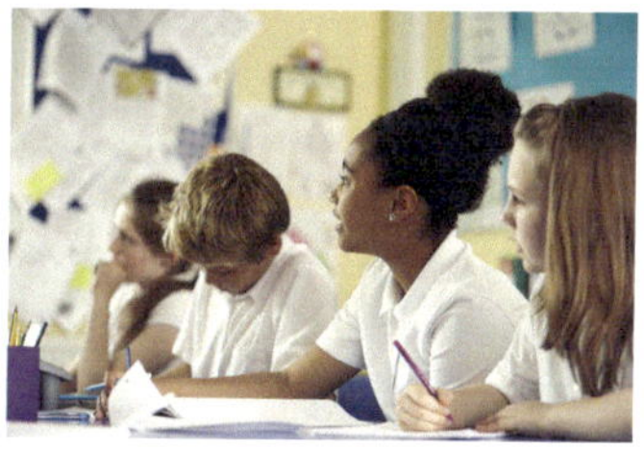

can look at the list of **Personal Goals** below to see whether you want to start achieving one or more of these in the next *week* or month. If you already do one of these just a little bit, you might want your **goal** to be that you do it more frequently.

____ I will listen to my teachers and follow their directions.

____ I will ask my teacher questions when I don't understand something.

____ I will check my work and fix mistakes I find.

____ I will take the advice my teacher gives me.

____ I will get better grades.

____ I will get my homework done on time.

____ I will learn the rules of a game or sport that I play at school.

____ I will wait my turn.

____ I will have good conversations with my friends.

____ I will learn to ____

____ I will ____

7.7 Some Great Personal Goals for Home Scenes

At home, think about your real-life home scene.

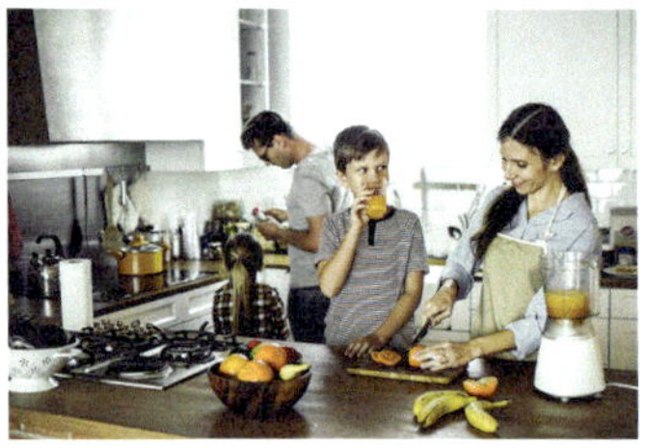

Think about what you want to accomplish in the next *week* or *month* to make your life better in your home. Look at the list of Personal Goals below and decide whether you want to start achieving one or more of them in the next *week* or *month*. If you already do one of these just a little bit, you might want your goal to be that you will do it more frequently.

____ I will ask for help when I need it.

____ I will listen to my parents and follow their directions.

____ I will ask my parents questions when I don't understand something.

____ I will clean up after myself.

____ I will take turns with the people in my family.

____ I will do more things by myself.

____ I will do my part to ensure a nice place to play and work.

____ I will have fun.

____ I will learn to ____

____ I will ____

7.8 Some Great Personal Goals for Friendship Scenes

Think about the real-life scene you have (or would like to have) with your friends. When you are with your friends, you work together so each of you feels safe with one another and trusts each other so you can share your ideas and have fun together.

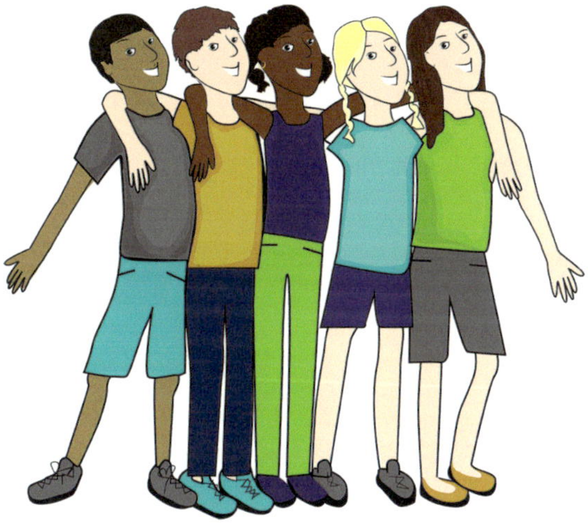

Think about what you want to accomplish in the next *week* or *month* to make your life better in your Friendship Scenes. Look at the list of Personal Goals below to see whether you want to start achieving one or more of these in the next *week* or *month*. If you already do one of these just a little bit, you might want your goal to be that you do it more frequently.

____ I will share with my friend(s).

____ I will take turns with my friend(s).

____ I will listen to what my friends are talking about.

____ I will do things with my friends that we all enjoy doing.

____ I will use self-control with my friends.

____ I will do things to help my friends.

____ I will learn to ____

____ I will ____

7.9 Examples of Goals That People Set for Themselves

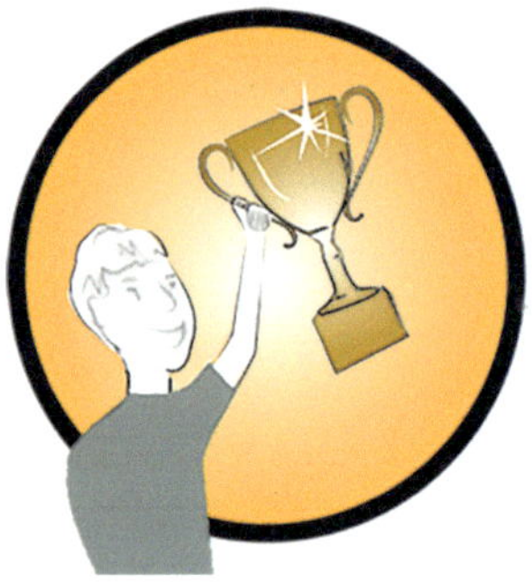

1. **John's Goal Area**: Completing assignments so I can be successful

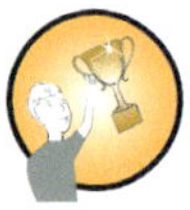

A. **John's Goal**: I will complete the assignments and tasks my teachers and guides ask me to do.

B. **Starting point/Baseline:** *Today* John does it this often:

Never sometimes half the time most of the time almost always

0 5 10 15 20 25 30 35 40 45 50 55 60 65 70 75 80 85 90 95 **100**

C. **Frequency/How Often?** John thinks he can realistically achieve this **goal** this often in the next week (he chose how far he can *realistically* move the arrow to the right):

Never sometimes half the time most of the time almost always

0 5 10 15 20 25 30 35 40 45 50 55 60 65 70 75 80 85 90 95 **100**

2. **Jessie's Goal Area**: Using a **self-control** strategy so I can stay calm and in control

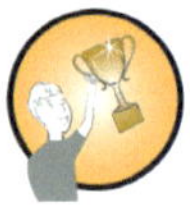

A. **Jessie's Goal**: I will use a self-calming strategy when I am starting to feel upset or frustrated.

B. **Starting point/Baseline:** *Today* Jessie does it this often:

Never sometimes half the time most of the time almost always

0 5 10 15 20 25 30 35 40 45 50 55 60 65 70 75 80 85 90 95 **100**

C. **Frequency/How Often?** Jessie thinks she can realistically achieve this **goal** this often in the next week: (She chose how far she can realistically move the arrow to the right):

Never sometimes half the time most of the time almost always

0 5 10 15 20 25 30 35 40 45 50 55 60 65 70 75 80 85 90 95 **100**

3. **Rob's Goal Area**: **Politely** Asking for Help

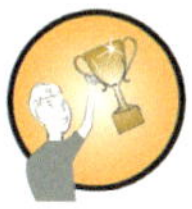

A. Rob's Goal: I will **politely** ask for help when I need it.

B. **Starting point/Baseline:** Today Rob does it this often:

Never sometimes half the time most of the time almost always

0 5 10 15 20 25 30 35 40 45 50 55 60 65 70 75 80 85 90 95 **100**

C. **Frequency/How Often?** Rob thinks he can realistically move the arrow to the right this much this week:

Never sometimes half the time most of the time almost always

0 5 10 15 20 25 30 35 40 45 50 55 60 65 70 75 80 85 90 95 **100**

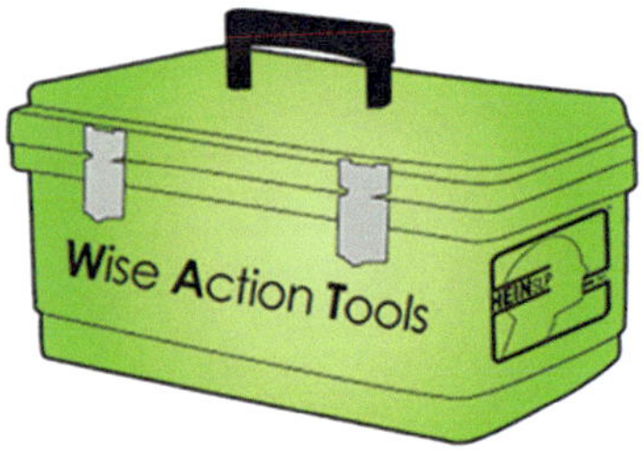

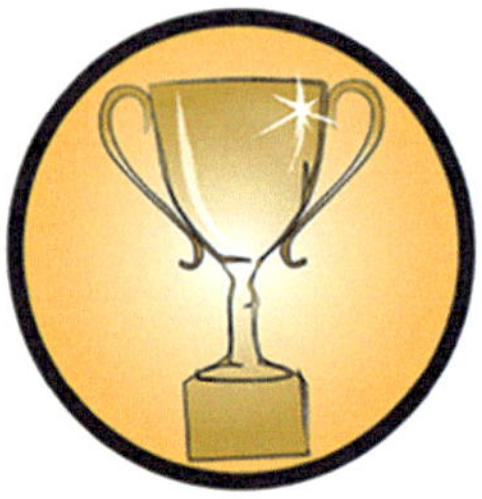

MY PERSONAL GOAL WORKSHEET

Today's Date: ______________________

Goal area: ____

My useful, realistic **goal** for the next week/month is: ____________________

____

A. Baseline: Circle how often I do it today.

Never sometimes half of the time most of the time almost always

0 5 10 15 20 25 30 35 40 45 **50** 55 60 65 70 75 80 85 90 95 **100**

B. My realistic **goal** for the next week/month is to do this ______________
(how often?)

Never sometimes half of the time most of the time almost always

My Goal : How often will I be able to do the action written in my goal
(circle how far you can *realistically* move to the right):

0 5 10 15 20 25 30 35 40 45 **50** 55 60 65 70 75 80 85 90 95 **100**

- -

Checking in: I am checking how I am doing on this date: ______________

How am I doing? ____

What am I doing well? ______________________________________

What can help me do **better**?_____________________________________

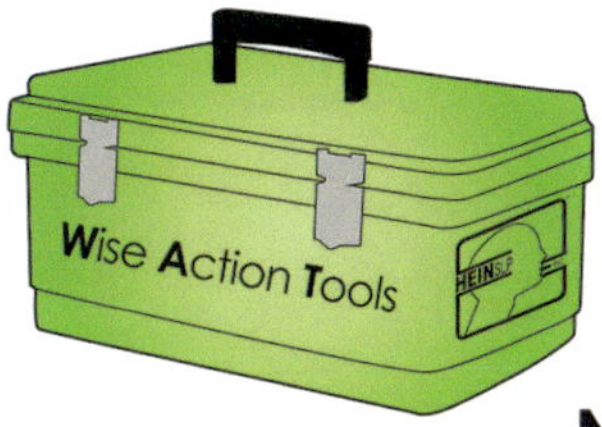

NOTING PROGRESS ON MY PERSONAL GOALS

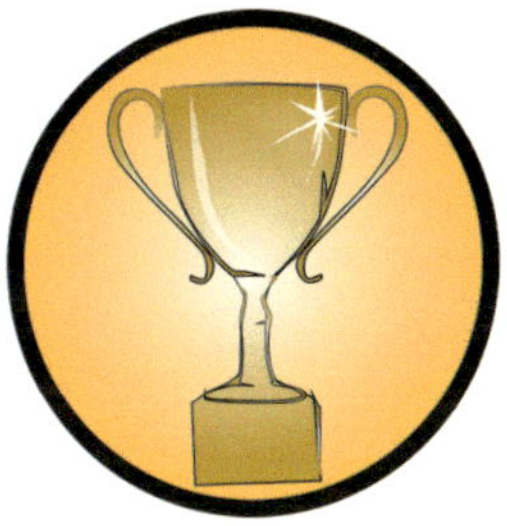

I am checking how I am doing on this date: ______________________________

How am I doing? What am I doing well? What can help me do better? __________

____

____

I am checking how I am doing on this date: ______________________________

How am I doing? What am I doing well? What can help me do better? __________

____

____

I am checking how I am doing on this date: ______________________________

How am I doing? What am I doing well? What can help me do better? __________

____

____

I am checking how I am doing on this date: ______________________________

How am I doing? What am I doing well? What can help me do better? __________

____

____

7.10 Take Positive Action to Take the Next Step Forward!

When you choose **goals**, you are making choices to keep yourself healthy and safe while you strive to make your life better. When you strive to do something, you keep working at it, no matter how hard it is! You don't give up! Keep taking the next small step that leads you closer to your **goal**. This is taking **positive** action. This is how to build your **best life**! You can take **positive** action and move **forward** with those on your Teams who are striving to do the same thing. As much as possible, everyone on each Team strives to take **positive** action with each step. Each small step **forward** taken by each person helps make our civilization great.

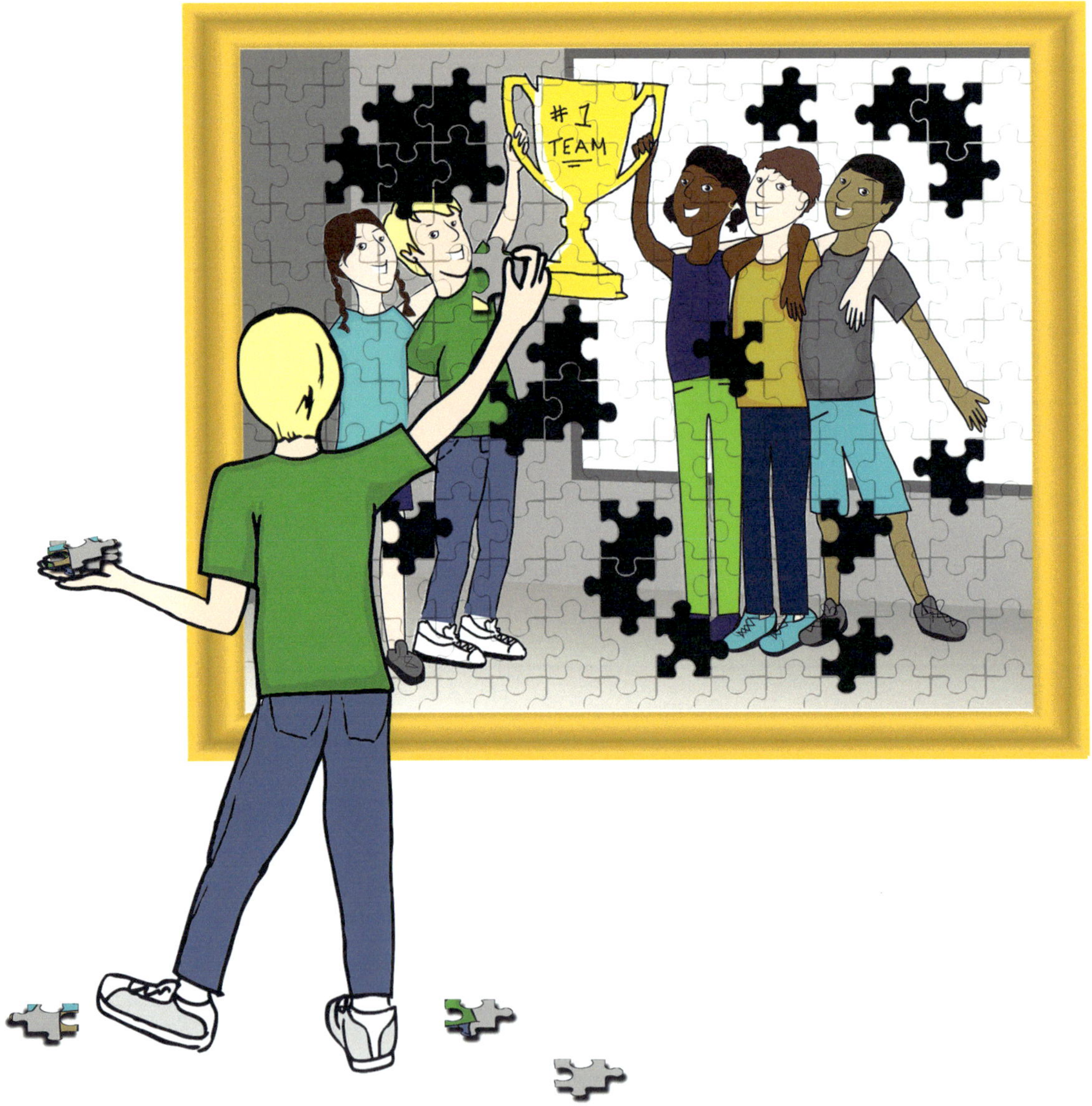

7.11 Survey the Scene: Positive or Negative Action in the School Scene

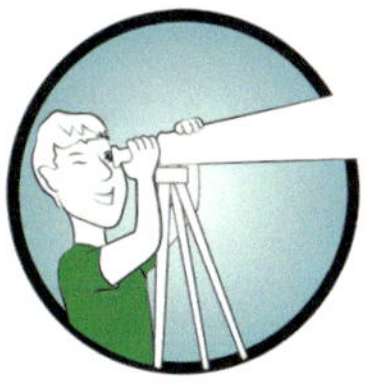

Directions: Survey the scene to see how Kendra acted in the two different scenes below. When do you think she was taking positive action and striving to meet a Personal Goal for School? When do you think she might have been giving up, doing nothing, or taking negative action to make her situation worse?

Draw a green circle around any words that show Kendra taking positive action to make things better at school. Draw a red circle around any words showing that Kendra's thinking or acting made her school situation worse.

1. Kendra got her assignment back from her teacher. There were four or five edits that the teacher had written on the paper to improve Kendra's writing. Kendra read her teacher's notes and did her best to make the **changes**. She asked for help when she did not understand something that the teacher had written.

   A. Kendra was taking positive action.

   B. Kendra was giving up, doing nothing, or taking negative action.

2. Kendra got her assignment back from her teacher. There were four or five edits that the teacher had written on the paper to improve Kendra's writing. Kendra saw her teacher's notes and could not believe that the teacher thought anything needed fixing. She thought her work was good enough. She did not read the notes and gave the paper back to the teacher without making any **changes**.

   A. Kendra was taking positive action.

   B. Kendra was giving up, doing nothing, or taking negative action.

Discuss: What do you think Kendra's Personal Goal for School was?

7.12 Survey the Scene: Positive or Negative Action in the Home Scene

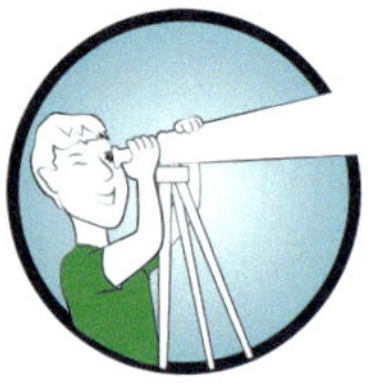

Directions: Survey the scene to see how Jonah acted in the two different scenes below. When do you think he was taking positive action and striving to meet a Personal Goal for home? When was he giving up, doing nothing, or taking negative action to make his situation worse?

Draw a green circle around any words that show Jonah taking a positive action to make things better at home. Draw a red circle around any words showing that Jonah's thoughts or actions made his home situation worse.

1. Jonah wanted to play a game on the family TV. His brother was already playing a game on the TV. Jonah yelled at his brother to get off the TV right away so he could use it. Jonah grabbed the TV controller. Jonah's brother got mad and tried to grab the controller back. No one got to use the TV because their father told them both to stop fighting and go to their rooms.

   A. Jonah was taking **positive** action.

   B. Jonah was giving up, doing nothing, or taking negative action.

2. Jonah wanted to play a game on the family TV. His brother was already playing a game on the TV. Jonah asked his brother if he could have a turn playing on the TV. Jonah's brother said he would finish his game in ten minutes. Jonah waited quietly and watched his brother play. Then, his brother gave Jonah the TV controller so Jonah could have his turn. Jonah thanked his brother.

   A. Jonah was taking **positive** action.

   B. Jonah was giving up, doing nothing, or taking negative action.

Discuss: What do you think Jonah's Personal Goal for Home was?

____

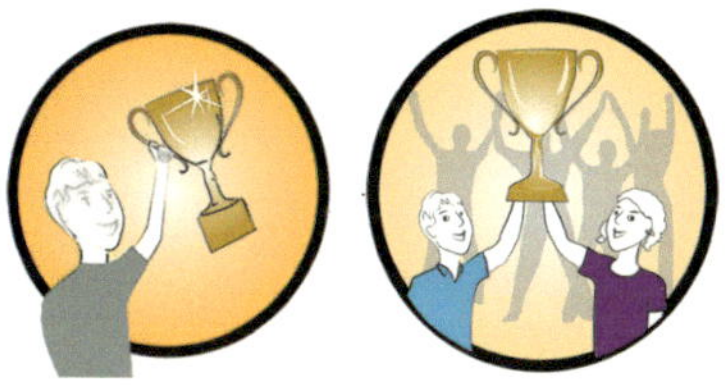

8 Achieving Personal Goals and Common Team Goals

8.1 Achieving Your Personal Goals and Common Team Goals!

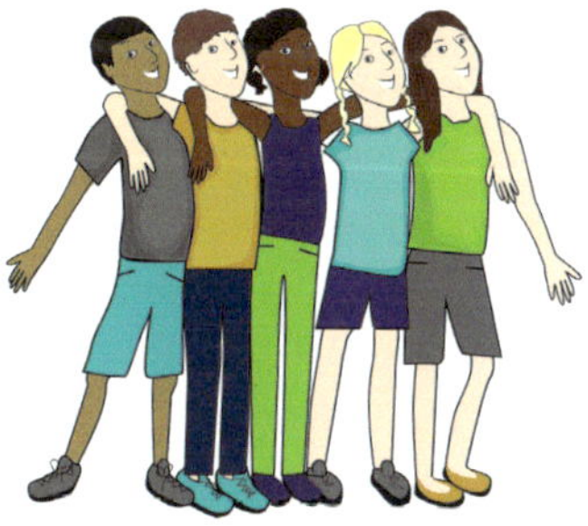

Survey the scene and notice who else is on your Team. Then you can use your positive power to try to make any situation better. 

You can use words and actions that help people get along better. This helps you achieve your Personal Goals while your Teams meet their Common Team Goals.

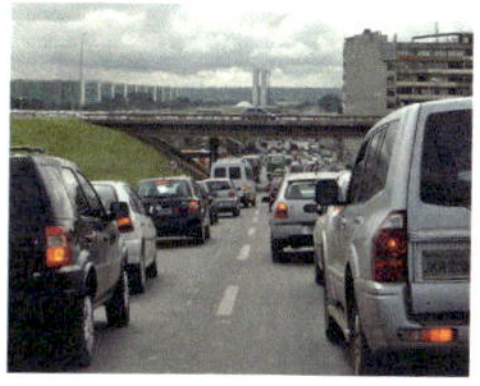

When you are on the same road or in the same room as others, you have interactions. This means you communicate with people and choose to do things with them.

You keep working on your own Personal Goal while you work with your Team on the Common Team Goal. Your actions have the power to meet both your Personal Goal and the Common Team Goal.

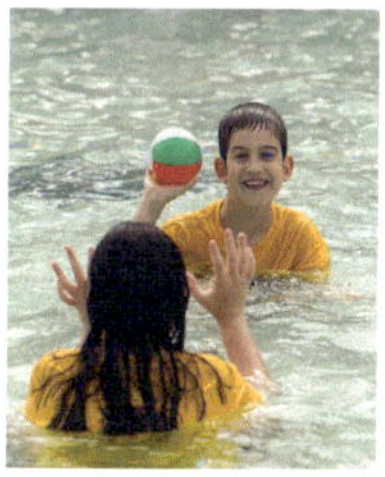

Think about the people on your Team. Consider how your words and actions will affect them. You can make helpful choices for the Team so it can be the best it can be. Whenever you communicate, you can do your best to help the Team reach its Common Team Goal.

Use your positive power to do your best in your next interaction with each of your Teams!

8.2 Survey the Scene: Basketball Practice at Home—Which Action Choices Let John Achieve Both Goals at Home?

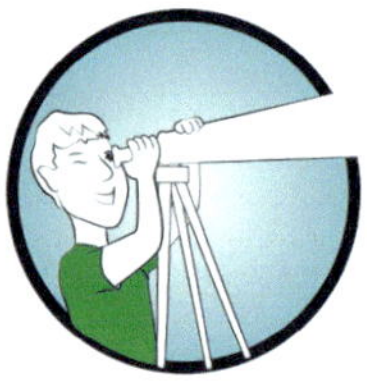

John and his Home Team act differently in Action Choice "A" and Action Choice "B." Which action helps John achieve both **goals**: his **Personal Goal** and the Home **Common Team Goal**?

Directions: Survey these scenes and decide whether John's Personal and Home Common Team Goals will both be met.

Use a green pencil to underline the actions that help the Team. Use a red pencil to underline the actions that block the Team from meeting its goal.

Action Choice A

John's **Personal Goal** is to play basketball better. The Home **Common Team Goal** is for everyone in the family to live in a peaceful place. John likes to dribble his basketball in the house when the rest of the family is sleeping. He likes to shoot the ball up to a target he made on the wall. He also likes to do this when the rest of the family is trying to sleep. His parents and his sister yell at him to stop making noise, but he does not stop.

1. Can John's **Personal Goal** be met by John's actions?

   yes no

2. Can the **Home Common Team Goal** be met by John's actions?

   yes no

3. Can both John's **Personal Goal** and the Home **Common Team Goal** be met by John's actions?

   yes no

4. Should John continue doing what he is doing?

yes no

5. Should John **switch** to doing a different action?

yes no

6. How could John help **change the scene** to make it **better** for everyone on the Team? ______________________________

____

Action Choice B

John's **Personal Goal** is to play basketball better. The Home **Common Team Goal** is for everyone in the family to live in a peaceful place. John's parents got him a basketball hoop for the driveway. John practices shooting baskets outside on the driveway after he finishes his homework. He only practices when the other people in the house are not trying to sleep.

1. Can John's **Personal Goal** be met by John's actions?

yes no

2. Can the Home **Common Team Goal** be met by John's actions?

yes no

3. Can *both* John's **Personal Goal** and the Home **Common Team Goal** be met by John's actions?

yes no

4. Should John continue doing what he is doing?

yes no

5. Should John **switch** to doing a different action?

yes no

6. How did John act in this scene to make it **better** for everyone on the Team, compared with Action Choice "A"? ______________________________

____

7. What did John's family do in this scene to make it **better** for John and the rest of the Home Team? ______________________________

____

8.3 Survey the Scene: Asking Questions—Which Action Choice Lets Trent Achieve Both Goals in Class?

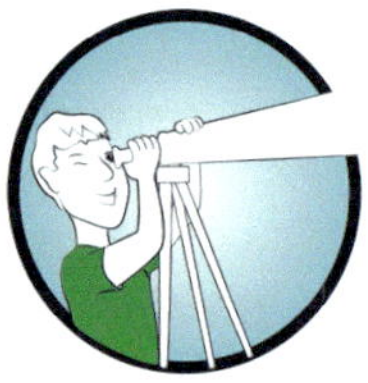

Trent and his Classroom Team act differently in the scenes below.

Directions: Survey these scenes carefully so you can decide whether Trent's Personal Goal and Common Team Goals for the classroom will be met.

Use a green pencil to underline the actions that help the Team. Use a red pencil to underline the actions that block the Team from moving forward with its goals.

Action Choice A

Trent's **Personal Goal** is to get good grades in class. The **Common Team Goal** for the classroom is for everyone in the class to learn together. Trent likes to ask questions in class but blurts out a lot of them without raising his hand. He does not give his classmates a turn to ask questions. His teacher does not answer his questions because he does not raise his hand. Trent gets frustrated and yells at his teacher. The other students in the class are not able to learn.

1. Can Trent's **Personal Goal** be met by his actions?

   yes no

2. Can the Classroom **Common Team Goal** be met by his actions?

   yes no

3. Can *both* Trent's **Personal Goal** and the Classroom **Common Team Goal** be met by his actions?

   yes no

4. Should Trent continue doing what he is doing?

   yes no

5. Should Trent **switch** to doing a different action?

   yes no

6. How could Trent help **change the scene** to make it **better** for everyone on the Team? ______________________________

   ____

Action Choice B

Trent's **Personal Goal** is to get good grades in his class. The **Common Team Goal** for the classroom is for everyone in the class to learn together. Trent likes to ask questions in class. He was forgetting to raise his hand to ask questions. The teacher gave him a reminder for his desk and gave him a signal to raise his hand if he forgot. Trent's teacher talked to him after class to let him know how important it was for his classmates to be able to ask questions, too. His teacher told Trent that he could answer some extra questions during his lunch break. By looking at the reminder card on his desk, Trent learned to raise his hand when he had a question. He let his classmates ask questions without interrupting them. He saved some of his questions to ask his teacher during his lunch break.

1. Can Trent's **Personal Goal** be met by Trent's actions?

   yes no

2. Can the Classroom **Common Team Goal** be met by Trent's actions?

   yes no

3. Can *both* Trent's **Personal Goal** and the **Common Team Goal** be met by Trent's actions?

   yes no

4. Should Trent continue doing what he is doing?

   yes no

5. Should Trent **switch** to doing a different action?

   yes no

6. What did Trent do in this scene that was **better** for everyone on the Team compared with *Action Scene "A"*? ______________________________

   ____

7. What did Trent's teacher do to help Trent meet his **Personal Goal** and the Classroom **Common Team Goal**? ______________________________

   ____

   ____

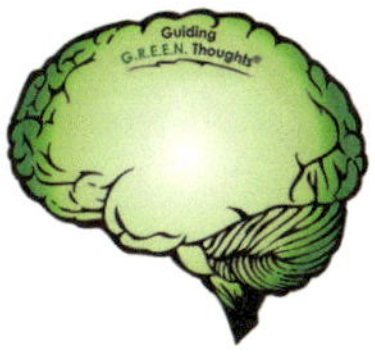

9 Getting Power from Guiding G.R.E.E.N. Thoughts®

9.1 What Is a Guiding G.R.E.E.N. Thought®?

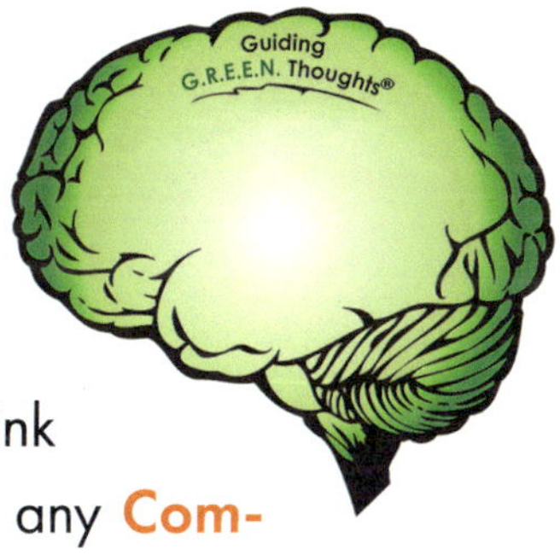

When you are in your home, school, or office—or on the playground, in the store, or in the car—you might be so busy concentrating on what you are doing that you forget to think about people around you. You may not be thinking about any **Common Team Goals**. You may need help in thinking more about the Team.

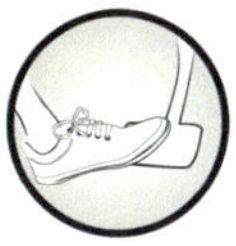

Tap on the brakes so you can Think First.

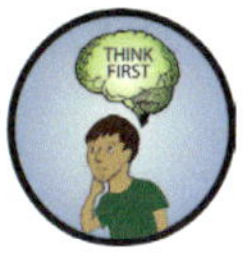

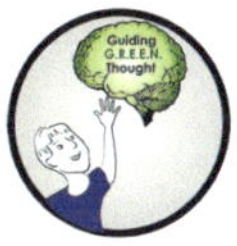

Reach up to your brain for a **Guiding G.R.E.E.N. Thought** so you can return to taking your best actions for the Team.

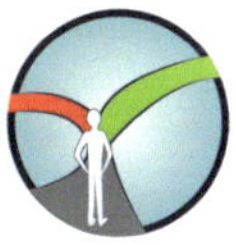

Guiding G.R.E.E.N. Thoughts® are **powerful** words that you can find in your brain. They remind you to guide yourself to make the best choices. With **Guiding G.R.E.E.N. Thoughts**®, you and your Team can achieve the **Common Team Goals**.

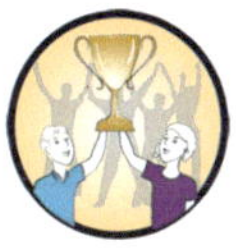

9.2 Reaching Up for a Guiding G.R.E.E.N. Thought

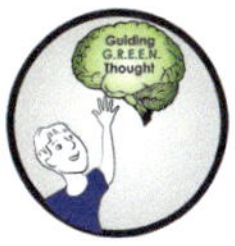

Reaching up for a **Guiding G.R.E.E.N. Thought**® is a Wise Action Tool that can help you act **positively**.

Wise Action Tools are strategies you can use to guide yourself to do your best to make wise action choices. They make life scenes **better** for yourself and the other people on your Teams.

To help you do the best for your Teams, you take time to Think First. Reach up to your brain for a **Guiding G.R.E.E.N. Thought** that will guide your actions. This thought will help you do and say things that make your life **better**, and it makes things **better** for your Teams, too.

This **Growing G.R.E.E.N. InterActions** Program provides many **Guiding G.R.E.E.N. Thoughts** for you to use in your life. When you think a **Guiding G.R.E.E.N. Thought**, it helps you act **positive**, **helpful, cooperative**, **useful**, and **kind**. You will have a chance to see that **Guiding G.R.E.E.N. Thoughts** help you and your Team reach **Common Team Goals**.

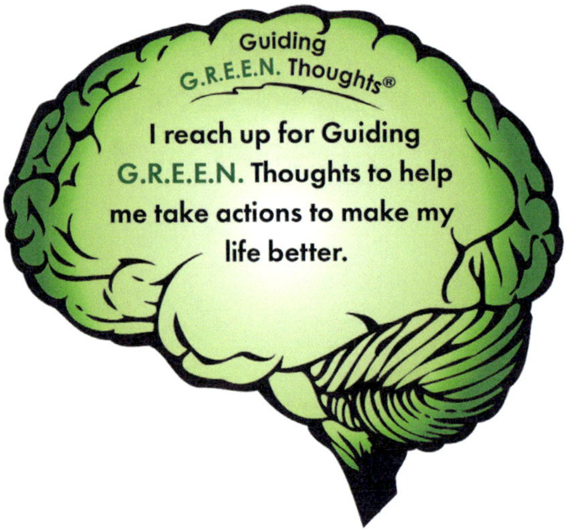

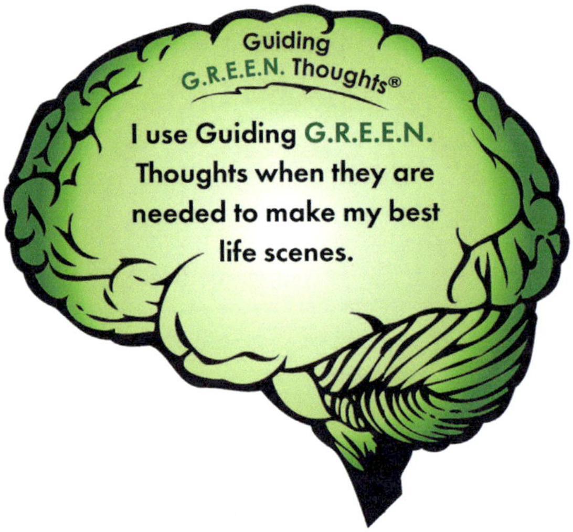

In this program, you will choose **Guiding G.R.E.E.N. Thoughts** that can help the characters you will be reading about. In the box of **Guiding G.R.E.E.N. Thoughts**, you will find thoughts to hold in your hand, read, and even carry with you! You can choose the ones most useful for you and keep them on your desk, in your binder, or even in your pocket.

Choose the most useful thoughts for the different scenes of your life. Remember to use these thoughts in the moments of your life when they are needed most. You will find that **Guiding G.R.E.E.N. Thoughts** help you make the best scenes or **change** scenes to make them **better**. Some **Guiding G.R.E.E.N. Thoughts** have blank spaces for you to write thoughts to guide yourself. Over time, there is no limit to the number of **powerful Guiding G.R.E.E.N. Thoughts®** you can use on your own. Your brain will help you be your **best self** so you can help make the **best world**!

Remember that in each scene of your life, you have the opportunity to choose words and actions that can help you and your Teams. An essential way to help your Team grow **better** is to act **G.R.E.E.N.** during your interactions.

9.3 Guiding G.R.E.E.N. Thoughts for G.R.E.E.N. Action

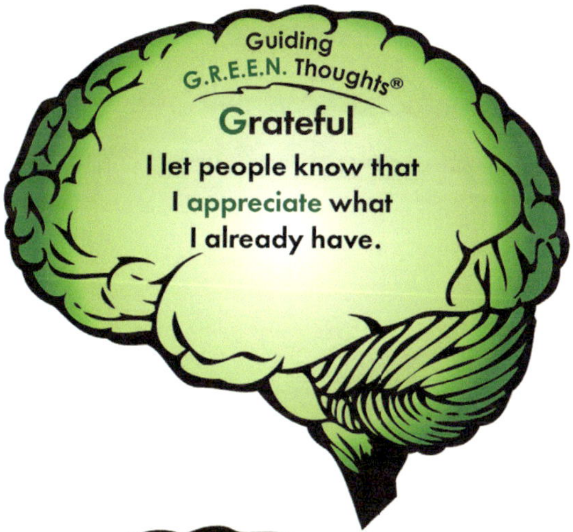

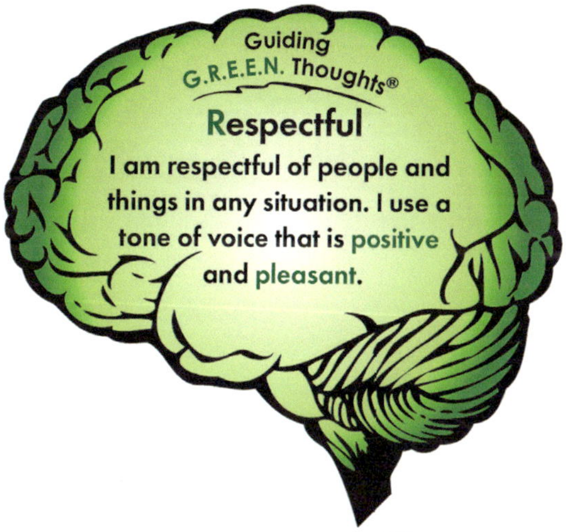

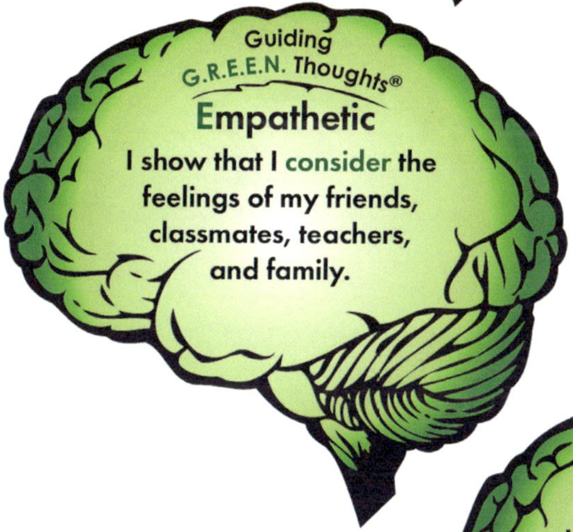

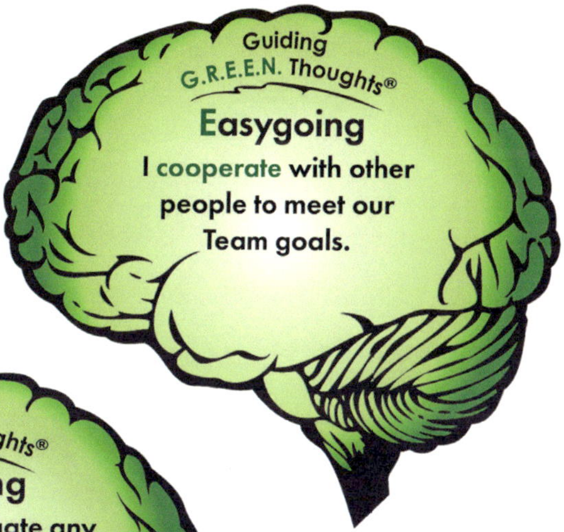

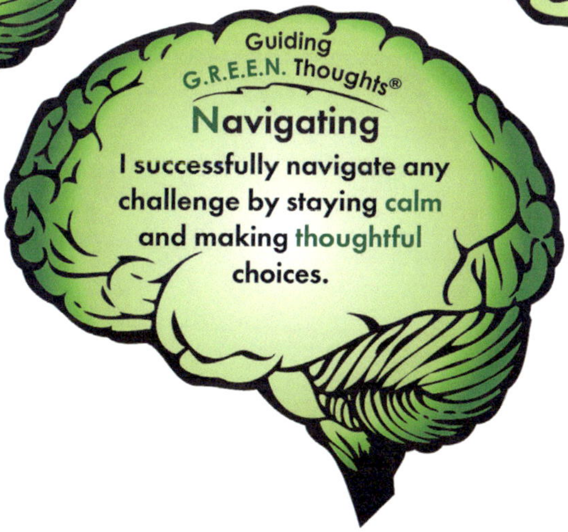

9.4 Practice Makes Perfect

When you learn something new, you become better at it by coaching yourself to think about it often and practicing it. **Guiding G.R.E.E.N. Thoughts** remind you that you have the **potential** to be a great Team member and have **thoughtful**, **helpful, powerful** interactions with other Team members. When you practice using your **Guiding G.R.E.E.N. Thoughts**, you will find it easier to meet both your **Personal Goals** and the **Common Team Goals**.

The more you practice acting G.R.E.E.N., the better you will become at acting G.R.E.E.N. When you practice, it becomes easier to act G.R.E.E.N. more often in real-life scenes with your real Teams.

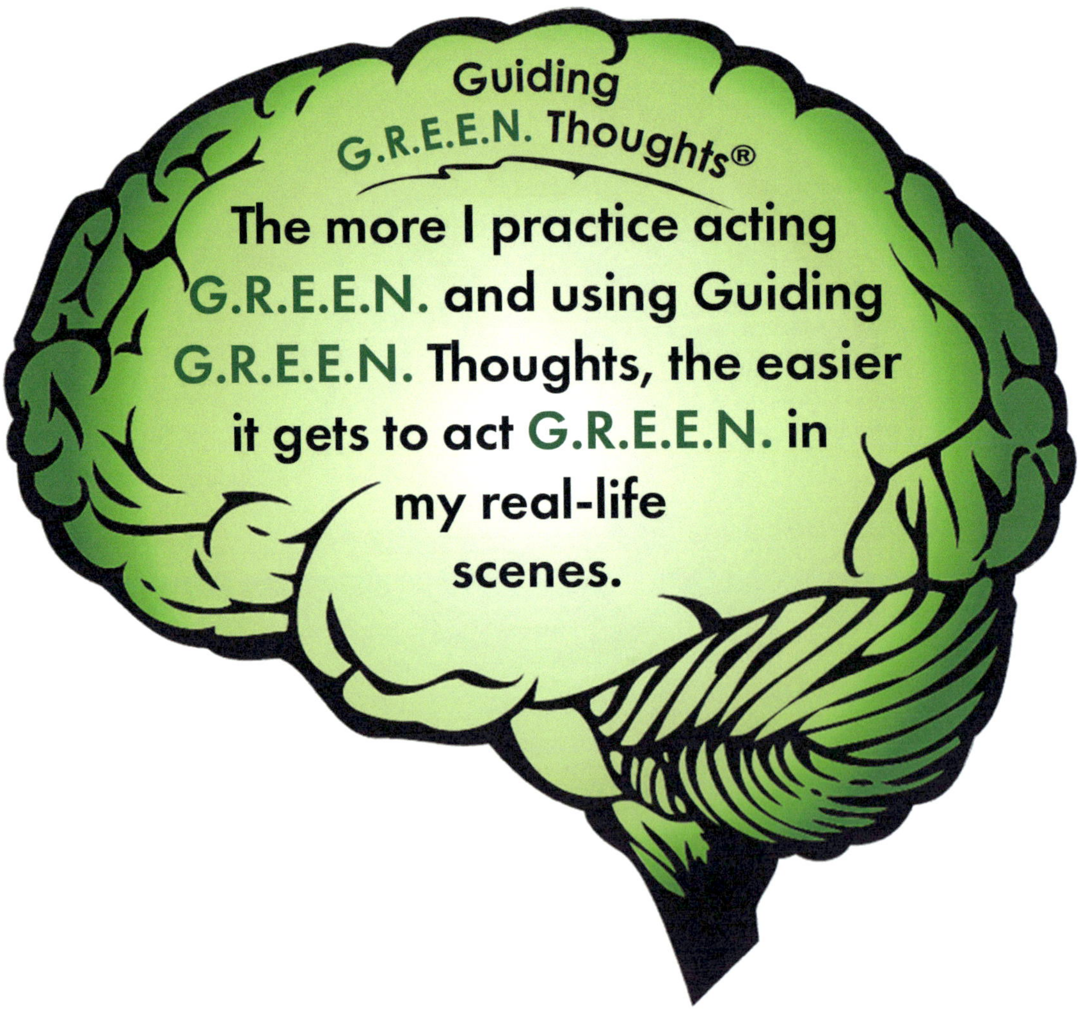

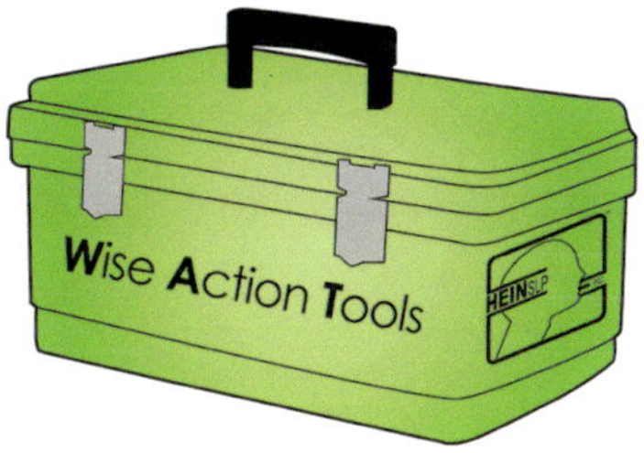

READY, SET, GOAL!

MY GOAL FOR RIGHT NOW

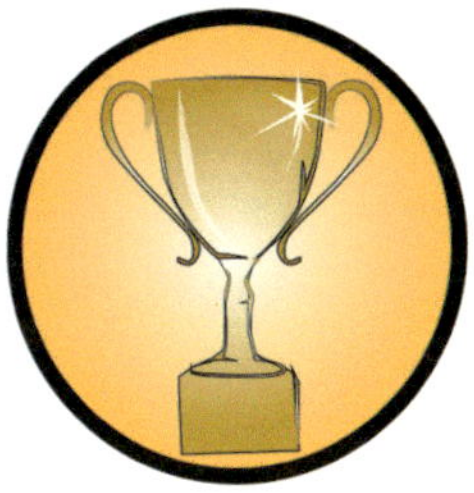

Name ______________________ Date ______________

1. The Team ______________________________

2. Common Team Goal to meet now ______________________________

____

3. My Personal Goal to meet right now ______________________________

____

4. Guiding G.R.E.E.N. Thought to help me meet my goal right now:

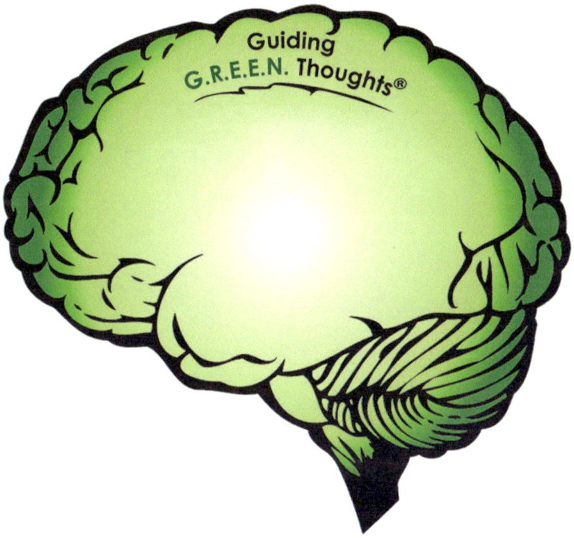

5. Take Action!

6. How did I do? ______________________________

   What did I do well? ______________________________

   What could I do next time to be even more successful? ______________________________

   ____

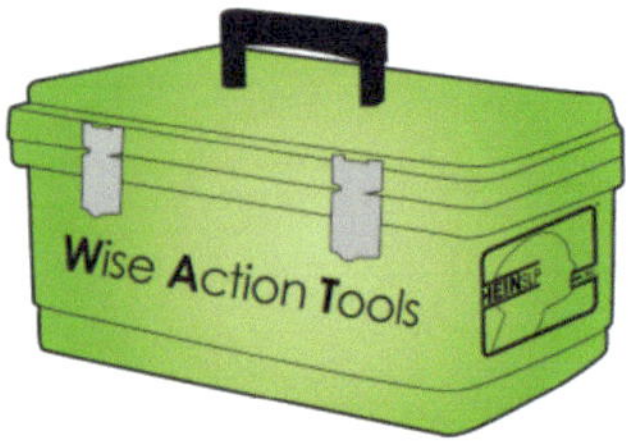

I DRAW MYSELF USING A GUIDING G.R.E.E.N. THOUGHT

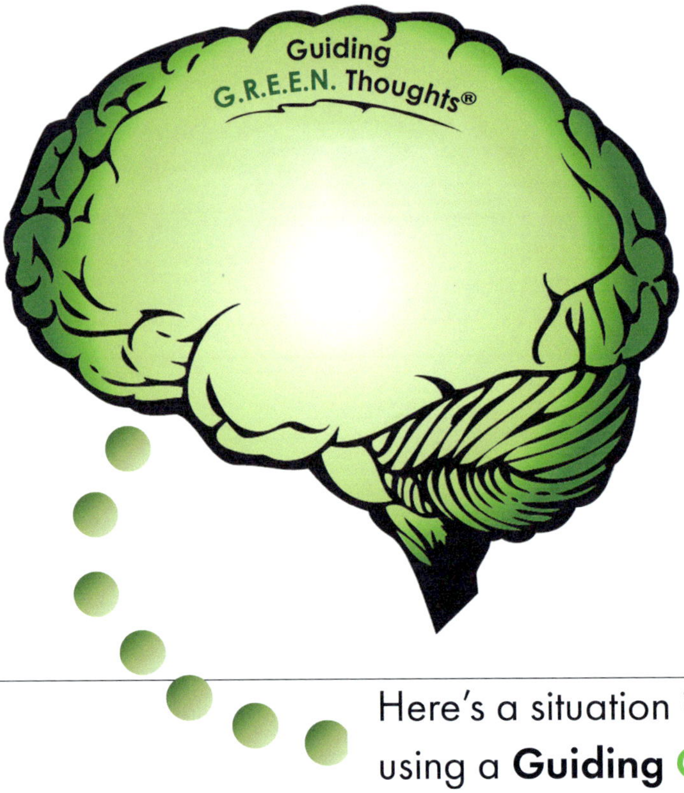

Here's a situation in which I am using a **Guiding G.R.E.E.N. Thought** so I can be the best I can be with my Team.

I am being my better self in a better world!

GUIDING G.R.E.E.N. THOUGHT SONG

A Song for **Guiding G.R.E.E.N. Thoughts**®

By Herb Hein

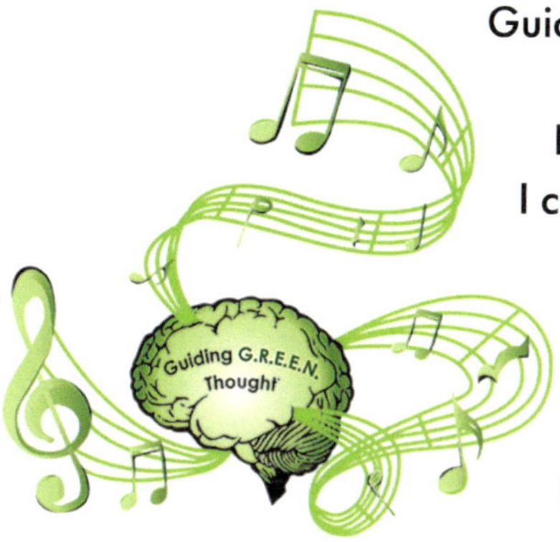

Guiding G.R.E.E.N. Thought...I can use one now.
It's an idea that can give me power.
I can be Grateful for what I've got, yeah!
I can be Grateful, whether it's a little or a lot.
Guiding G.R.E.E.N. Thought...
I can use one now.
It's an idea
that can give me power.
I can be Respectful with the words I say.
Choosing the way to treat you right
gives us a good foundation.
Guiding G.R.E.E.N. Thought...I can use one now.
It's an idea that can give me power.
I can be Empathetic and care to know how you're feeling.
I can be Empathetic to help you on your way!
Guiding G.R.E.E.N. Thought...
I can use one now.
It's an idea
that can give me power.
I can be easy to get along with.
I can be Easygoing so we can meet our goals.
Yes, I can be easy to get along with,
sharing and taking turns are things that I can do.
Guiding G.R.E.E.N. Thought...
I can use one now.
It's an idea
that can give me power.
I can be Navigating around obstacles.
Makin' changes in direction helps me movin' forward.
Guiding G.R.E.E.N. Thought...
I can use one now.
It's an idea
that can give me power.
It's an idea that can
give me power now!

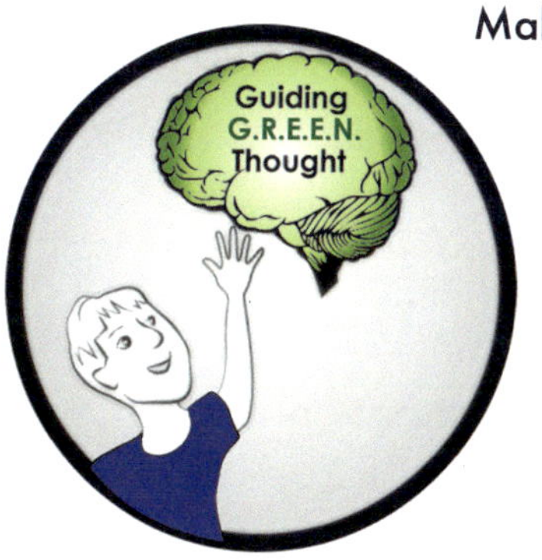

9.5 Strategy: Challenge Your Memory for Guiding G.R.E.E.N. Thoughts

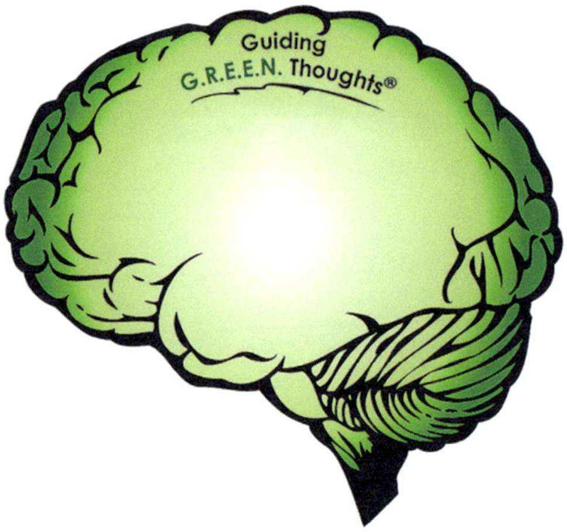

As you learn which **Guiding G.R.E.E.N. Thoughts** are most important for you, you can challenge yourself to remember them. This will help you use them wherever you are.

Read one and try to remember it without looking at the words. Find one or two "key" words that help you picture the whole thought.

Then work on adding another **Guiding G.R.E.E.N. Thought** to your memory. Find one or two "key" words that help you picture the second thought. Challenge yourself to remember the first and second thoughts by picturing their "key" words.

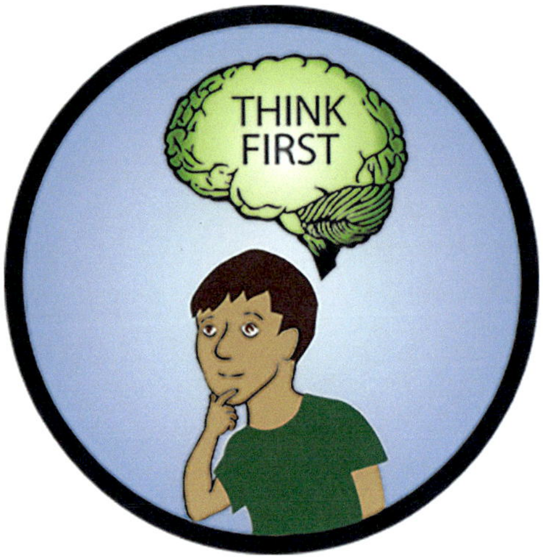

If you try to use more **Guiding G.R.E.E.N. Thoughts** at once, you will remember them better if you add just one new thought at a time. Read it, choose "key" words for it, then try to say it without looking.

This **Guiding G.R.E.E.N. Thought** memory challenge strategy will help you use these thoughts in your real-life scenes.

As you improve your memory for these **Guiding G.R.E.E.N. Thoughts**, you will find yourself using them as you Think First and make the best action choices with your Teams.

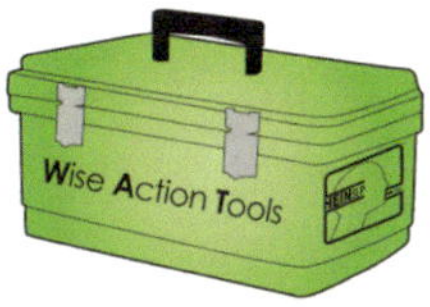

GUIDING G.R.E.E.N. THOUGHT MEMORY CHALLENGE

Choose your most important **Guiding G.R.E.E.N. Thoughts**®. After reading them a few times, challenge yourself to write out what they are without looking at them. Write a "key" word from each thought that helps you picture the whole idea. Keep challenging yourself to remember all your important **Guiding G.R.E.E.N. Thoughts**. This will help you use them when needed.

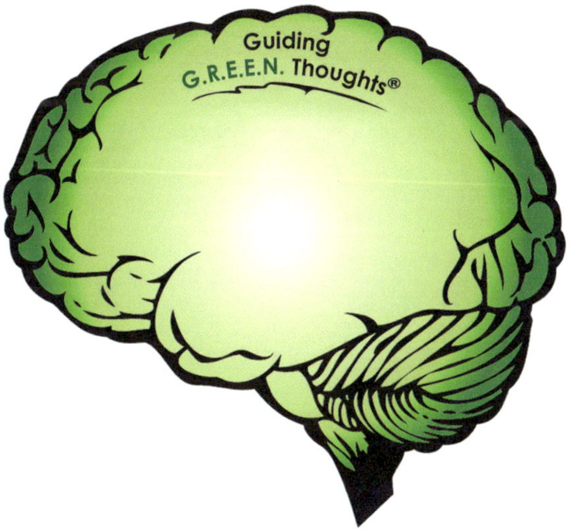

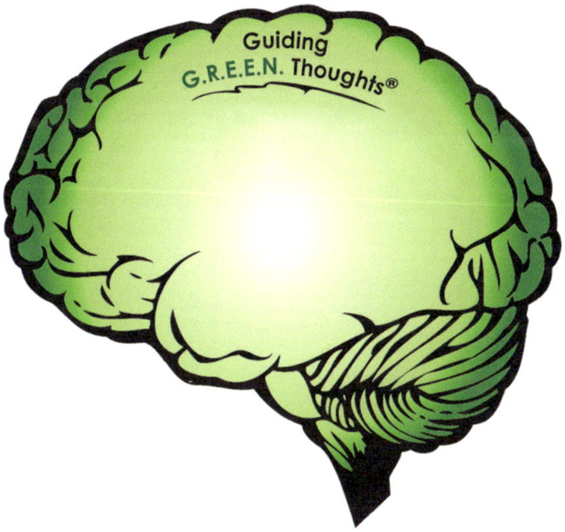

1. Key word ________________

2. Key word ________________

3. Key word ________________

4. Key word ________________

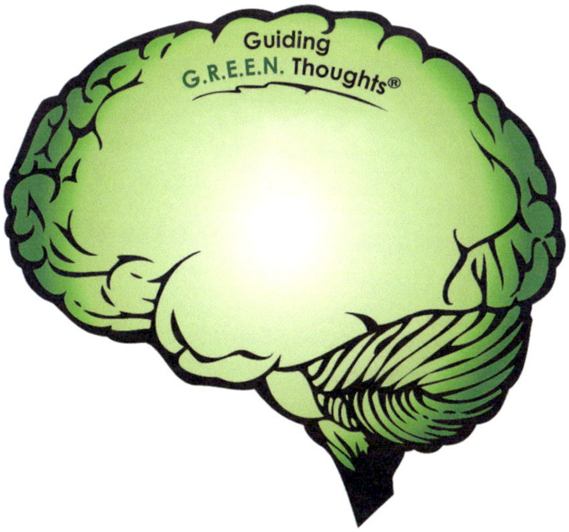

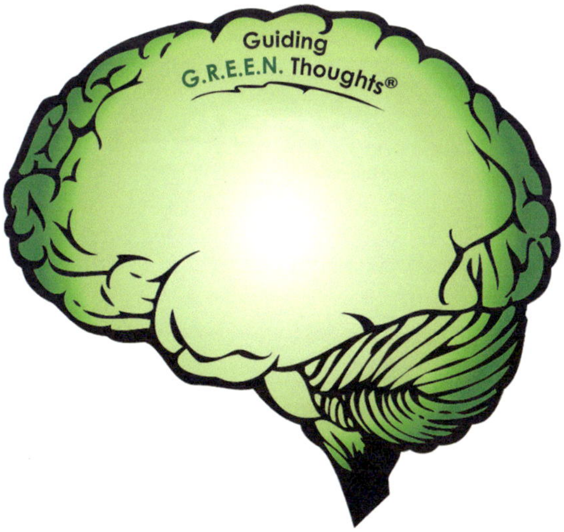

10 Examples of Guiding G.R.E.E.N. Thoughts® to Use

GRATEFUL

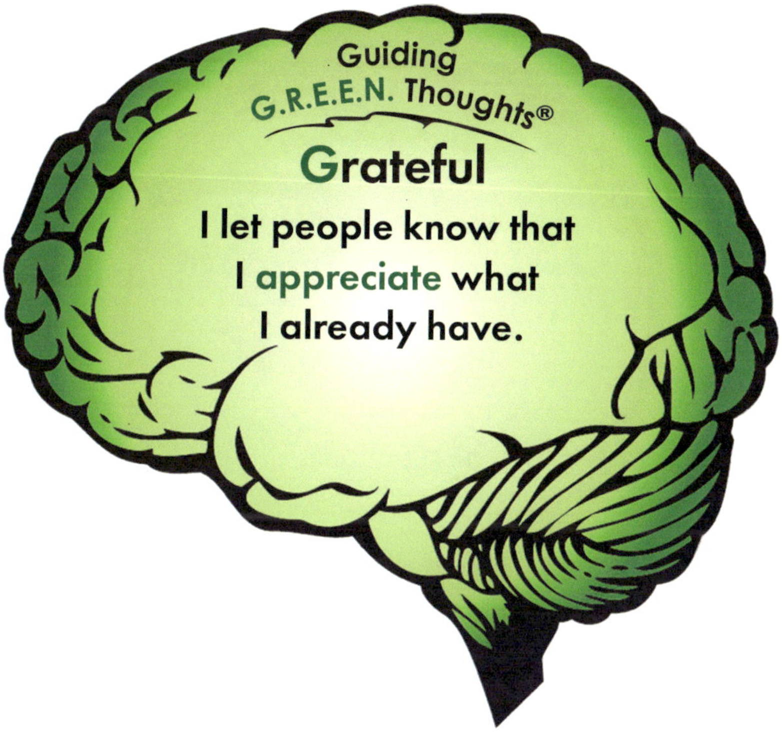

- I say "Thank you" when someone helps me.
- I say "Thank you " when someone gives me something.
- I am satisfied with having some of what I want and do not need to always have more.
- If someone offers me more than what I need, I say, "No thank you, I already have enough."

RESPECTFUL

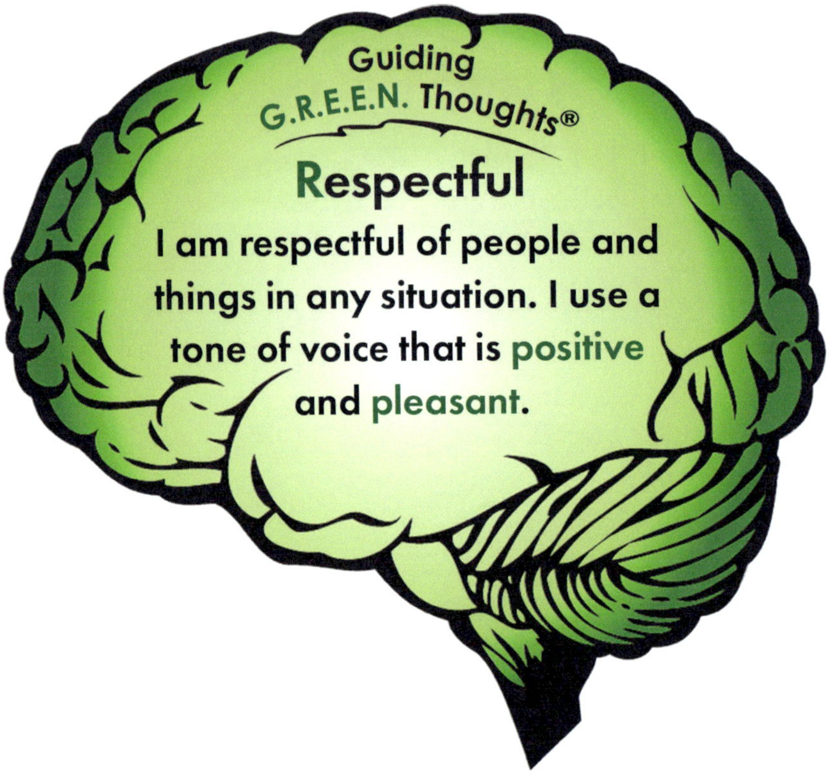

- I **respect** people in all situations.
- I treat animals and property with **respect**.
- I look at you when you are talking to me.
- I use a tone of voice that shows I am interested in what you are saying.
- I answer you immediately and with a **positive** tone.
- I have conversations about topics that other members of my Team want to talk about.
- I tell the truth when I am talking with other people on my Teams.

EMPATHETIC

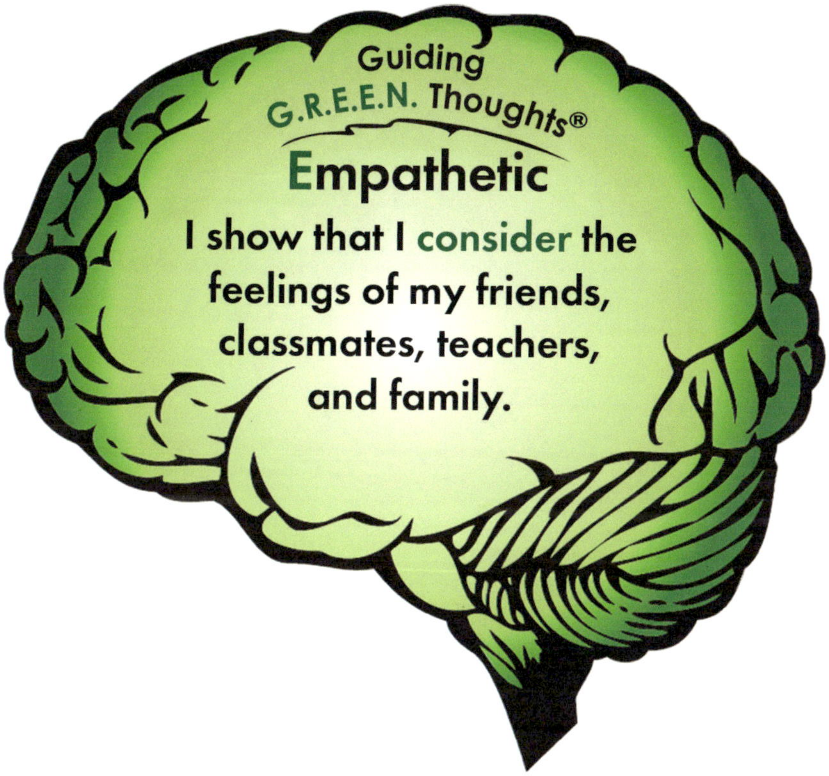

- I **survey the scene** to guess how people are feeling.
- In addition to focusing on my needs, I focus on what other people on my Team need.
- My words and actions show others that I **care**.
- When my Team member seems upset, I stay calm and listen to their point of view.

EASYGOING

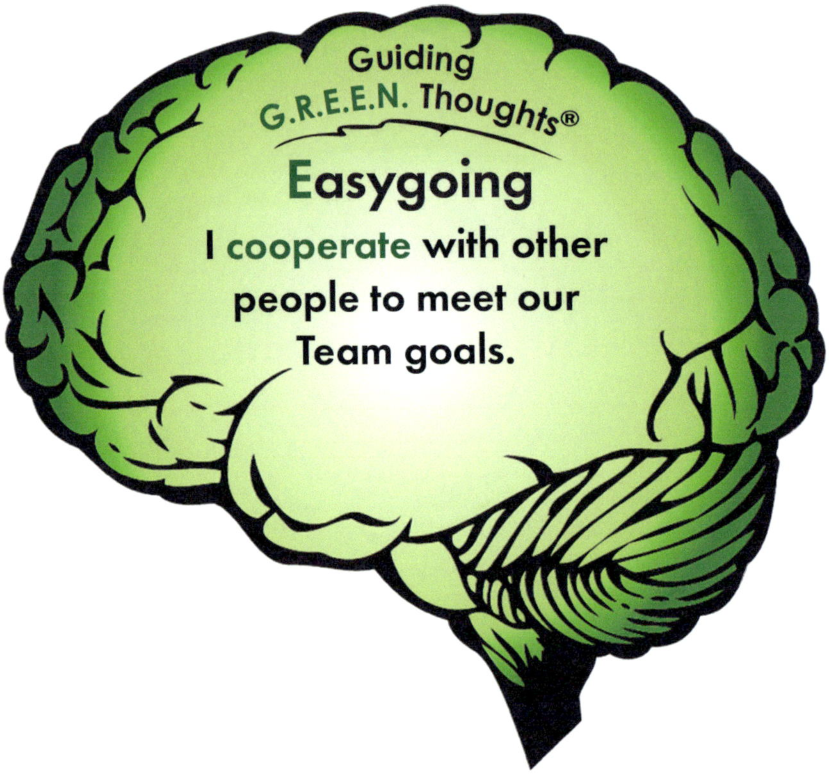

- I listen to directions and follow them.
- I share with others.
- I **take turns**.
- I choose to act in a way that is **safe**, **logical**, and **good for all**.
- I have a **positive** attitude.
- I have **cooperative conversation**s.

NAVIGATING

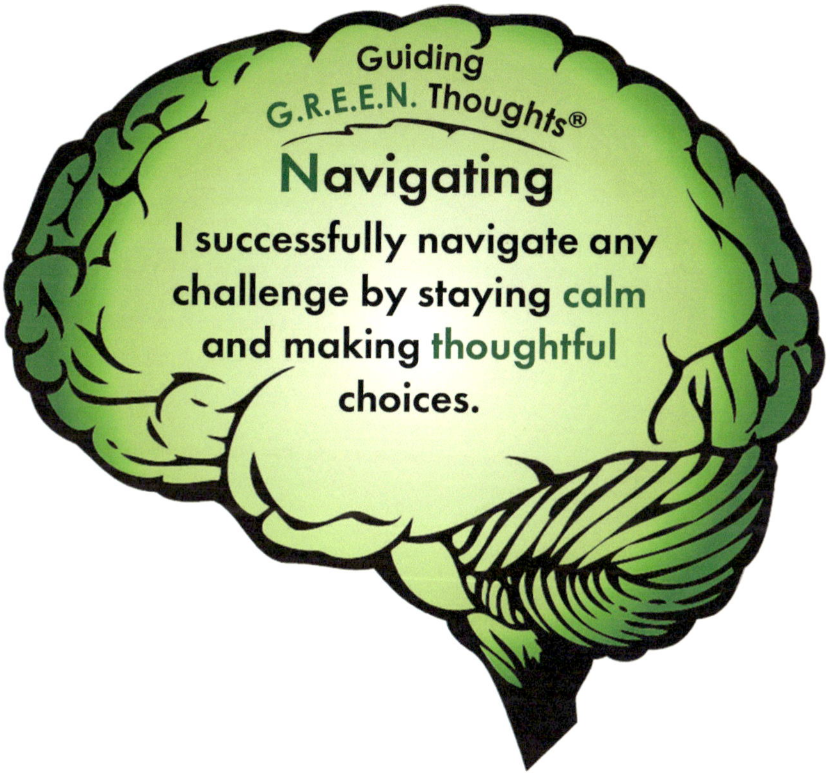

- I am open to new thoughts and accept feedback from others.
- I use **self-control** to make the best choices.
- I wait for the best time to act.
- I understand and accept when someone tells me "no."
- I ask for help when I need it.
- I allow myself to be flexible and change my action to **better** ones.

11 Thinking First to Make the Best Choices

11.1 Read and Discuss: You Have the Power to Make Your Team Great

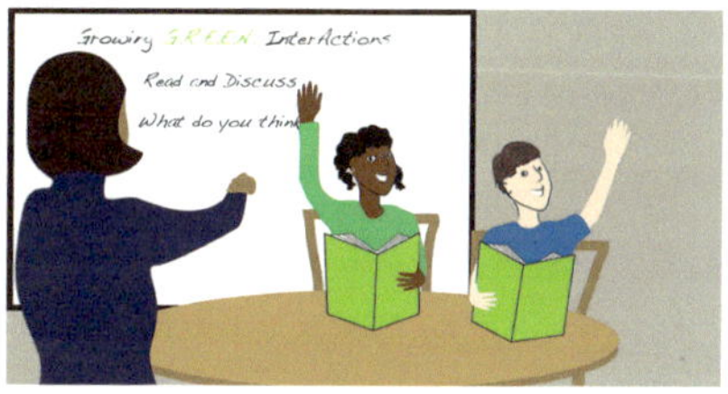

Have you noticed that your human brain gives you the **power** to make great choices? You have the **potential** to do this when you Think First before acting. Having **potential** means that it is possible for you to do something. You can decide the best choice and take that action.

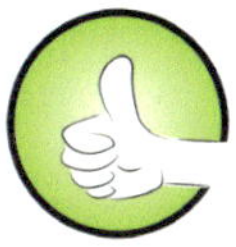

It is possible to make a negative choice to act without thinking about the people around you. You could act like you are living by yourself on your own island. This might be fun for a little while, but after some time you might miss being with other people. You also would not be using your **potential** to do great things with others. Things might not move **forward** and could get worse if you don't help the Team.

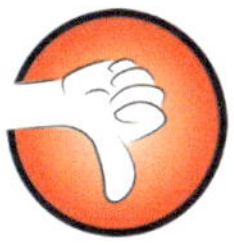

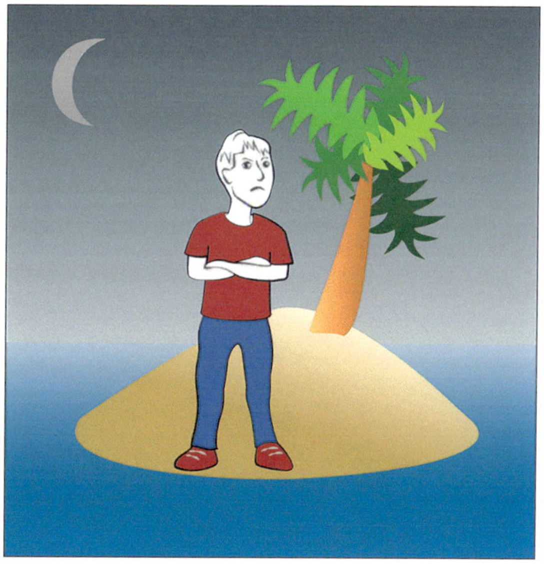

When you look around you and **survey the scene**, you will see that you are not living on an island by yourself.

There are people around you in almost every situation. You may not always want to be with other people, but you are still on the same Team with them. This is true when you are at home, school, work, and play. You can make the best choices when you remember that when people are in your life scene, they are on your Team.

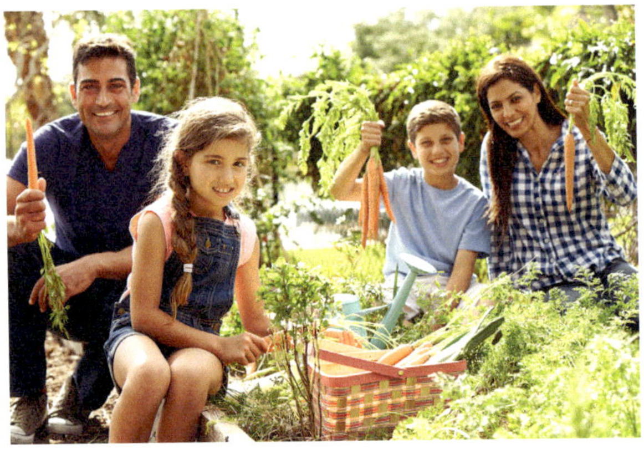

Use your **potential** to be a **thoughtful**, **caring**, **kind** Teammate. Other people also have the **potential** to take **positive**, **helpful** action to be **supportive** Teammates for you. This helps everyone make **mutually beneficial** action choices. You all have the **potential** to be **thoughtful**, **caring**, **kind**, and **helpful** Teammates.

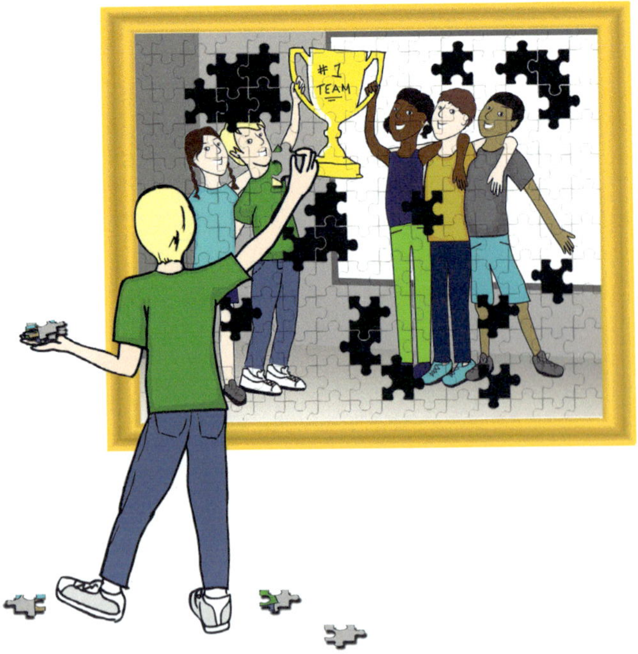

Instead of acting as if you are living alone and caring only for yourself, you can choose to take **positive** action with your Teammates. Use your **potential** to make the best choices with others, and you will find that **powerful** things start to happen.

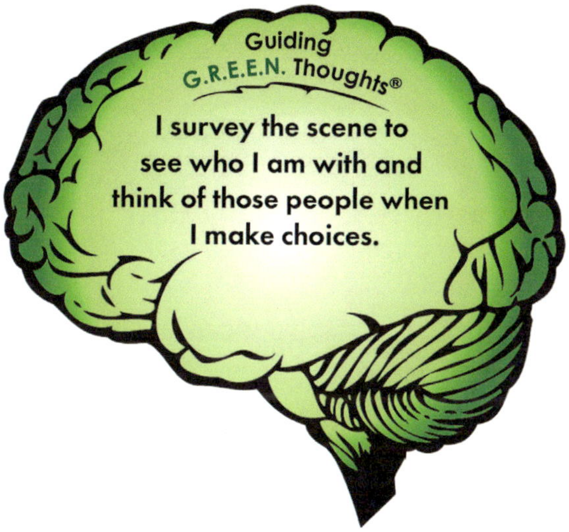

11.2 Positive and Negative Consequences of Your Actions

When you choose actions, it is important to understand the positive and negative consequences that may come from the actions you choose.

Positive consequences mean that things get better.

Negative consequences mean that things get worse.

Our actions have consequences—what we say and do matters when we interact with other people.

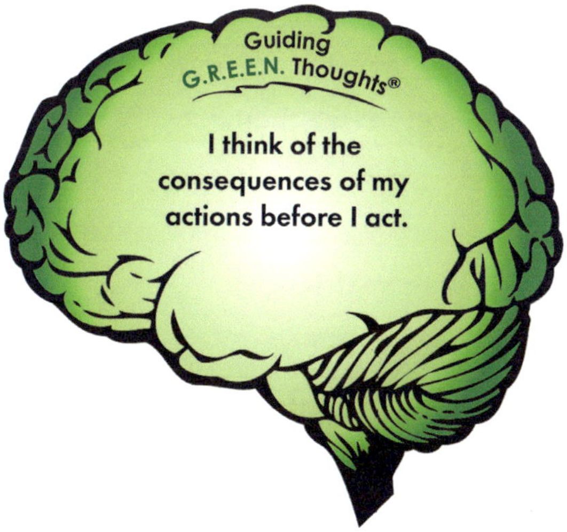

11.3 Survey the Scene: Will These Actions Lead to Positive or Negative Consequences?

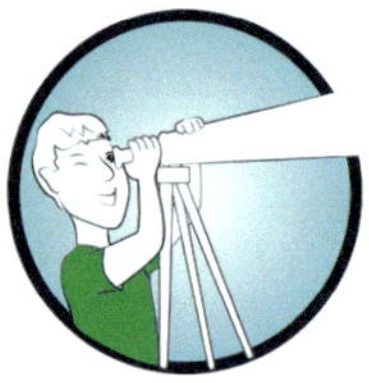

Directions: The following are some actions a person might take. Circle whether you think there will be positive or negative consequences from each action.

1. I pay attention to the teacher in my class.

   Positive consequences   Negative consequences

2. I listen to my mother.

   Positive consequences   Negative consequences

3. I yell at my classmate and hit him during class.

   Positive consequences   Negative consequences

4. I share with my friend.

   Positive consequences   Negative consequences

5. I *don't* take turns with my friends.

   Positive consequences   Negative consequences

WHAT'S BEST FOR THE TEAM?

A Song for **Guiding G.R.E.E.N. Thoughts®**

by Herb Hein

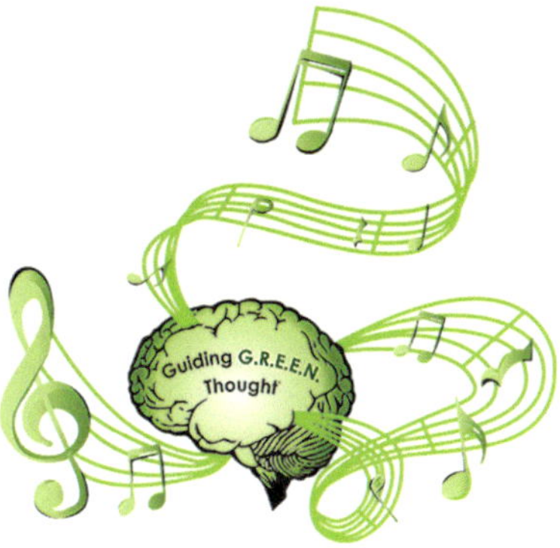

This life's real, It's not a video game,
So what we do *does* matter,
And we have the power
to make good choices in every scene.
Positive or negative consequence,
Our actions change the scene!
Positive or negative consequence,
What's best...for the Team?
What are the choices? I ask...what are the choices?
We get to choose...what's best for the Team!
Positive or negative consequence,
Our actions change the scene!
Positive or negative consequence,
What's best...for the Team?
What's best...for the Team?
Let's make the best choice for the Team
'cuz this life's real!
This life's real.

11.4 Read and Discuss: What Is a R.E.D. Interaction?

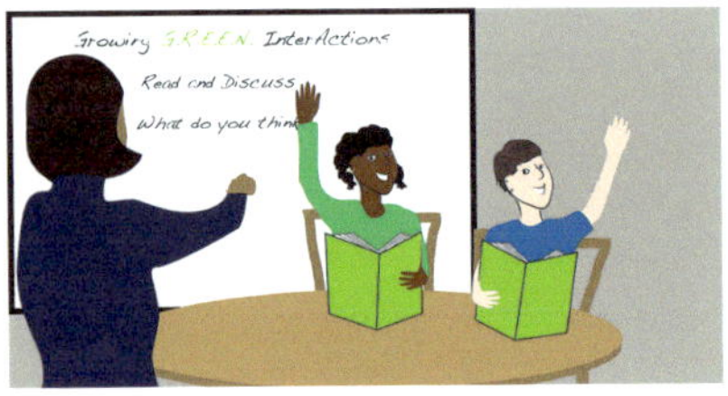

When we follow the rules, we do our part to move ourselves and our Teams **forward**. If we do not follow the rules, people will think our actions are the opposite of **G.R.E.E.N.** They will think we are acting **R.E.D.**

Acting **R.E.D.** is the opposite of acting **G.R.E.E.N.**! **R.E.D.** is an acronym for the behaviors we should avoid when interacting with others. When we act **R.E.D.**, we are probably not Thinking First to **survey the scene** to see what others around us might want or need. We may not remember our **Personal Goals** and are probably not taking time to think about **Common Team Goals**. When we act **R.E.D.**, we hurt ourselves and our Teams.

R.E.D. stands for:

Rude

Egocentric

Disruptive

These three words describe actions that are *not* **helpful** to yourself and others on your Teams. When you act **R.E.D.**, you are *not* Thinking First to **survey the scene**. You are *not* noticing what others around you want or need. You might *not* remember your **Personal Goals** and you are *not* taking time to think about the **Common Team Goals**.

Here are some **R.E.D.** behaviors to avoid:

Rude: When you are rude, you do *not* care about others and their feelings. You are rude when you neglect the needs of your Team. When you neglect something, you ignore it and act as if it is not even there. It is rude to neglect the people on your Teams. Being rude might keep your Team from meeting its **goals**.

Egocentric/Selfish: When you are rude, you are *not* acting **kind** or **helpful** to others. You are thinking only about yourself. When you think only of yourself and no one else, you act egocentric and selfish. Being egocentric and selfish keeps your Team from reaching its **goals** because you act as if the Team does *not* matter to you. Think First to **survey the scene** and see what others on your Team might want or need, too.

Greedy: When you want everything for yourself and do *not* want to **share**, you act as if you do *not* **care** whether other people have what they need. This means you are acting greedy. Notice whether you are **sharing** with others or acting greedy. Think First to **survey the scene** and determine whether you can help the others on your Team get what they want or need, too.

Disruptive: When you are disruptive, you disturb other Team members. Whether you know it or not, your actions can cause trouble that keeps you and the Team from moving **forward** together. Disruptive actions may be distracting, confusing, or upsetting and keep the Team from feeling safe and calm enough to do its best to achieve **Common Team Goals**. Your disruptive behavior has negative consequences for the people and things around you. When you act this way, you are *not* being **flexible** because you are *not* thinking of how to act more **peaceful** and **good for everyone**. It is important to learn how to **change** so that you are no longer disruptive. You can learn some **self-control** strategies and make some **transformations** to help the scene become **better**. You can learn about **self-control** strategies and **transformations** in other parts of this program.

Choose to Act G.R.E.E.N.!

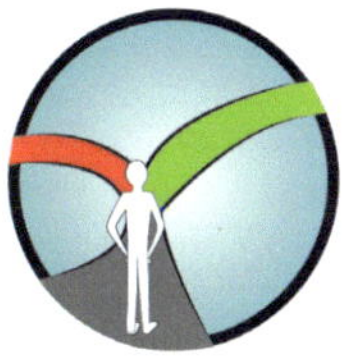

As a **powerful** human, you can think about the choices you make. You can choose to act either **G.R.E.E.N.** or **R.E.D.** You can work to have your actions result in **positive** consequences or choose to *not* control your actions and suffer negative consequences. Most people feel better when their actions have **positive** consequences.

Reach for a **Guiding G.R.E.E.N. Thought**® to help you make the best choices. This program helps you increase your **power** to act **G.R.E.E.N.** as often as possible.

11.5 Survey the Scene: Is This Action G.R.E.E.N. or R.E.D.?

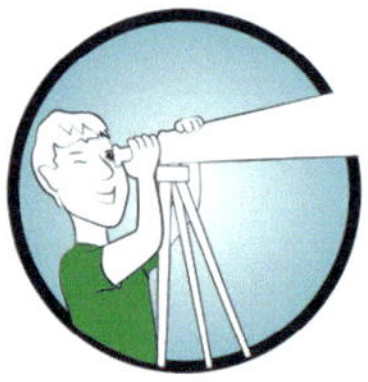

Directions: Let's see if you can recognize the difference between G.R.E.E.N. and R.E.D. action. Underline a G.R.E.E.N. action with a green pencil. Underline R.E.D. action with a red pencil. Which side has the words you can choose to describe the action? Circle the words (G.R.E.E.N. or R.E.D.) that match the action.

1. Katrina thanked her teacher for his help.

Grateful	
Respectful	**Rude**
Empathetic	**Egocentric**
Easygoing	**Disruptive**
Navigating	

2. Katrina's mother stopped at the yogurt store to get Katrina and her brother some frozen yogurt. When Katrina got her yogurt, she complained that she was not happy because she wanted more toppings than she and her brother already had.

Grateful	
Respectful	**Rude**
Empathetic	**Egocentric**
Easygoing	**Disruptive**
Navigating	

3. Carl said "Good morning!" to his father after his father said, "Good morning" to him.

Grateful	
Respectful	Rude
Empathetic	Egocentric
Easygoing	Disruptive
Navigating	

4. Carl interrupted when his brother was telling their mother what happened at school. Carl did not let his brother finish his story because Carl kept talking about a movie that he liked.

Grateful	
Respectful	Rude
Empathetic	Egocentric
Easygoing	Disruptive
Navigating	

5. After Audrey's friend Sarah said that last night her dog ran out of the front gate and did not return home, Audrey said, "I'm sorry that happened. I hope you find him."

Grateful	
Respectful	Rude
Empathetic	Egocentric
Easygoing	Disruptive
Navigating	

6. When Audrey's friend Mark said that he was worried about the math test they had to take on Friday, Audrey said, "I'm really good at math! I'm not worried at all!"

Grateful	
Respectful	**Rude**
Empathetic	**Egocentric**
Easygoing	**Disruptive**
Navigating	

7. John realized that he and his sister, Monica, wanted to go to different restaurants for dinner. He thought for a minute, and then suggested they could go to the place that she wanted tonight. Then they could go to the place that he wanted next week.

Grateful	
Respectful	**Rude**
Empathetic	**Egocentric**
Easygoing	**Disruptive**
Navigating	

8. When John's mother said they were going out to eat, John yelled that he was not going to go unless they went to his favorite restaurant. He then went in his room and slammed the door.

Grateful	
Respectful	**Rude**
Empathetic	**Egocentric**
Easygoing	**Disruptive**
Navigating	

11.6 Read and Discuss: Drivers Learn to Take G.R.E.E.N. Actions on the Road

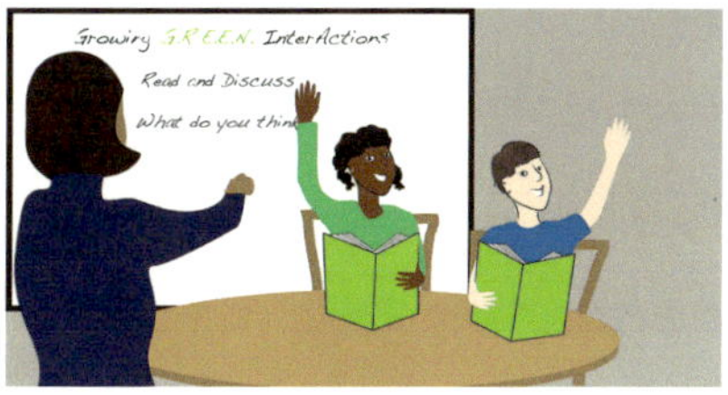

When cars were first invented, workers built roads for people to get from one place to the other safely and easily. Everyone on the road **shared** a **goal**—to get to their **destinations** safely. As increasingly more people traveled on the roads, driving rules were created so that people would not crash into each other!

People worked to make the roads safe so cars could drive in different directions without crashing. Everyone had to follow the rules of the road to get to where they wanted to go. People needed to know when to stop and when to go. People needed to read signals and signs!

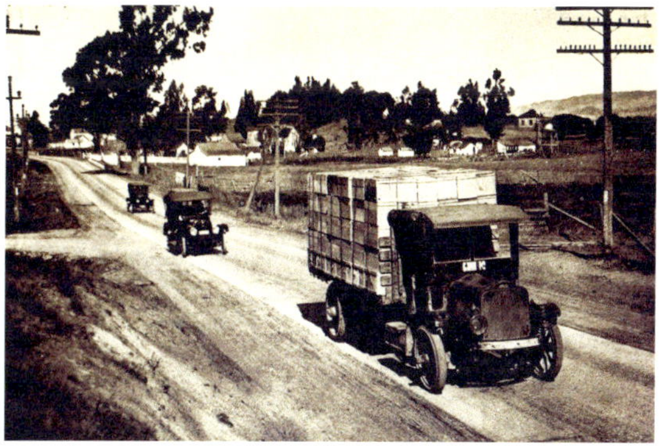

Today, we have even more cars on our roads. Everyone on the road wants to get somewhere. Many rules of the road help us act **safe**, **logical**, and **good for everyone** on the road. If you want to get a driver's license, you must know the rules of the road and pass tests to prove it. You must learn to follow road signs and signal when **changing** direction. If everyone on the road knows the rules, follows them, **pays attention to signals and signs**, and knows how to signal and drive safely around other drivers, everyone can get to their **destinations**.

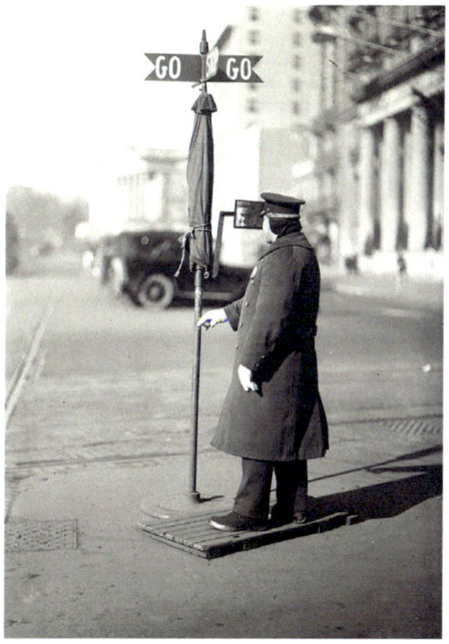

A basic, important rule of the road is to stop at red lights and go at **green** lights.

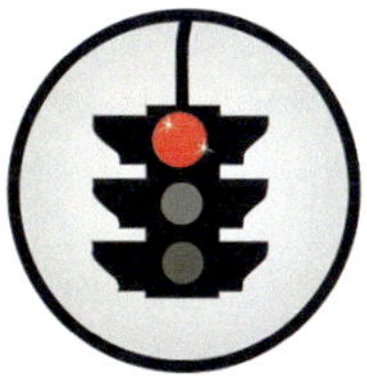
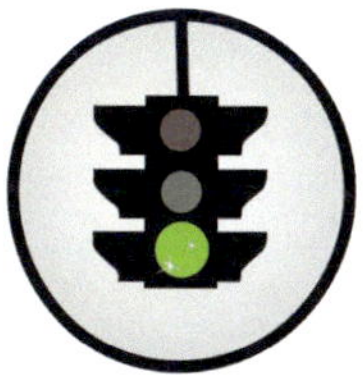

It is *not* a **safe** or **logical** idea to go when you are supposed to stop. If we go when we are supposed to stop, it is *not* **safe** and it is *not* **good for everyone**.

We have the human **power** to make the choice to *not* crash. How do we do this? We can learn to step on our brakes if we are headed in the wrong direction.

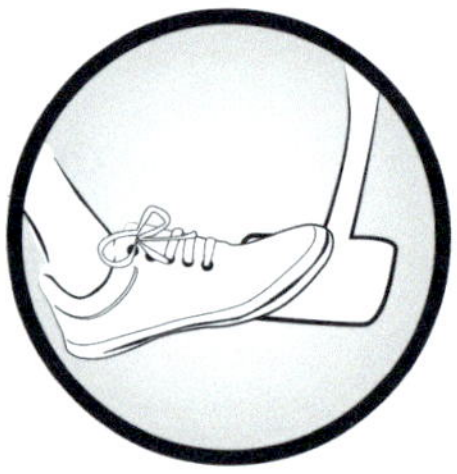

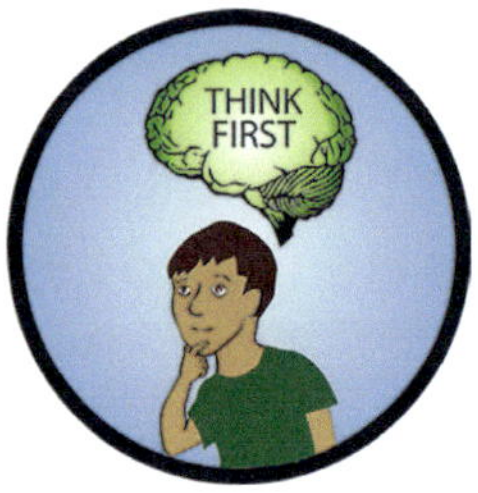

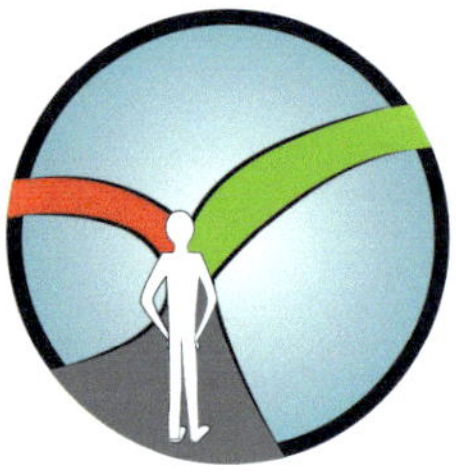

We can learn to step on our brakes to think of **better** choices for ourselves and those around us.

11.7 Read and Discuss: Red Lights and G.R.E.E.N. Lights Are in Your Brain!

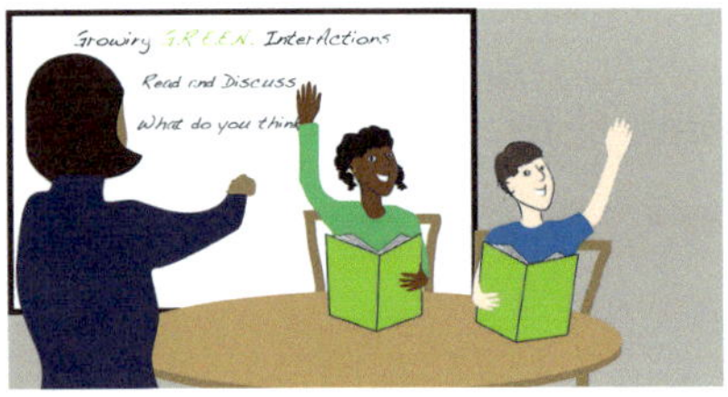

Red lights and **green** lights on roads tell you whether to stop or go. Your brain also has red and **green** lights. They don't look the same, but they act much the same.

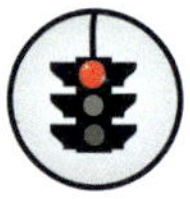

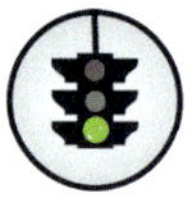

The red lights and **green** lights in your brain help you regulate or control what you do.

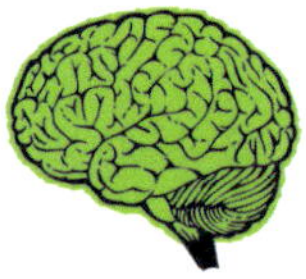

When you use **self-control**, your brain tells you when to stop doing something that could hurt you. It can tell you to step on the brake to stop going in the wrong direction with your actions. Then you can **change** to go in the **right** direction!

You see a stoplight in your brain that helps you make **positive** 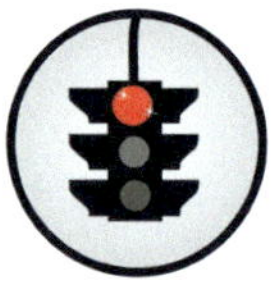 choices with your actions.

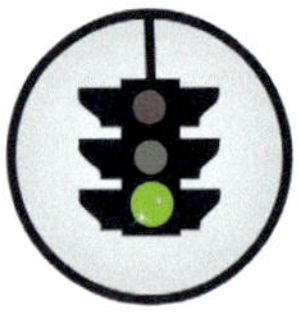

Your brain also can give you signals to encourage you to get excited about making **good** choices that lead in **good** directions. Your brain can remind you to take **positive** actions and keep taking them! Special brain chemicals and brain connections help you work these control signals. These control signals work best when you Think First and **pay careful attention to what is going on around you**. Then the special brain chemicals and special connections in your brain help you move in the **right** direction to meet your **goals**.

Just like building electrical connections in a house, your brain learns by building new connections between its cells. Brain cells are called neurons. The brain connections between neurons are called synapses.

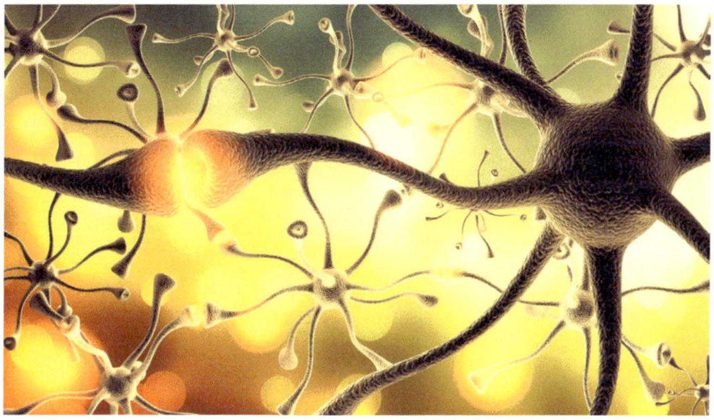

When you take action, you make stronger connections between the neurons in your brain. When you choose **positive** actions, you make it easier to do the same thing the next time. Each time you take action, the connection gets stronger. This means you have the **power** to control your brain! You can practice making good choices that strengthen the connections in your brain. With more practice, **positive** choices become easier to make.

You will have many opportunities to practice making good action choices in the **Growing G.R.E.E.N. InterActions** Program.

An earthworm can be trained to pick a certain path to avoid an electric shock. This means an earthworm's brain can tell it to make good choices for its path.

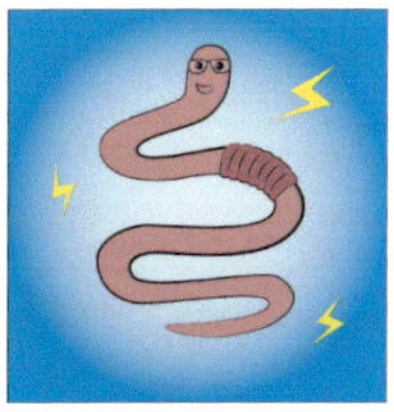

An earthworm's brain helps it learn by experience. Your brain can help you learn from your experiences, too. You can choose good paths and actions that help you move **forward** in a **positive** direction.

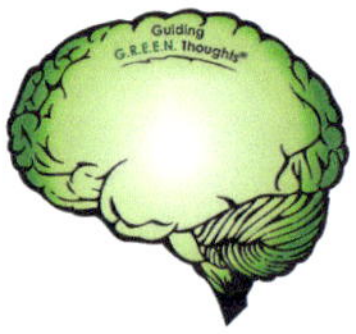

As you move **forward** in a **positive** direction, you become more able to control yourself. **Pay attention to your actions**. Show yourself and others that you have the **self-control** to make the best choices. This is **self-regulation**. The ability to **self-regulate** is an important function of your brain. When you want to achieve a **goal** for yourself or your Team, you act **positively**. This requires you to **self-regulate** by using your **powerful** brain.

You can be in charge of stepping on the brake to stop or inhibit negative actions. When you step on the brake, you stop yourself from **R.E.D.** actions that won't help you or other people on your Team.

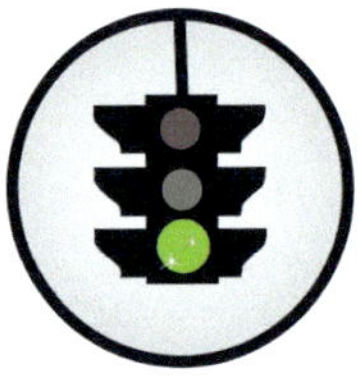

You can turn on the **green** light and think **helpful Guiding G.R.E.E.N. Thoughts** that will help you act **positively** so things can get better. You can think **powerful** thoughts that will help you take **G.R.E.E.N.** actions that will help you reach your **goals**.

1. What can "**green** lights" help you do in your brain? ____________________

   ____

2. What can "red lights" help you do in your brain? ____________________

   ____

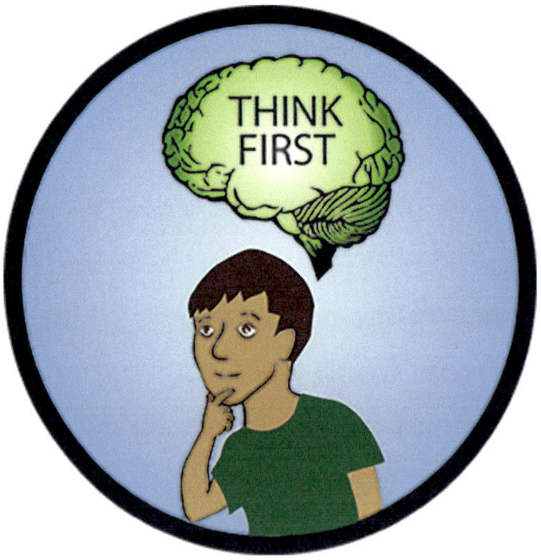

11.8 You Can Think First with Your Powerful Brain!

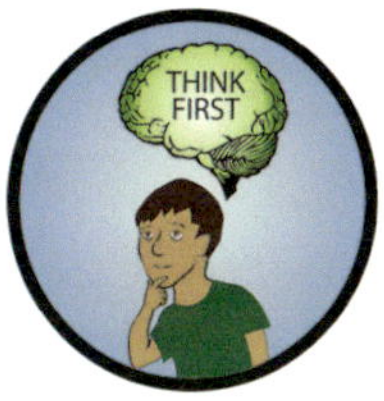

Because you have a human brain, you can *think* about your *thinking*!

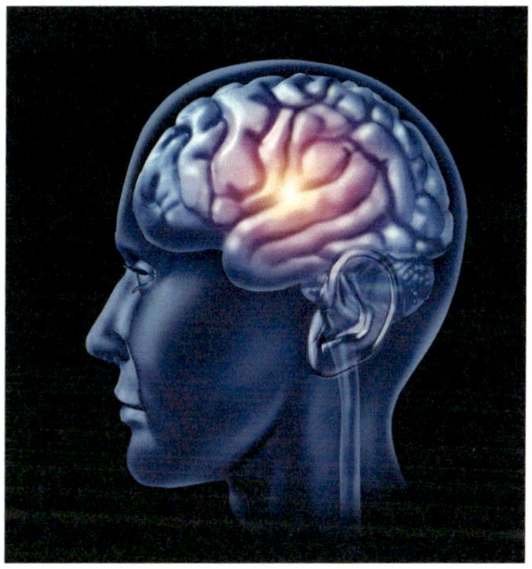

This means you can think to yourself and ask, "Am I thinking thoughts that help me?"

You can also think about your actions! This means you can think to yourself and ask, "Is this action going to help me?"

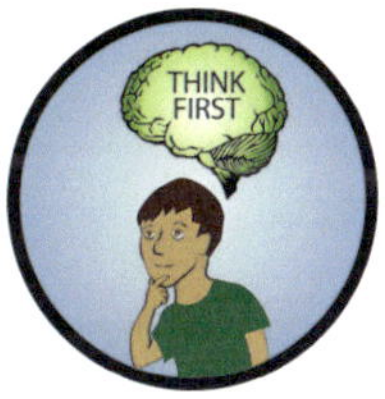

With your human brain, you can learn to Think First about your thoughts and about what you are going to do *before* you take any action.

Thinking First keeps you from acting in an impulsive way.

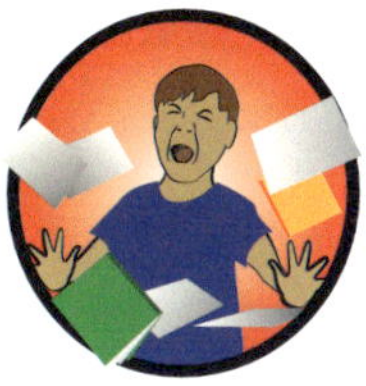

Many other animals often act impulsively, meaning they take action *without any thinking at all*!

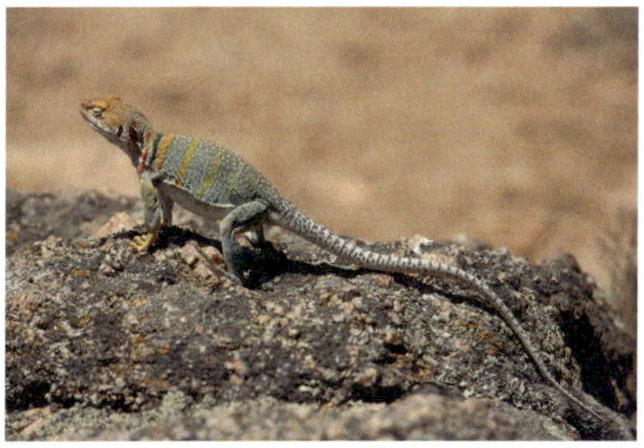

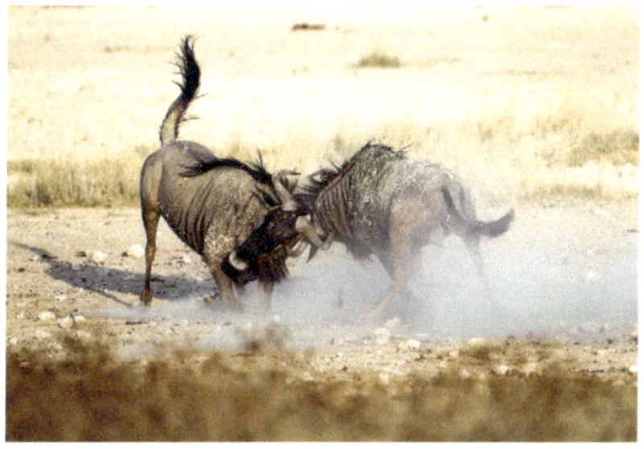

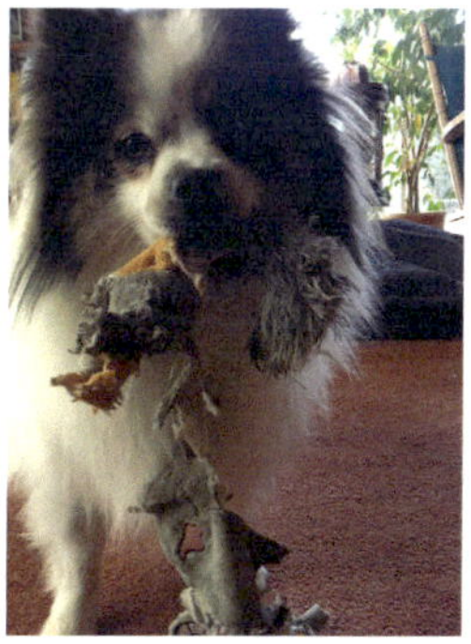

11.9 Do You Think First or Do You Act Impulsively?

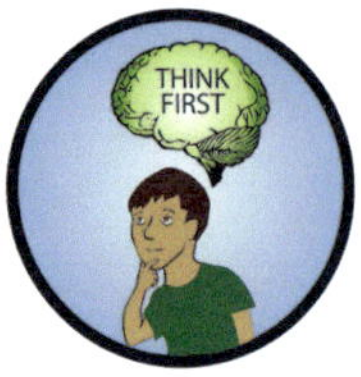

1. How often do you Think First before doing something?

   10% 20% 30% 40% 50% 60% 70% 80% 90% **100%**

2. How often do you act impulsively *without* Thinking First?

   10% 20% 30% 40% 50% 60% 70% 80% 90% **100%**

When you act *without* thinking, you are being impulsive!

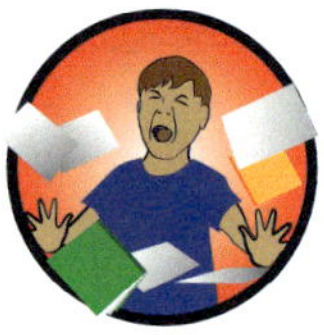

After you use some ideas in this book, you will find that you Think First more often.

11.10 Survey the Scene: Is This Action Thoughtful or Impulsive?

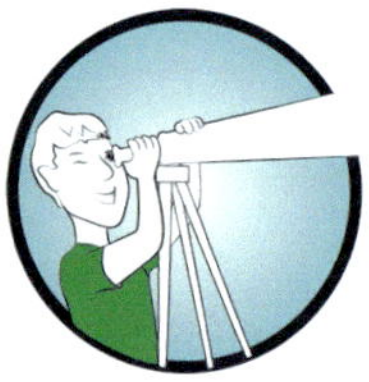

Survey the scenes below to determine whether these people are acting thoughtful or impulsive. Who is Thinking First before acting? Who is not Thinking First before acting?

Directions: Underline thoughtful actions with a green pencil and impulsive actions with a red pencil. Then circle whether the action is thoughtful or impulsive. Explain your answers to a partner.

1. Alex looks around the classroom to decide whether it is work time or break time. He sees that it is a break time, so he gets out of his seat to go to his classmate to ask about the interesting thing that his classmate brought from home.

   thoughtful **impulsive**

2. Eddie looks to see that his mother is busy taking something hot out of the oven. He waits until she takes a break and then he asks her to look at a picture of the toy he would like for his birthday.

   thoughtful **impulsive**

3. Alex gets out of his seat without permission during a classroom math lesson to pick up something that catches his attention on someone else's desk.

   thoughtful **impulsive**

4. Eddie sees a picture of something that he wants for his birthday. He runs into the kitchen and puts the picture in front of his mother's face while she is taking something hot out of the oven. Then he shouts, "This is what I want for my birthday! When can I get it? "

   thoughtful **impulsive**

11.11 Using the Civilized Choice Checker to Make the Best Choices for the Team

When you take the time to Think First, it is possible to see the different actions you can take. The Civilized **Choice Checker** helps you **survey the scene**, get the main idea about what is happening, and think about the important features of your different choices. Take the time to be **thoughtful** to compare these features, and you will see which choice wins as the best choice for you and your Team. You can use the Civilized **Choice Checker** to compare these features:

1. Is the action choice logical? Does it make sense by helping things get better?
2. Does this choice allow people and things to be safe? Does this choice keep people from getting hurt and things from getting broken?
3. Is this action choice **good for everyone**? Does this choice help make things better for everyone in this scene?
4. Does this choice show good **self-control**? Does this choice help you use **patience** and **cooperation** to reach **Common Team Goals**?

As you continue through this program, you will learn more about these feature words and other important ways to Think First and make your best action choices.

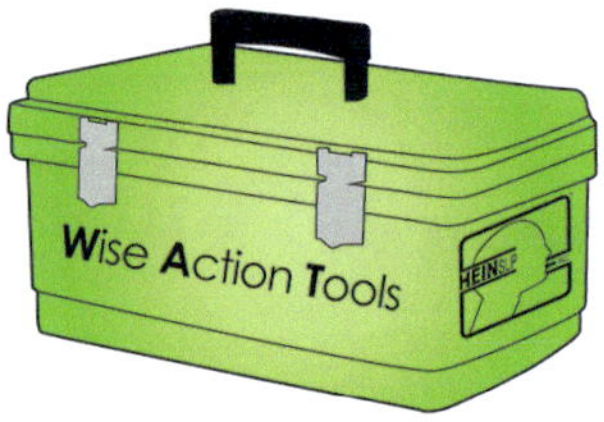

CIVILIZED CHOICE CHECKER

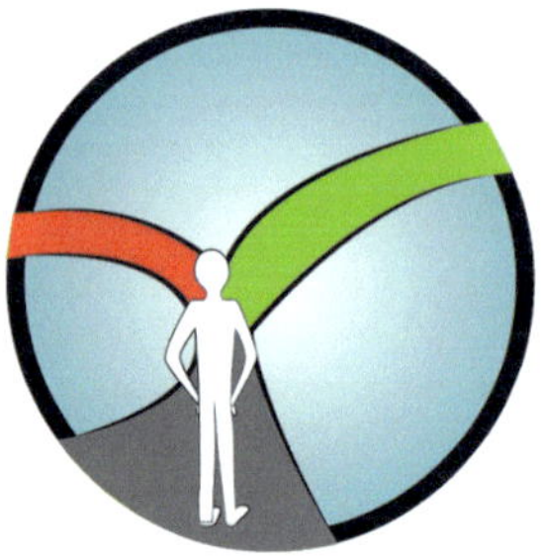

When I **survey this scene**, I think this is happening:

____

This is one way to act (**Choice A**): ______________________________

____

This is another way to act (**Choice B**): ____________________________

____

	Write "+" for yes and "-" for **no**	
	Action Choice A	Action Choice B
1. This is a logical choice. Things will get better instead of worse.		
2. This is a safe choice. People will *not* get hurt. Things will *not* get broken.		
3. This choice is good for everyone. Things will be better for *everyone* in the scene.		
4. This choice uses good self-control to meet the goals.		
Total score: Add up the + signs to see which choice is the best. Which choice wins?		

11.12 Making Choices That Are Logical, Safe, and Good for Everyone

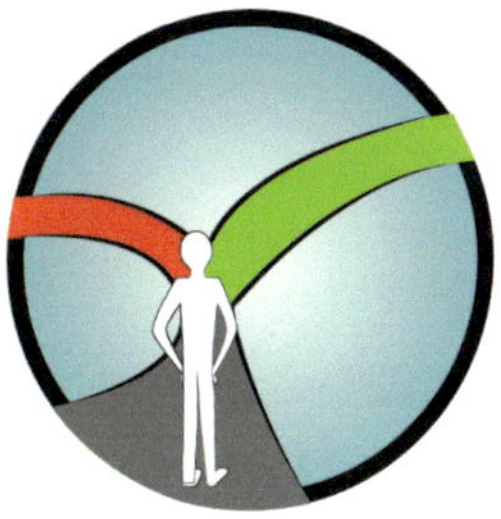

Because you have a **powerful** human brain, you can Think First and choose to act in certain ways. You can use your **power** and choose to act in **logical**, **safe** ways that are **good for everyone**. Let's review what these words mean to help you make these choices.

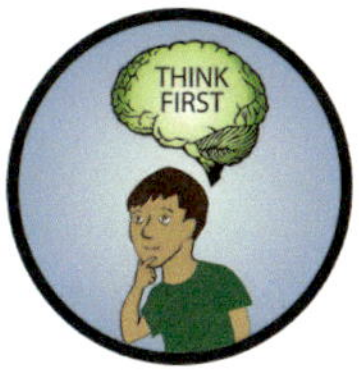

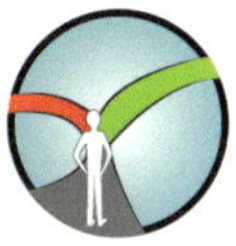

Making Logical Choices

You can choose to act **logically** or illogically.

To act **logically** is to carefully think about how things are going right now in a situation and what to do next that makes sense.

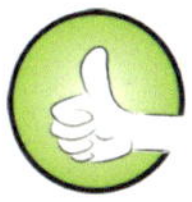

You can choose to either:

1. act in ways that **make sense** so that things get **better**, or
2. act in ways that don't make sense so that things get worse.

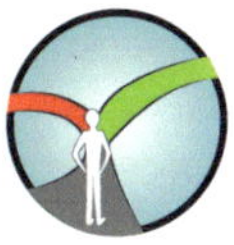

Making Safe Choices

With your **powerful** human brain, you can choose to act **safely**!

To act **safely** means to act carefully so you *don't* get hurt and you *don't* hurt the people or things around you.

You can choose to either:

1. be **safe** and act **safely** with others, or
2. be unsafe and act in ways that hurt other people and things.

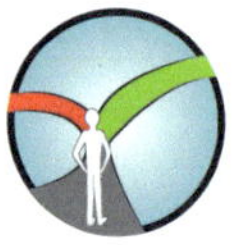

Making Choices That Are Good for Everyone!

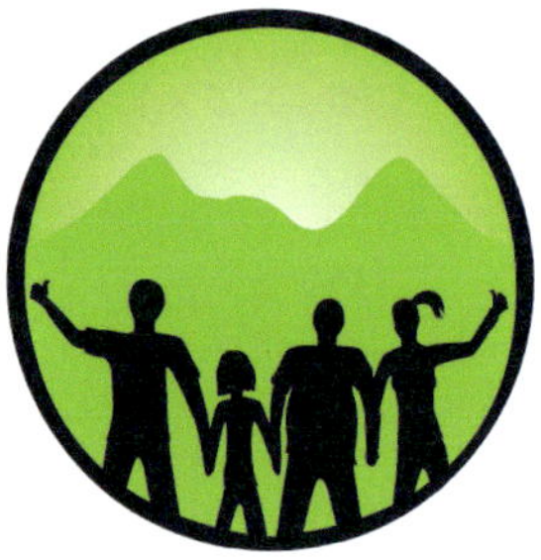

Because you have a **powerful** human brain, you can choose to act well so everyone on your Team benefits. This means you help yourself and other people at the same time. You get to make choices that help other people move in the **best direction**, too.

Acting **good for everyone** shows that you are thinking of **positive**, **helpful** actions for you and the people you are with. You can help make things **better** for everyone. Everyone involved can win!

You can choose to either

1. do things in a way that is **good for you and good for the people around you**, or
2. do things in a way that is selfish and only good for you.

You have the **power** to Think First and take the time to use a **Guiding G.R.E.E.N. Thought**. This can help you choose **logical**, **safe** actions that are **good for everyone**.

11.13 Logical or Illogical?

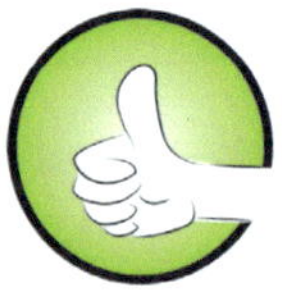

Because you have a **powerful** human brain, you can choose to act **logically**. This means you can do things that **make sense** and **make things get better** for yourself and others.

When your actions do *not* **make sense**, making things worse for yourself and others, you are acting illogically. You may *not* have considered the negative consequences of your actions. To move **forward** and have your **best life**, it is best to Think First and act **logically**.

Let's compare **logical** and illogical actions:

Directions: Write an *L* if the sentence is about being logical. Write an *I* if the sentence is about being illogical.

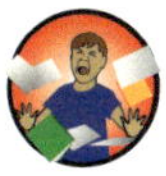

__ 1. Doing things to make things **better**.

__ 2. Doing things that **make sense**.

__ 3. Doing things to make things worse.

11.14 Survey the Scene! Are These Actions Logical or Illogical?

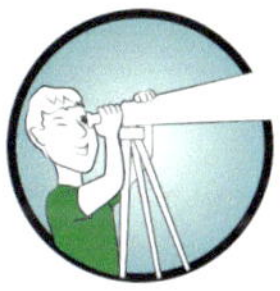

Directions: Circle whether the actions below are **logical** or illogical: Explain why you made your choice.

1. Drinking when you are thirsty

   + logical – illogical

2. *Not* stopping to drink when you are thirsty

   + logical – illogical

3. Hurting yourself on purpose

   + logical – illogical

4. Taking care of your body so you can live a healthy life

   + logical – illogical

5. Yelling when the teacher is trying to teach class

   + logical – illogical

6. Paying attention when the teacher is trying to teach class

   + logical – illogical

7. Breaking something that you need

   + logical – illogical

8. Being careful with necessities

   + logical – illogical

What do you think? Answer the following questions:

1. What does it mean to be **logical**? Being **logical** means to do or say things that ______________________________

   ____

2. What happens when you act illogically? If you act illogically, ______________

   ____

3. Are you helping yourself or your family or your class when you act illogically?

   yes no

   Why or why not? ______________________________

4. Are you helping yourself or your family or class when you act **logically**?

   yes no

   Why or why not? ______________________________

5. What would other people in your family or your classroom think about you when you acted in an illogical way? ________________________________

____

6. What would you do if someone told you they thought you were acting in an illogical way?

____

7. What can you do to help yourself be logical in your actions? ____________

____

11.15 Survey the Scene: Are the Actions in These Scenes Good for Everyone?

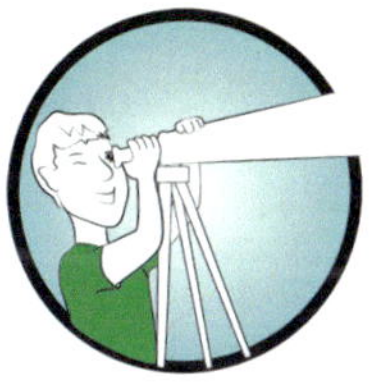

Directions: Survey the scenes that follow and determine whether the people's actions are good for everyone in the scene.

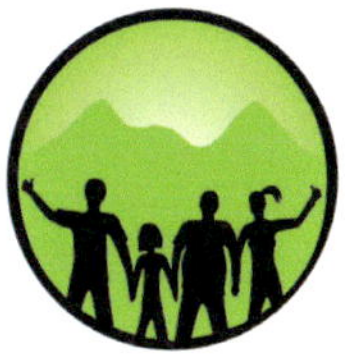

As you read the scenes, circle in green pencil when someone acts helpful. Circle in red pencil when someone acts unhelpful, hurtful, or selfish.

Scene #1

The situation: John and Brianna's mother had to visit their grandmother in the hospital. She asked them to help each other out while she was gone.

John fed the dog while Brianna made two sandwiches. Brianna packed the sandwiches and some water in a backpack. John packed a water dish for the dog. John walked the dog to the park and Brianna walked with them, carrying the backpack. John and Brianna enjoyed a little picnic while the dog ran and played. When they were done, Brianna packed up their things while John threw out their trash.

1. Did both people act to make things **good for everyone**?

   yes no

2. Could this scene be any **better**?

   yes no

   How? ____

Scene #2

The (same) situation: John and Brianna's mother had to visit their grandmother in the hospital. She asked them to help each other out while she was gone.

Briana asked John to feed the dog. John said he was too busy watching TV. Because the dog needed to be fed, Brianna gave him his food. Brianna asked John to help make lunch. John said he did not want to. Brianna made sandwiches for both of them, but she decided she would not do anything else for John until he did something to help her out. Brianna asked John to walk the dog. He said he did not feel like it. Brianna packed up her sandwich and drink, as well as a water dish for the dog, and walked the dog to the park. When John and Brianna's mother came home, John complained that Brianna made a terrible sandwich. Brianna told her brother he was lucky that she made him anything to eat. She told her mother the ways that her brother did not help.

1. Did both people act to make things **good for everyone**?

   yes no

2. Could this scene be **better**? How? ______________________________

3. Which scene had actions that were **good for everyone**?

   Scene 1 Scene 2

11.16 Guiding G.R.E.E.N. Thoughts for Actions That Are Logical, Safe, and Good for Everyone

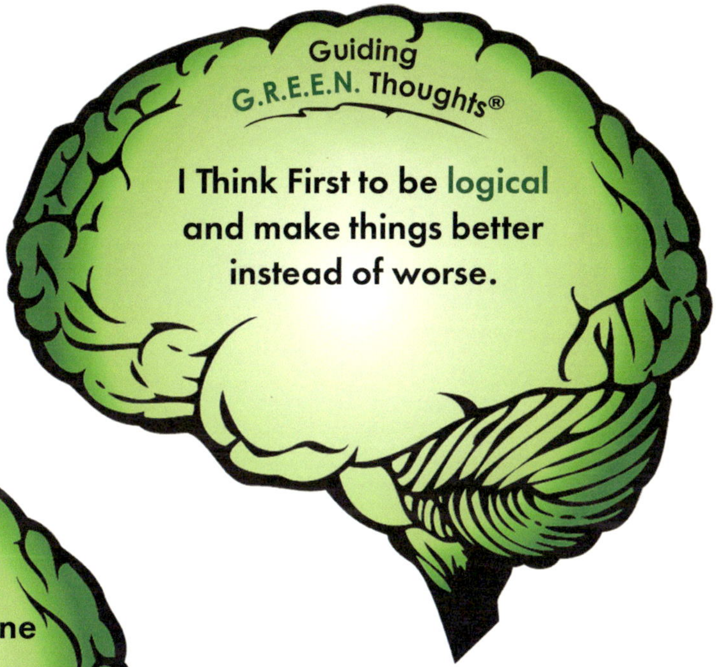

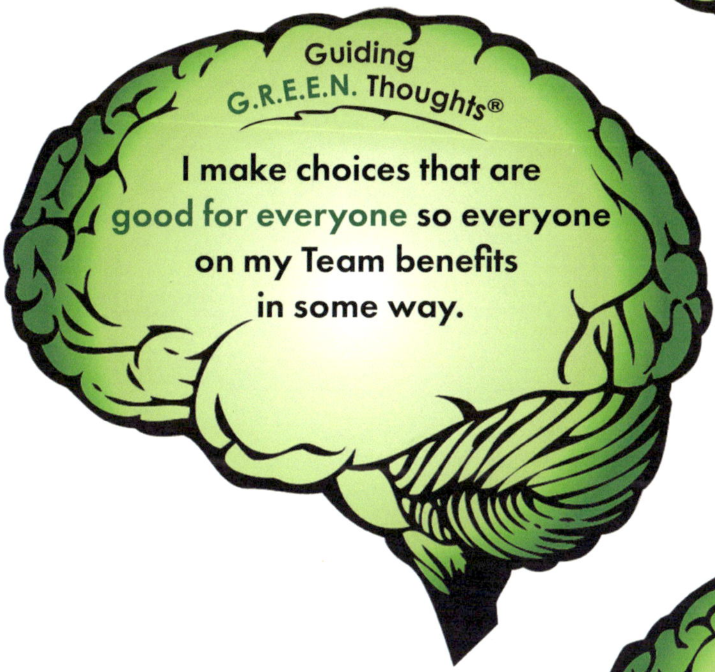

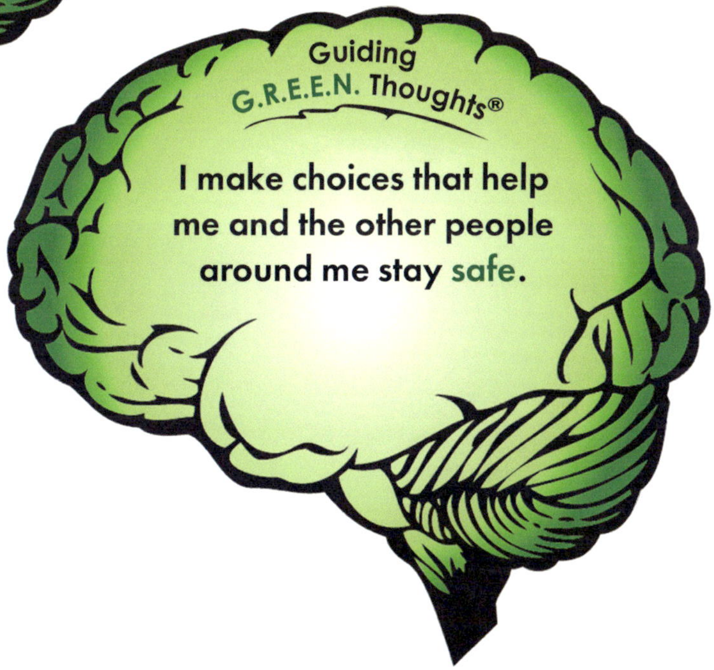

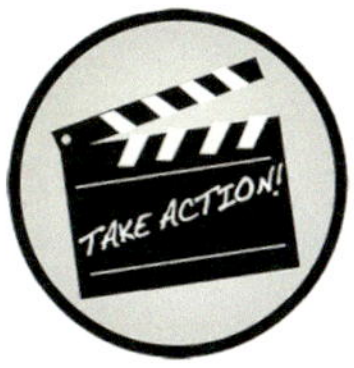

12 Getting Ready for G.R.E.E.N. Scene Action

12.1 Why Are We Acting in G.R.E.E.N. Scenes?

Learning to interact successfully with others on your Teams can be challenging. This program teaches you some important **Guiding G.R.E.E.N. Thoughts** that will help you make the best choices for your Teams. It also helps you choose words for the best Team interactions. You will practice using these guiding thoughts, choose the best words, and act to make the best G.R.E.E.N. Scenes. This makes it easier for you to use these skills with your real-life Teams. In G.R.E.E.N. Scenes, you experience the positive consequences of your choices and feel what it is like to "Act G.R.E.E.N. for the Team."

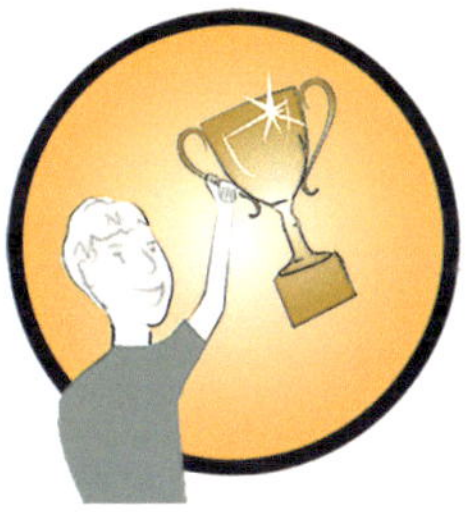

In G.R.E.E.N. Scenes, you practice acting in positive ways on different Teams in many situations. After you practice these G.R.E.E.N. Scenes, you will understand what to look for and say in real-life scenes. You will learn how to achieve your Personal Goals along with Common Team Goals.

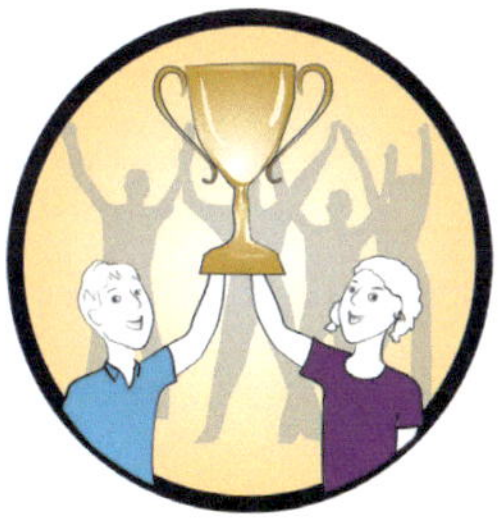

12.2 Making the Best G.R.E.E.N. Scenes

Guiding G.R.E.E.N. InterActions will help you practice G.R.E.E.N. Scenes for your Home, School, and Friendship Teams. The following is a list of steps to take and tools to use when acting in G.R.E.E.N. Scenes:

1. Use Warm-Ups for Acting G.R.E.E.N. These will help you get ready to play your part on your Acting Team. You may want to use a self-calming strategy, such as taking some slow, controlled breaths to get ready to do your best.

2. Think First and **survey** the G.R.E.E.N. Scene. Listen to and read the scene first. Find clues to help you answer the questions on the Wise Action Tool called "**Surveying the Scene before Taking Action**" that can be found on the next page. Decide who is in the scene, where the scene is taking place, and what each person needs.

3. Think First of the **Common Team Goal.** As you **survey the scene**, make your best guess about the **Common Team Goal**. What would everyone in the scene want to have as a **goal**? ______________________________________

4. Choose **Guiding G.R.E.E.N. Thoughts** for the G.R.E.E.N. Scene. Think of the most important **Guiding G.R.E.E.N. Thoughts** that the characters in the scene could choose. Choose from the ones provided to you or think of a **Guiding G.R.E.E.N. Thought** of your own.

5. Take Action! Now it is time to act out the G.R.E.E.N. Scene. You can perform the same scene more than once to see whether you and your Team can get better each time.

6. Use the G.R.E.E.N. Scene Review Form. If you observed the scene, give **honest**, **supportive**, and **helpful** feedback to the people on the Acting Team.

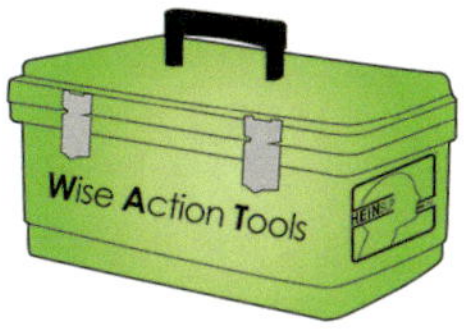

SURVEYING THE SCENE BEFORE TAKING ACTION

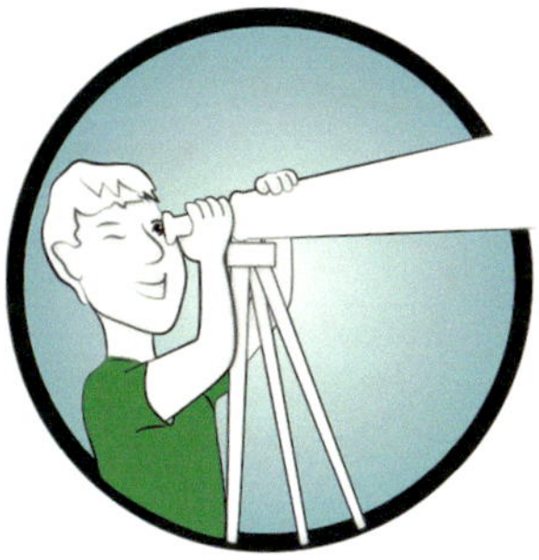

Directions: As you read each G.R.E.E.N. Scene, find clues to help you answer the following questions. This will help you know how to act in the scene.

1. The name of this G.R.E.E.N. Scene is ______________________________

2. What is the setting (where is this scene happening)? ______________________________
____

3. Who are the characters (who is in this scene)? ______________________________
____

4. What kind of Team is in this scene? Home Team School Team Friendship Team

5. What does each character in this scene want or need? ______________________________
____
____

6. What do you think is the Common Team Goal in this scene? ______________________________
____

7. What would be a positive consequence of everyone in the scene doing their best to act G.R.E.E.N.?
____

12.3 Rules for Acting in G.R.E.E.N. Scenes

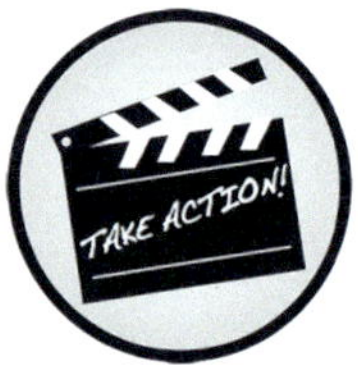

Rules for Taking Action!

Just as rules help civilizations be their best, rules can help the Acting Team be its best.

Here are the rules for acting in a G.R.E.E.N. Scene. If everyone on the Team follows these rules, everyone will achieve their **Personal Goals** of acting in a G.R.E.E.N. way. At the same time, the whole Team will get to reach the **Common Team Goal** of working together well.

Team Rules

1. We use **self-control** strategies.
2. When we speak, our words and tone are **respectful**.
3. We Think First and **survey the scene** before acting in order to see who else is on the Acting Team. This helps us work together to act out a great scene.

12.4 Using the G.R.E.E.N. Scene Review Form

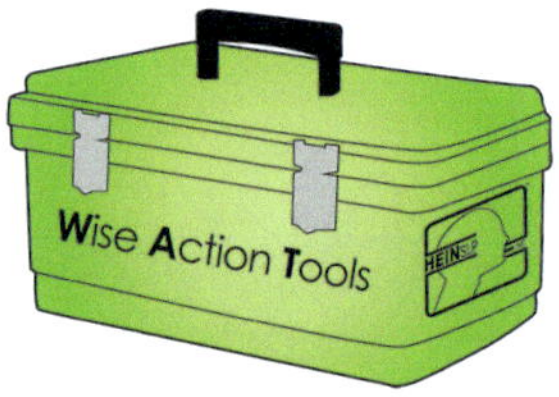

If observers are in the audience watching the scene being acted out, have them fill out the G.R.E.E.N. Scene Review Form.

1. The audience can judge whether the actors are showing that they are **G**rateful for getting the help and cooperation they need.
2. The audience can judge whether the actors are **R**espectful in their choices of words and tone.
3. The audience can judge whether the actors showed that they were **E**mpathetic and cared about one another.

4. The audience can judge whether the actors are **Easygoing** and **cooperative** with one another.

5. Members of the audience can judge whether the actors displayed good **Navigating** skills.

12.5 G.R.E.E.N. Scene Warm-Ups

Check to see if you are ready to do your best by taking **G.R.E.E.N.** warm-up action!

__ 1. I can tell who else is on my Team right now.

Question: *Who is on your Team right now?*

Answer: Name the others on your Acting Team.

__ 2. I am able to make eye contact with the Scene Director for at least a count of five.

Direction: *Look at me so I know you are ready to get started.*

Action: Look at the Scene Director for a count of five.

__ 3. If I need to get calm and focused, I am able to take a Five Break with five slow, full breaths.

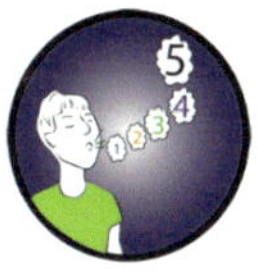

Direction: Let's make sure we are calm and focused in order to do our best, by taking a Five Break.

Action: Slowly breathe in (1...2...3...4) and out (1...2...3...4) five times

__ 4. I know the **Common Team Goal** of this Acting Team.

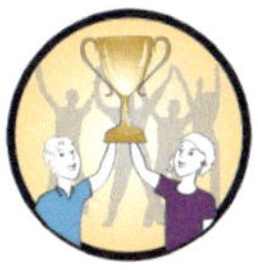

Question: *What is the* ***Common Team Goal*** *for the acting Team?*

Answer: *"We help each other do our best to act* ***G.R.E.E.N.*** *in this scene."*

__ 5. I can choose a **Guiding** G.R.E.E.N. **Thought** to use right now.

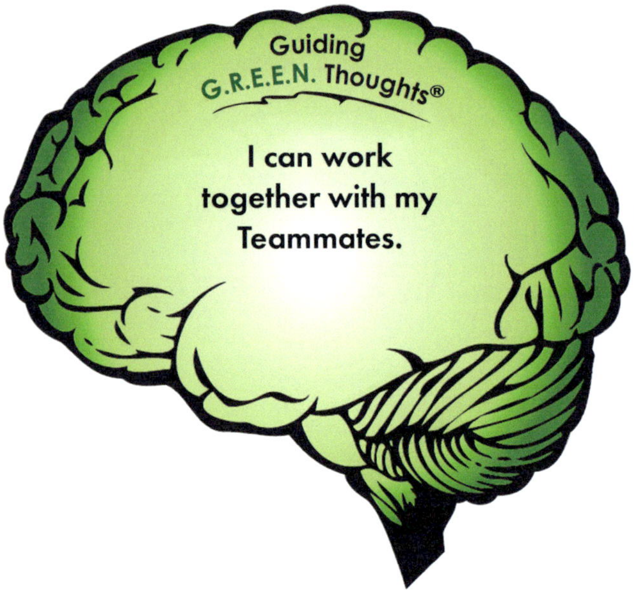

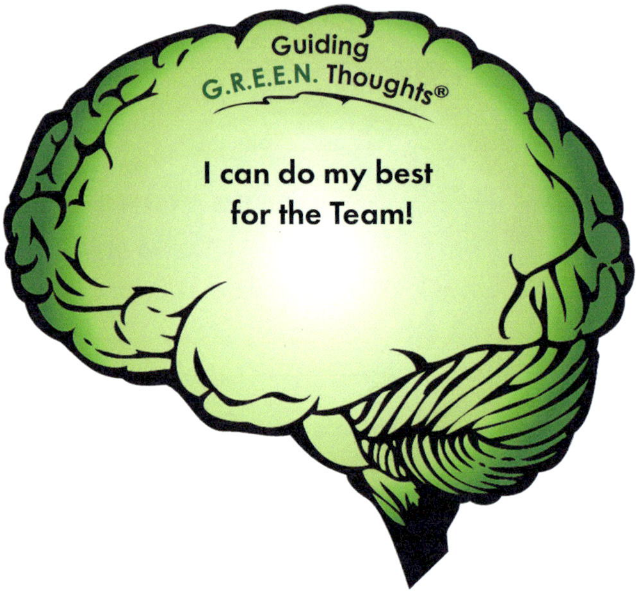

Question: What important **Guiding** G.R.E.E.N. **Thought** would be helpful right now?.

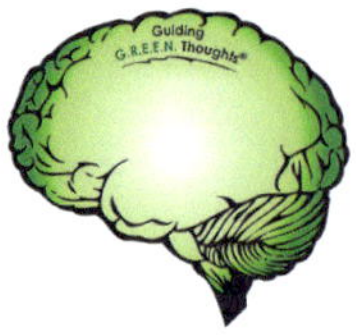

Action: Point to a useful **Guiding** G.R.E.E.N. **Thought** and read it aloud.

__ 6. When I am asked if I am ready to take G.R.E.E.N. action, I can answer "I am ready!"

Question: *Are you ready to act G.R.E.E.N. in this scene?*

Answer: *Yes, I'm ready to act G.R.E.E.N.!*

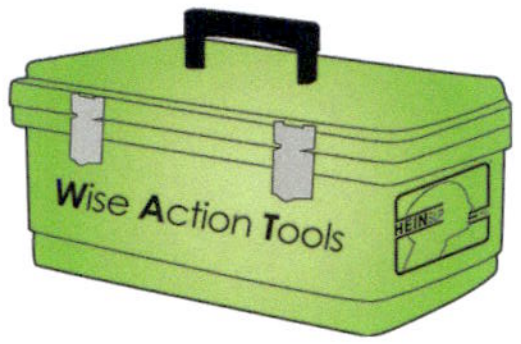

G.R.E.E.N. SCENE REVIEW FORM

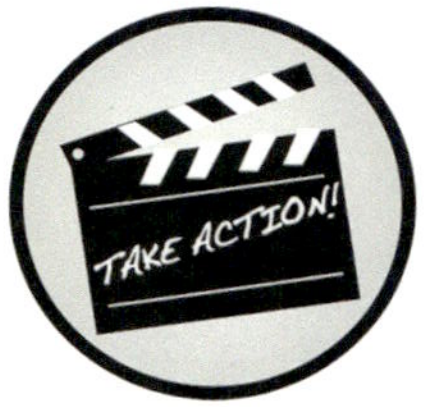

Date ______________________ Name of Reviewer ______________________

Name of G.R.E.E.N. Scene/Situation ______________________

The goal of this "Team" ______________________

G.R.E.E.N. SCENE TEAM MEMBER	ROLE IN THIS SCENE	G Grateful said "thank you" or otherwise showed appreciation	R Respectful used polite words and tone of voice	E Empathetic acted as if they cared about the other people	E Easygoing acted cooperatively to help achieve the TEAM goal	N Navigating stayed calm and handled a challenging situation
1.						
2.						
3.						

Comments—extra "takes" or cues needed? ______________________

12.6 Start with Quick G.R.E.E.N. Scenes

Quick G.R.E.E.N. Scenes

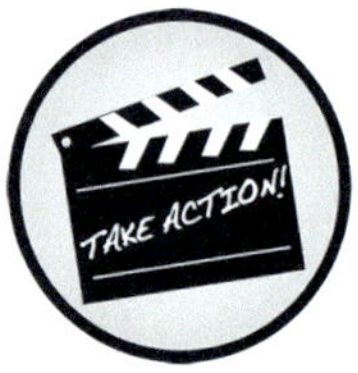

The first scenes to act out will be Quick G.R.E.E.N. Scenes, which will help you see how well you can keep the most important **Guiding G.R.E.E.N. Thoughts** in your brain. By acting out these Quick G.R.E.E.N. Scenes, you will learn what to say in situations that often occur in your real life. Once you learn to act G.R.E.E.N. in these quick, short scenes, you will be ready to practice acting in longer, more complicated G.R.E.E.N. Scenes. You and your guide will choose which G.R.E.E.N. Scenes will help you the most as you strive to act more G.R.E.E.N. in your real life.

12.7 Directions for Quick G.R.E.E.N. Scenes

Each Quick G.R.E.E.N. Scene includes a Person #1 and Person #2. Person #1 will say something to Person #2. Person #2 will then say something back to Person #1. When you are asked to be Person #2, please say words that show that you are acting G.R.E.E.N. Scripts are provided for you if you cannot think of G.R.E.E.N. words to say on your own.

Person #1 and Person #2 can switch roles so each has a chance to see the scene from the other's point of view.

Directions:

1. Get set with the G.R.E.E.N. Scene Warm-Up.
2. Get the G.R.E.E.N. Scene clapboard.

3. Choose two actors for each Quick **G.R.E.E.N.** Scene.
4. The script is reviewed so everyone knows what to say.
5. The Acting Team is asked what the **Common Team Goal** is for the scene. They are given some help if they are unable to answer.
6. For each scene, the Director says "Quiet on the Set!" to signal that it is time to pay attention to the scene.
7. The Director "claps" the clapboard and says, "Action." Person #1 says the printed line. Person #2 responds using words and a tone that show the best possible effort at acting **G.R.E.E.N.**
8. After Person #2 has had a chance to respond, the Director claps the clapboard again and says, "Cut!"
9. The actors are given feedback about whether they acted **G.R.E.E.N.**
10. If the scene is not successful, Person #2 can try again, with the Director saying "Take Two!" Write T 2 next to the clapboard for any scene that needs a second take.
11. The roles in the scene can be switched.

12.8 Quick G.R.E.E.N. Scene Score Sheet—Basic G.R.E.E.N. Skills

How Do You Get Points?

- Give yourself a **G.R.E.E.N.** plus (+) for telling the Scene Director the **Common Team Goal**.
- Give yourself a **G.R.E.E.N.** plus (+) for telling the Scene Director the **Guiding G.R.E.E.N. Thought** most useful for Person #2 in each scene.
- Give yourself a **G.R.E.E.N.** plus (+) for acting **G.R.E.E.N.** on the first "take." Count your action as a half point (1/2) if you needed to have a second "take" to act **G.R.E.E.N.** in the scene. If you needed more than one "take," you will have a chance to get points the next time you act.

12.9 Basic G.R.E.E.N. Skills Score Sheet:

What Is Your Score?

My name ____

Total your plus marks (+++++) at the end of these Quick G.R.E.E.N. Scenes.

If you did not get all the points this time, what can you do to improve your score next time?

Date: ______________________________

G. __________ + R. _________ + E. _________ + E. _______ + N. _______ = ______

My total score for these Quick G.R.E.E.N. Scenes is ______________________

Date (if scenes are acted out a second time): ____________________________

G. __________ + R. _________ + E. _________ + E. _______ + N. _______ = ______

My total score for these Quick G.R.E.E.N. Scenes is ______________________

12.10 Quick Grateful G.R.E.E.N. Scene

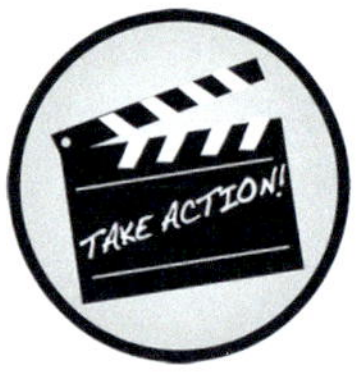

The Scene: It is math class. Person #2 has been having trouble solving a math problem. Person #1 is the teacher who has come to help Person #2.

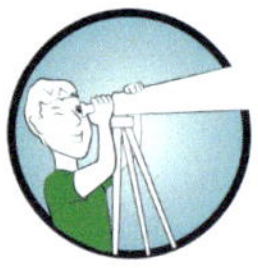

What is the **Common Team Goal** for this Classroom Team?

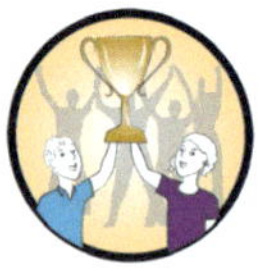

____ +

____

(**Students will learn how to solve math problems**.)

What is the **Guiding G.R.E.E.N. Thought** that can help Person #2 act G.R.E.E.N. in this scene? +

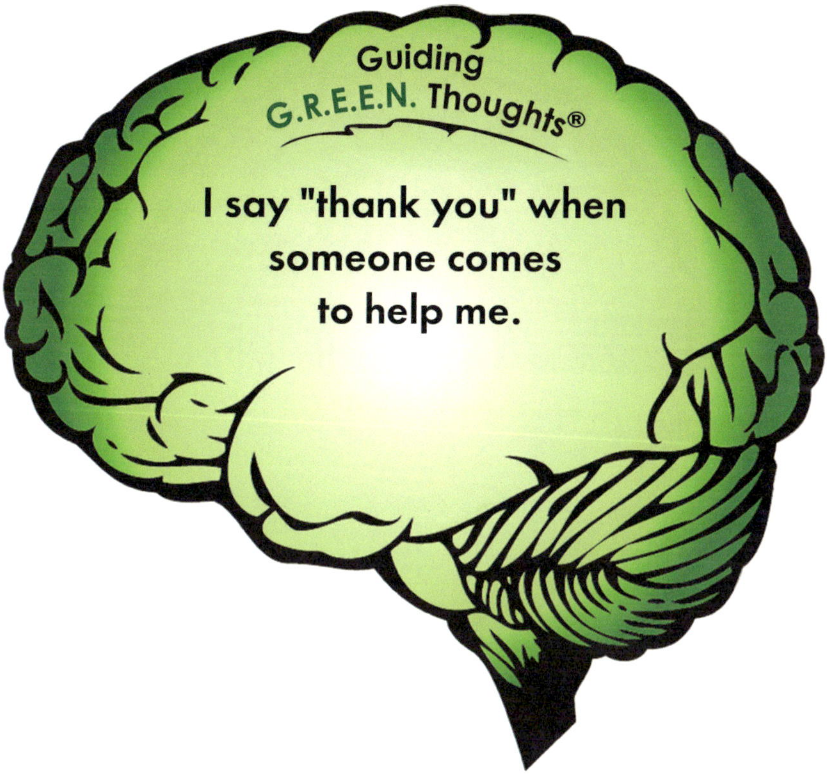

Person #1, the teacher: *I am here to help you solve your math problem.*

Person #2: *Thank you for coming to help me.* +

How G.R.E.E.N. was this scene? Total number of plus marks = ________________

____ Great Take the first time.

____ Second Take was needed (T-2).

____ G.R.E.E.N. Scene could not be acted out successfully on this date.

12.11 Quick Respectful G.R.E.E.N. Scene

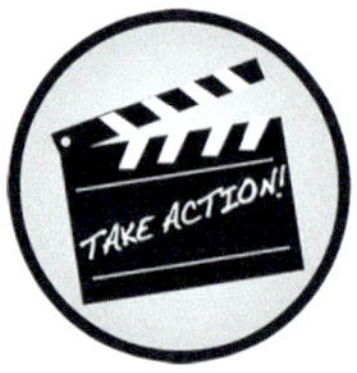

The scene: It is the morning. Person #2 has just come into the kitchen where Person #1 has been making breakfast. Person #1 is the mom or dad.

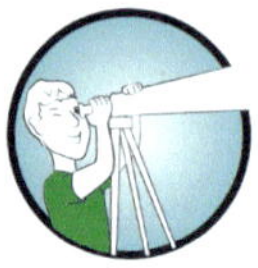

What is the **Common Team Goal** for this Home Team?

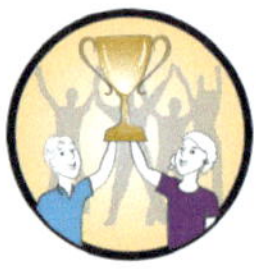

____ +

(**Everyone will feel that they are important to one another.**)

What is the **Guiding G.R.E.E.N. Thought** that can help Person #2 act **G.R.E.E.N.** in this scene? + 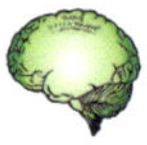

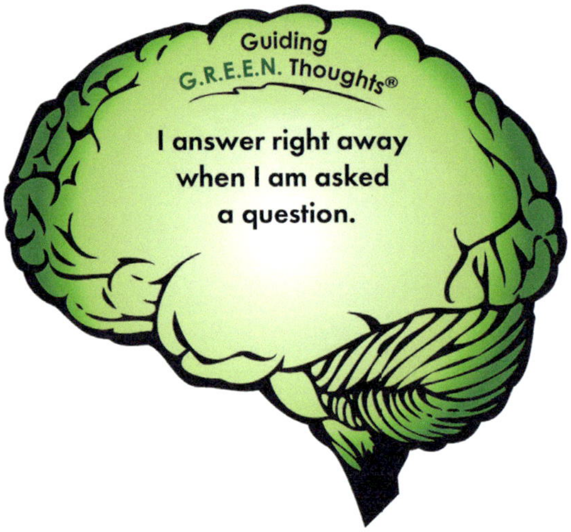

 **Person #1, the parent**: *Good morning. How are you today?*

 **Person #2**: *I'm* ______________________________. *How are you?* +

How **G.R.E.E.N.** was this scene? Total number of plus marks = ____________

____ Great Take the first time.

____ Second Take was needed (T-2).

____ **G.R.E.E.N.** Scene could not be acted out successfully on this date.

12.12 Quick Empathetic G.R.E.E.N. Scene

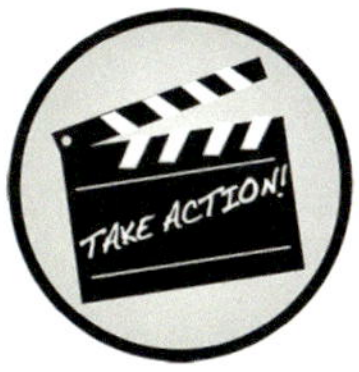

The scene: It is recess time at school. Person #1 is a friend of Person #2. Person #2 is good at shooting baskets. Person #1 is on the basketball team, and is good at passing and dribbling the ball, but is having trouble getting the ball into the basket.

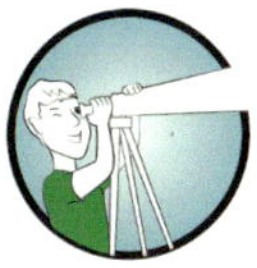

What is the **Common Team Goal** for this Friendship Team?

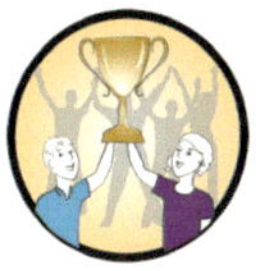

____ +

(**We show that we care about one another**.)

What is the **Guiding G.R.E.E.N. Thought** that can help Person #2 act **G.R.E.E.N.** in this scene? +

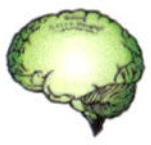

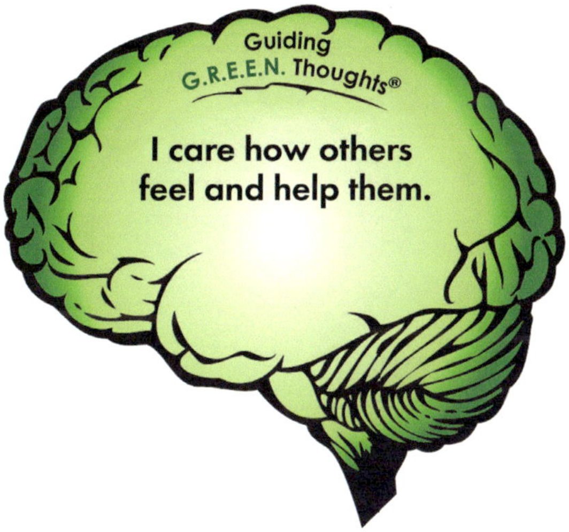

Person #1: *I just can't get the ball into the basket. I think our team is losing because of me.*

Person #2: *I'm sorry you feel that way. Do you want to practice shooting baskets with me? Maybe I can help you get better.* +

How **G.R.E.E.N.** was this scene? Total number of plus marks = ________________

____ Great Take the first time.

____ Second Take was needed (T-2).

____ **G.R.E.E.N.** Scene could not be acted out successfully on this date.

12.13 Quick Easygoing G.R.E.E.N. Scene

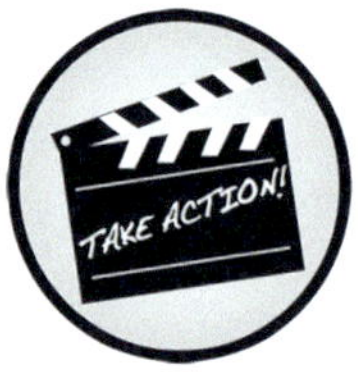

The scene: It is the night to bring the trash down to the curb so the trash truck can pick it up in the morning. Several trash cans need to be brought down to the curb. Person #1, the parent, would like some help with the chore. Person #2, the son or daughter, is relaxing on the couch.

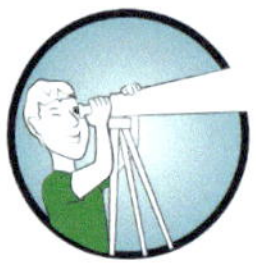

What is the **Common Team Goal** for this Home Team?

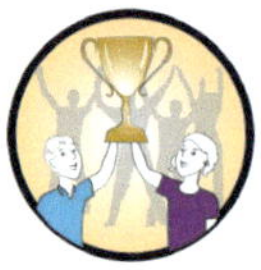

____ +

(**We help one another do the things that need to get done**.)

What is the **Guiding G.R.E.E.N. Thought** that can help Person B act **G.R.E.E.N.** in this scene? +

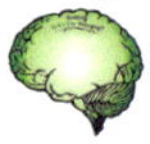

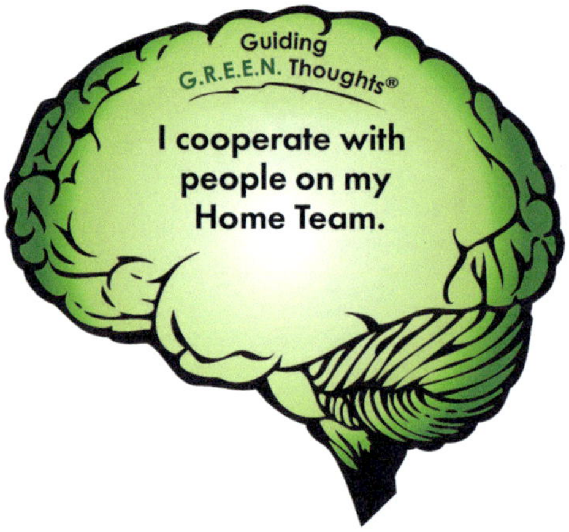

Person #1, the parent: *Can you please help me bring down the trash?*

Person #2: *Yes. I will be right there to help you after I put on some shoes.* +

How **G.R.E.E.N.** was this scene? Total number of plus marks = ______________

____ Great Take the first time.

____ Second Take was needed (T-2).

____ **G.R.E.E.N.** Scene could not be acted out successfully on this date.

12.14 Quick Navigating G.R.E.E.N. Scene

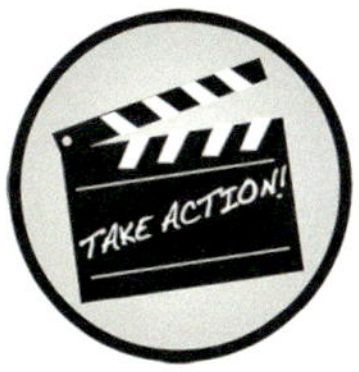

The scene: Person #1, the teacher, is explaining something new to the class. Person #2 keeps moving in his seat and tapping his pencil on the desk. He has a fidget to squeeze but is not using it. Person #2 is distracting the teacher and the rest of the class.

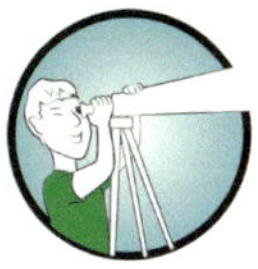

What is the **Common Team Goal** for this Classroom Team?

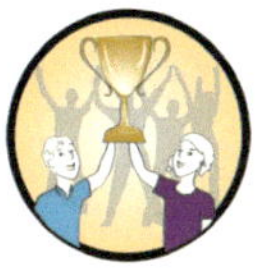

____ +

(**We use self-calming strategies in order to pay attention during lessons.**)

What is the **Guiding G.R.E.E.N. Thought** that can help Person #2 act **G.R.E.E.N.** in this scene? +

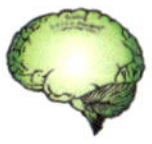

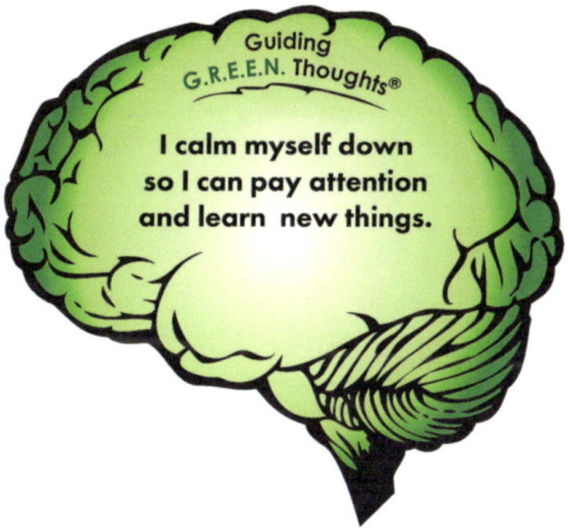

Person #1, the teacher: *Please stop tapping your pencil and squeeze the fidget ball instead so you can get your body calm. Then you and the rest of the class can **pay attention to what I am saying**.*

Person #2: *OK, I will stop tapping and use the fidget instead. Sorry for being distracting.* +

How **G.R.E.E.N.** was this scene? Total number of plus marks = ________________

____ Great Take the first time.

____ Second Take was needed (T-2).

____ **G.R.E.E.N.** Scene could not be acted out successfully on this date.

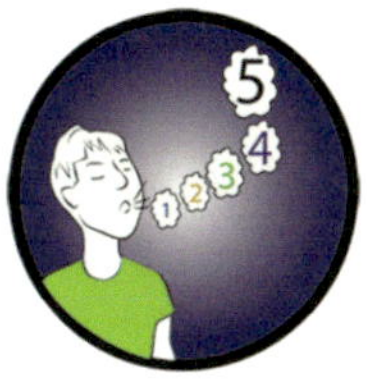

13 Self-Calming Strategies

13.1 Learning How to Get Calm

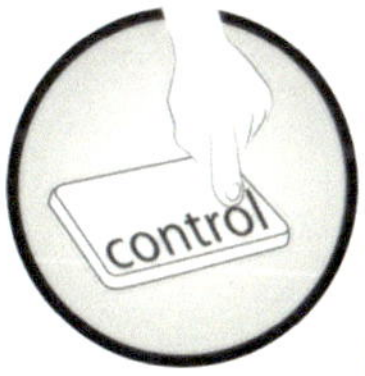

You will find that it is important to learn how to get yourself to feel calm. When you are calm, you can keep yourself in good control. When you have good **self-control**, you can Think First about any scene you are in and the possible consequences before you take any action.

When you are calm, it helps you use your brain to focus on what is going on around you so you can then choose the best words and actions to **navigate** the scene you are in. So, take the time to learn this important strategy of **self-calming** so you can act successfully in any challenging **G.R.E.E.N.** Scene or in any scene in your real life.

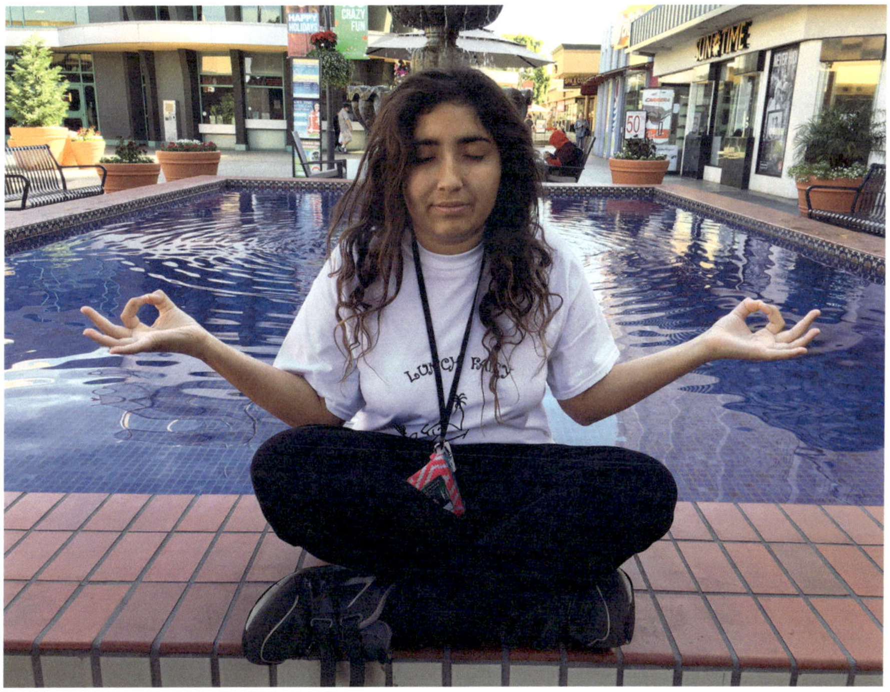

13.2 Check Yourself! Are You Calm Enough to Think First?

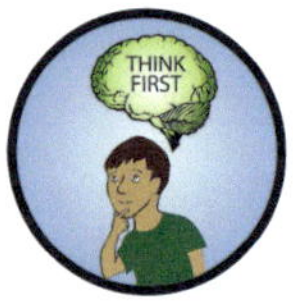

In order to make the best choice in a scene, **survey the scene** really closely. This includes taking a **look at *yourself***!

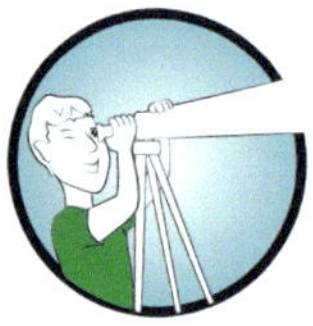

Ask yourself these questions:

- *Am I calm enough right now to Think First?*

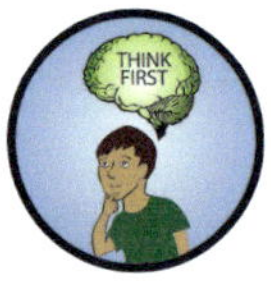

- *Am I calm enough to listen to others?*

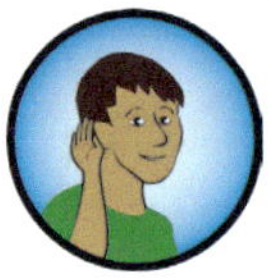

- *Am I calm enough to make* **safe** *choices that are not impulsive?*

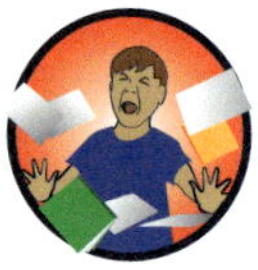

When you **survey the scene** and ask yourself these questions, **pay attention to feedback** that you get from the people on your Teams and from your own body. When your body sweats, it tells you that you feel hot. When your body shivers or you get goose bumps, it is telling you that you are probably cold. Your body also gives you signals or feedback when you are getting upset, frustrated or nervous. Learn to understand the signals your body is giving you about how you feel. You also can be aware of signals from people around you. Their feedback can give you information about how they think you are acting.

Sometimes your brain or body is giving you clues to **flip the switch** 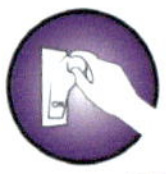 and do something different so you can successfully **navigate** through a scene. This feedback can let you know that you need to make a **change** in how you act. **Navigating** through a scene in your life is like driving on the road. When you are not paying attention to your actions and the direction you are headed, it is like drifting off the road or taking the wrong one! There would be a negative consequence. Instead, you might need to carefully pull off the road to stop and step on the brakes. You then take a short break so you can be calm and figure out what **change** you need to make to get on the right road again.

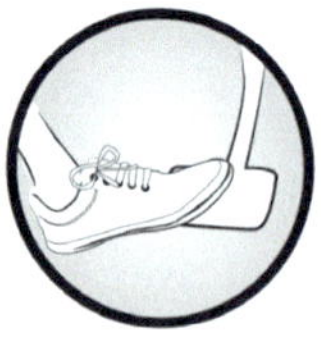

When you get feedback from yourself or others that you are not Thinking First right now, perhaps it is a good time to Brake to Take a 5 Break. This means you move to where you can stop and step on the brakes for a short

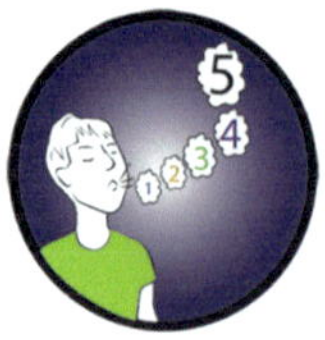

time. You then give your body and your brain a break to use the strategy of slowly and carefully breathing in and out at least five times to help you get ready to return to the right road.

When you feel calm enough to drive on the right road again, you can take the best actions with the people you are with. Whether you get feedback clues from your own body or from others, it is useful to know when to use a **self-control** strategy and how to use one or more that work for you!

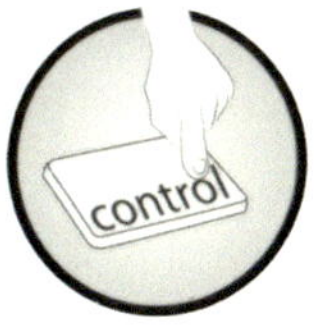

13.3 Guiding G.R.E.E.N. Thought: I Use Feedback to Get Calm

Use the self-coaching strategy of being alert to any feedback around you. Here are some **Guiding G.R.E.E.N. Thoughts** to coach yourself to get calm and stay calm.

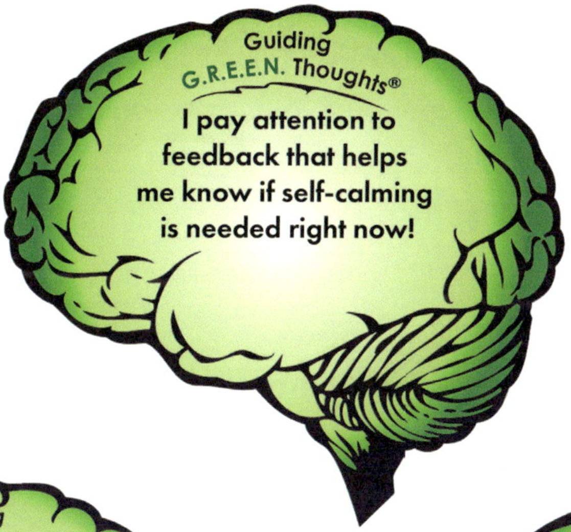

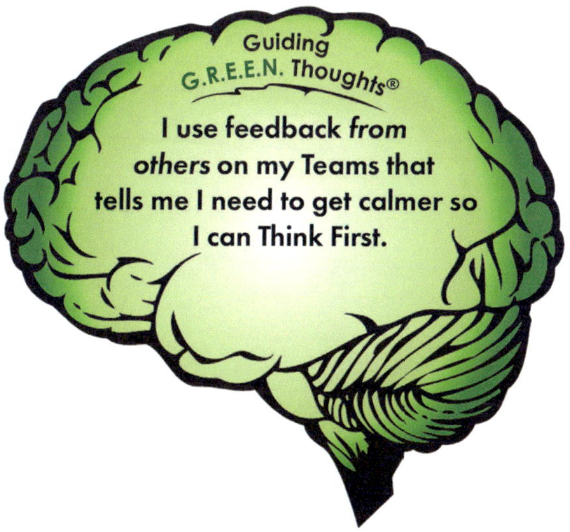

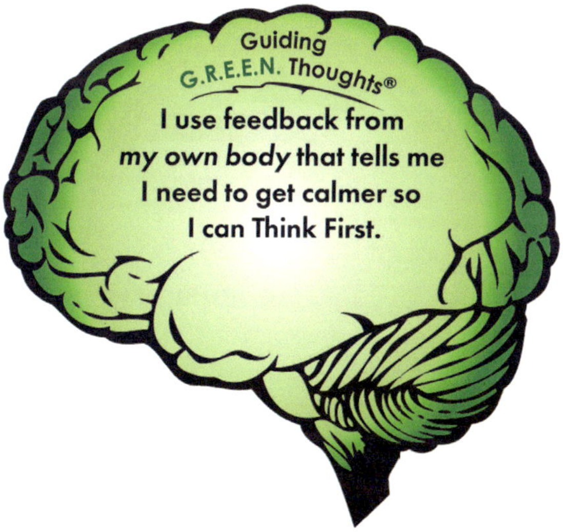

13.4 Powerful Self-Calming Strategies

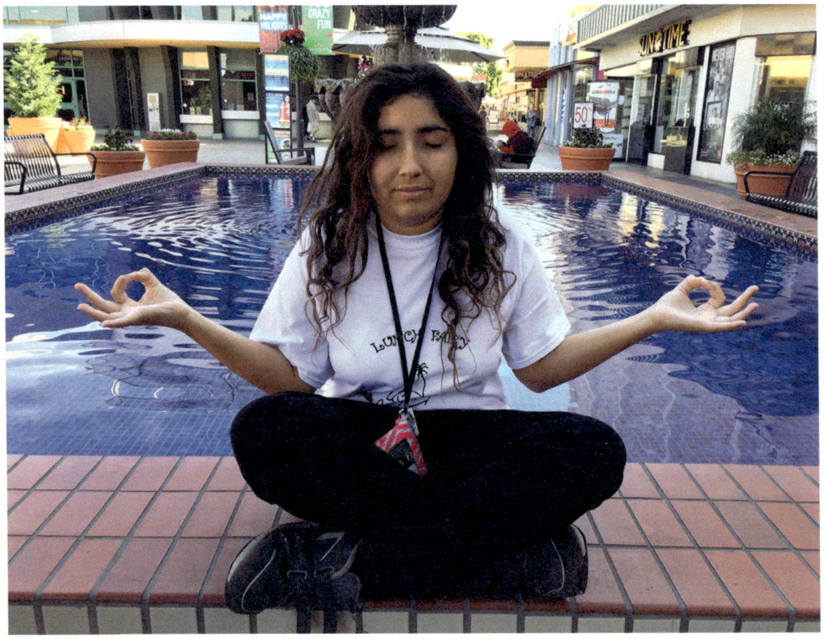

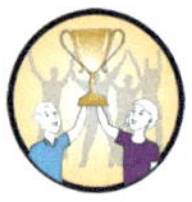

1. Remember that you have **Personal Goals** and **Common Team Goals**. Find the **power** to remember your **goals** and the reason you want to calm yourself to reach those **goals**.

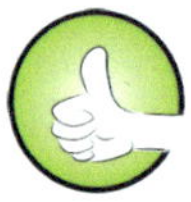

2. Think about the **positive** consequences when you stay in control.

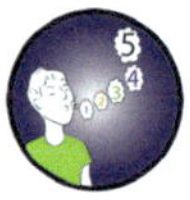

3. Use the strategy of controlled breathing when you Brake to Take a 5 Break to help you calm your body and your mind!

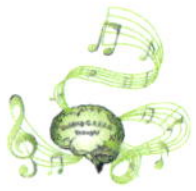

4. You can listen to the song "Brake to Take a 5 Break" to help you use the controlled breathing strategy to calm your body and your mind.

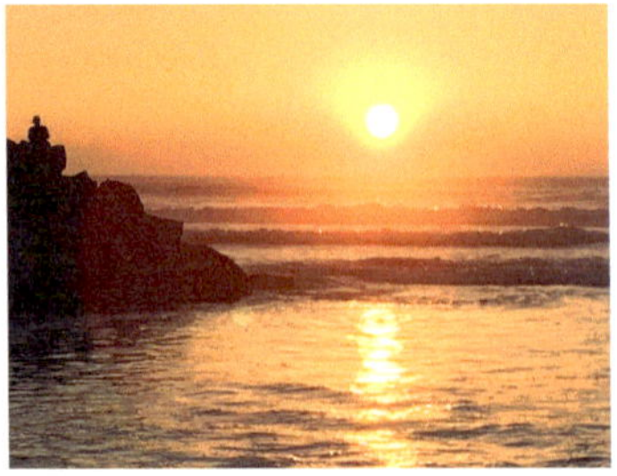

5. Use the strategy of "visualization" to picture a peaceful place and become calmer.

After you have become calm again, you will be ready to do your best for yourself and the Team.

BRAKE TO TAKE A 5 BREAK

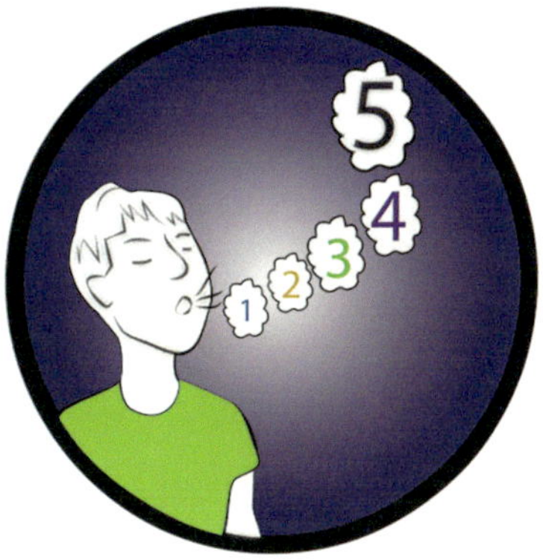

These are the steps for Braking to Take a 5 Break:

1. First, tell yourself to step on the brakes so you can avoid heading in the wrong direction. This will give you time to **flip the switch** and change your direction.

2. Next, stop what you are doing so you can get ready to Take a 5 Break.

   Let your brain give your body a red light signal to avoid doing something without thinking. When you have stopped, you can remind yourself of your goals. When you become calm, you will survey the scene and move forward in the direction best for yourself and those around you.

3. You are ready for a 5 break.

   Concentrate on taking 5 controlled breaths. This is a powerful way to become calm. The only important thing for a few seconds is your breathing. You calm yourself by focusing all your attention on your breathing. You breathe in and out slowly 5 times. Start with at least 5 controlled breaths and repeat if you need to.

I breathe in slowly through my nose like just like I am breathing in the smell of fragrant flowers.

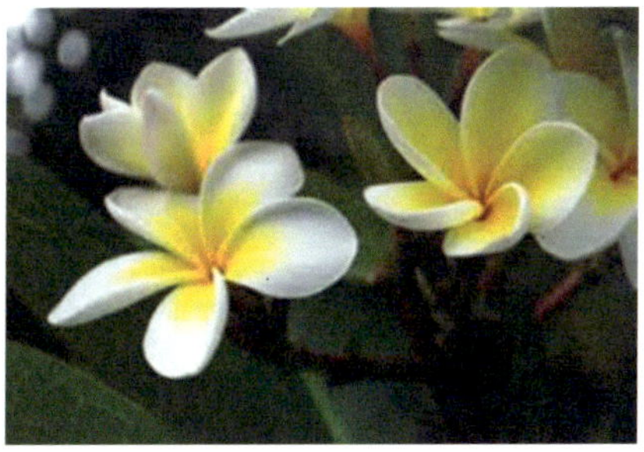

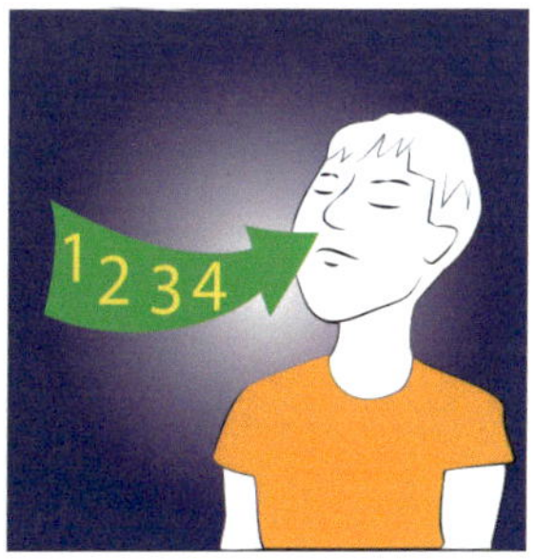

I count slowly to four: 1 . . . 2 . . . 3 . . . 4

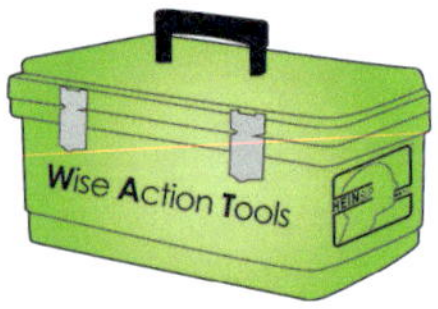

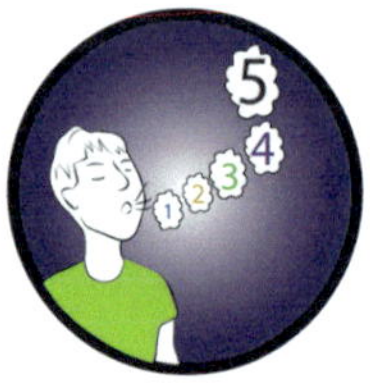

Then I breathe out slowly through my mouth as if I am blowing out many birthday candles.

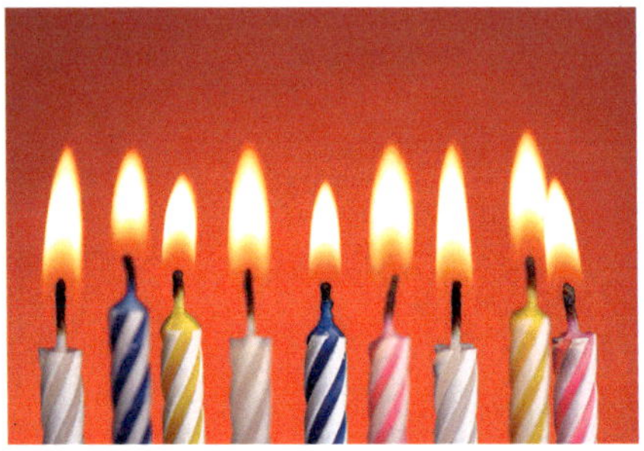

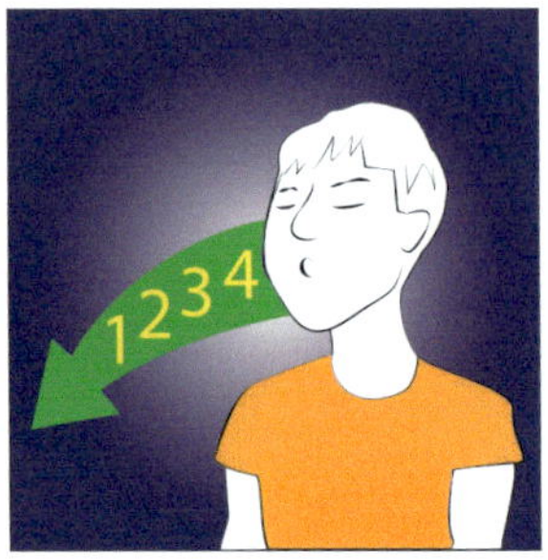

I count slowly to four: 1 . . . 2 . . . 3 . . . 4

4. When you listen to the "Brake to Take a 5 Break" song, it will help you do your controlled breathing with a calming rhythm. Each time you do this, you will get better at concentrating on the slow rhythm so it helps you get calmer:

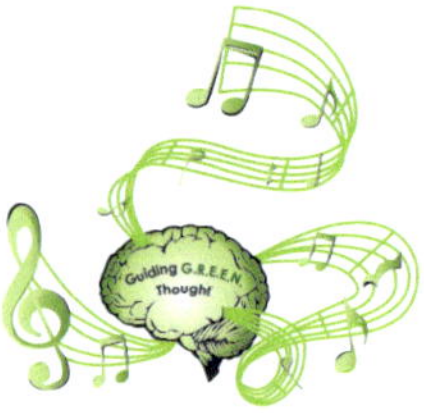

1. BREATHE in . . . 2 . . . 3 . . . 4 BREATHE out . . . 2 . . . 3 . . . 4

2. BREATHE in . . . 2 . . . 3 . . . 4 BREATHE out . . . 2 . . . 3 . . . 4

3. BREATHE in . . . 2 . . . 3 . . . 4 BREATHE out . . . 2 . . . 3 . . . 4

4. BREATHE in . . . 2 . . . 3 . . . 4 BREATHE out . . . 2 . . . 3 . . . 4

5. BREATHE in . . . 2 . . . 3 . . . 4 BREATHE out . . . 2 . . . 3 . . . 4

5. While doing your controlled breathing, you may do some other things with your body to help you get even more calm:

   a. Count on your fingers while taking each of the five full breaths.

   OR

   b. Give yourself a full body hug while taking the five full breaths.

   OR

   c. Press your hands together while taking the five full breaths.

   (Try each self-calming body movement to see which one helps you calm down the most.)

6. Once you feel calmer, you will be able to reach for **Guiding G.R.E.E.N. Thoughts** to successfully navigate the scene.

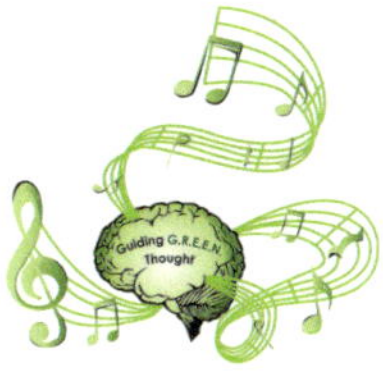

BRAKE TO TAKE A ⑤ BREAK

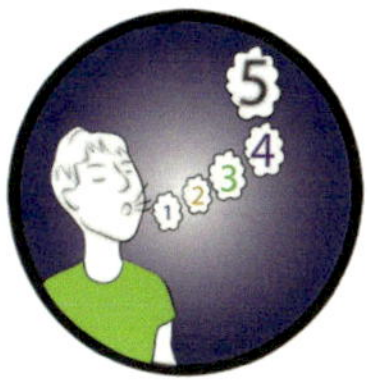

A Song for **Guiding G.R.E.E.N. Thoughts®**

by Herb Hein

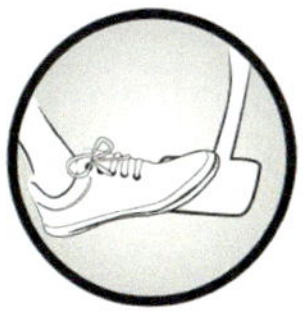

BRAKE TO TAKE A ⑤ BREAK
BRAKE TO TAKE A BREAK FOR ⑤
BRAKE TO TAKE A ⑤ BREAK
BRAKE TO TAKE A BREAK FOR ⑤

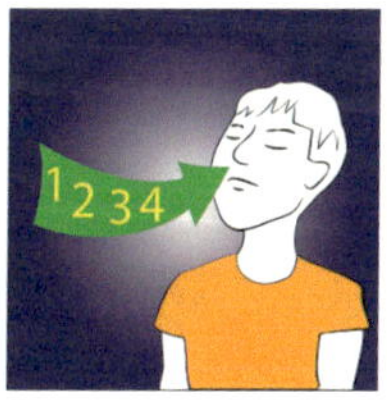

(BREATHE IN.2.3.4.)...(BREATHE OUT.2.3.4.)
(BREATHE IN.2.3.4.)...(BREATHE OUT.2.3.4.)
(BREATHE IN.2.3.4.)...(BREATHE OUT.2.3.4.)
(BREATHE IN.2.3.4.)...(BREATHE OUT.2.3.4.)
(BREATHE IN.2.3.4.)...(BREATHE OUT.2.3.4.)

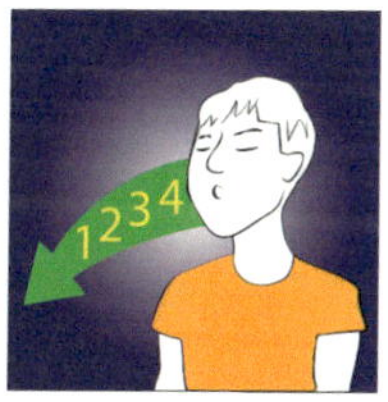

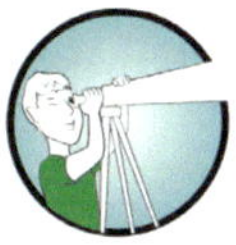

Survey the scene: Who else is on my Team?

What are the goals? What are we trying to do here together?

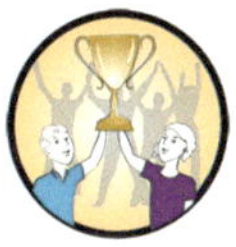

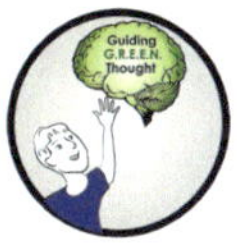

Reach up for a thought.

There's a Guiding G.R.E.E.N. Thought for me to choose!

Start the change. Make a powerful transformation.

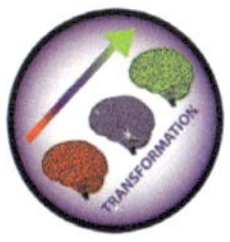

Take action! Do what I need to say or do.

Take action! Do what I need to say or do.

Take action!..., Ready, set, go!

13.5 You Can Think First after Your Calming Break!

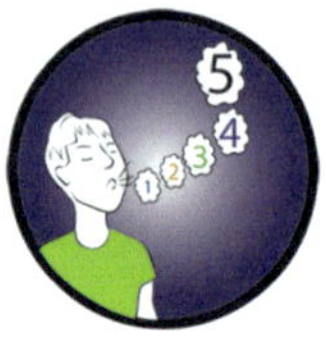

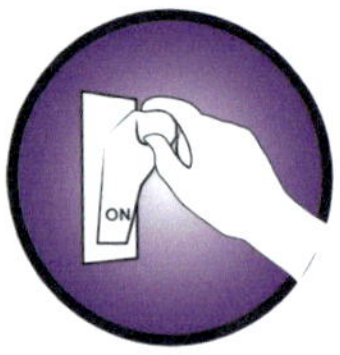

Congratulations! You used the feedback from yourself and others to **flip the switch** to **navigate** a challenging situation! You took action to get yourself calmer! This is a great first step in learning to **navigate** around obstacles.

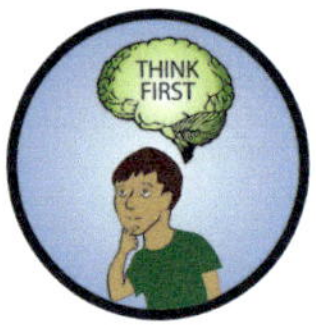

Now you are ready with a **positive** attitude to Think First and continue **navigating** well:

1. 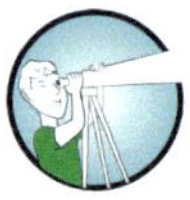 **Survey the scene** to see who else is on your team.

2. Ask yourself, "What are the **goals** of this Team? What are we trying to do here together?" 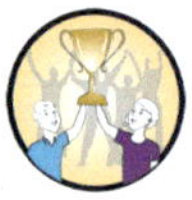

3. 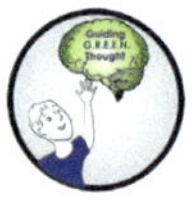 Choose a **Guiding G.R.E.E.N. Thought** that helps you move in the right direction.

4. Do your best to think about any **changes** you want to make in your thoughts or actions to help you move **forward**. You can think about how you can make a **powerful change** or **transformation** to help you head in the best **direction** with your Teams. 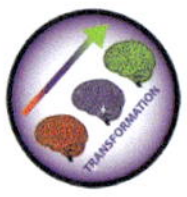

5. 

Take Action! Do whatever you need to do and say whatever you need to say to make the scene **better** for yourself and the others around you.

You have learned "controlled breathing" as one strategy to **calm yourself** as you Brake to Take a 5 Break. Look at some other **self-calming** Wise Action Tools on the next pages. With your **powerful** human brain, you can use "visualization" as another **self-calming** tool. This means you will make pictures in your imagination. For example, you can imagine being in a place where you feel comfortable, safe and at peace. Visualization is a **powerful** tool for **self-calming**.

13.6 Picture a Peaceful Scene to Help Yourself Stay Calm

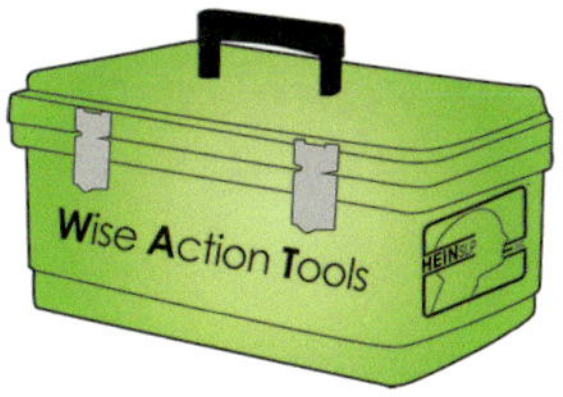

When you Brake to Take a 5 Break, you can picture yourself in a calm, peaceful place that you choose. With each breath you can get more relaxed thinking about that peaceful scene. You can draw a calming picture on your own or you can choose pictures on the next page or any picture, drawing, or photo that you like.

Whenever you need to, you can Reach Up for a **Guiding G.R.E.E.N. Thought** to think about this calming scene that will help you act G.R.E.E.N. with others on your Teams. Whenever you need to, you can imagine that you have taken a trip to be within one of your calming pictures for a while. Then you can take this calm, relaxed feeling with you wherever you go and use it in any situation! You can keep this feeling with you when you are with others on your Teams.

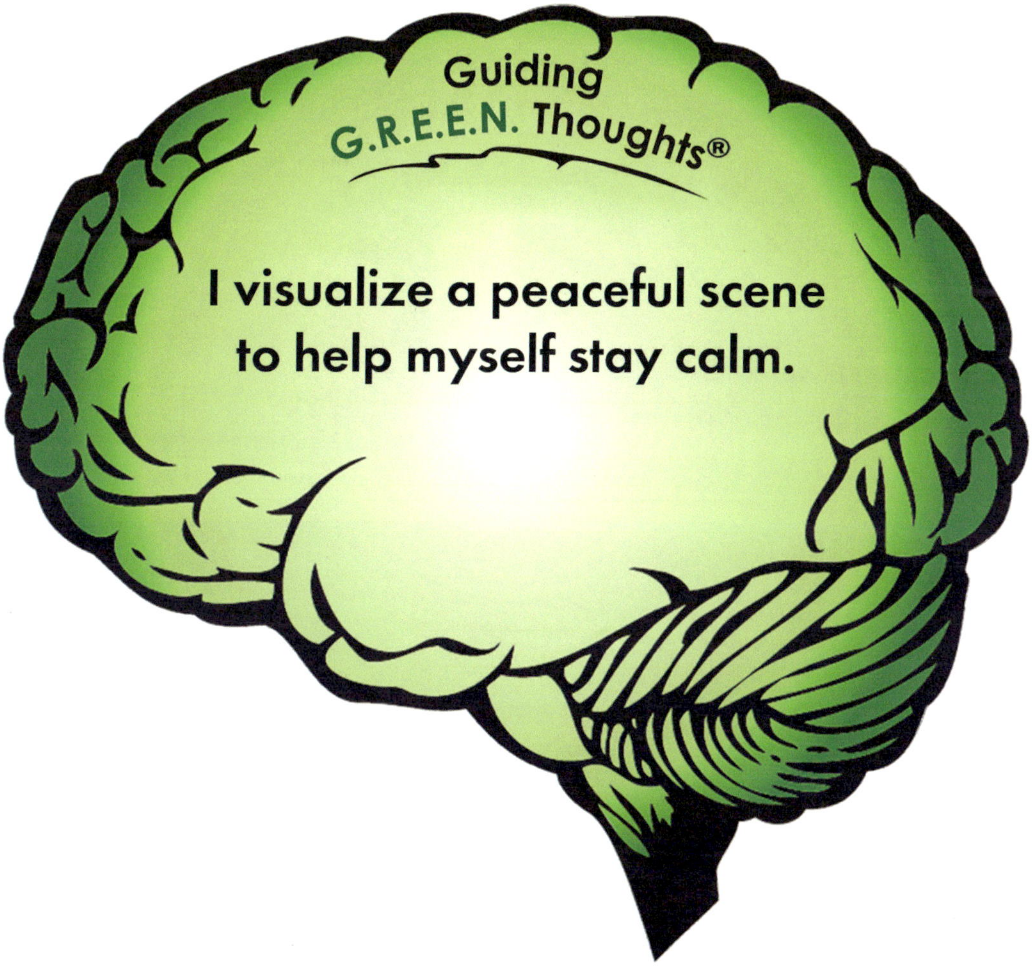

PEACEFUL SCENES TO HELP ME STAY CALM

I feel more calm when I look at these pictures. I can think of these pictures at any time and any place when I want to **self-calm** and stay calm.

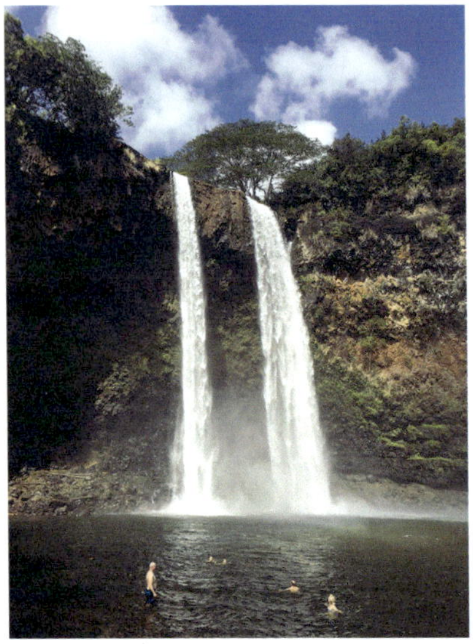

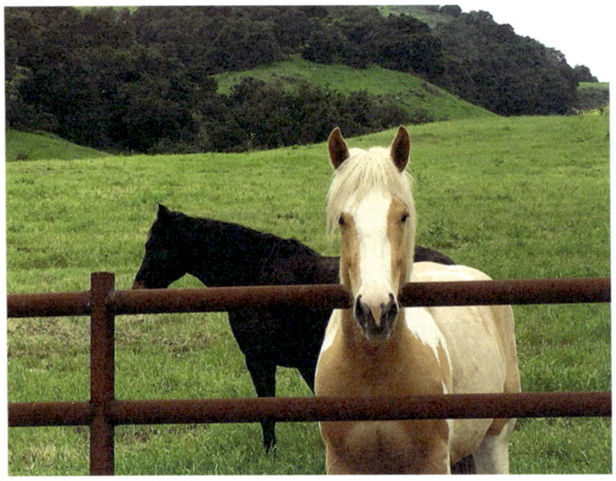

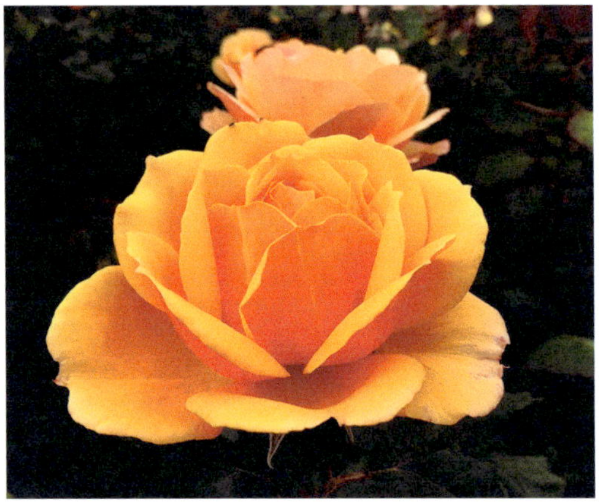

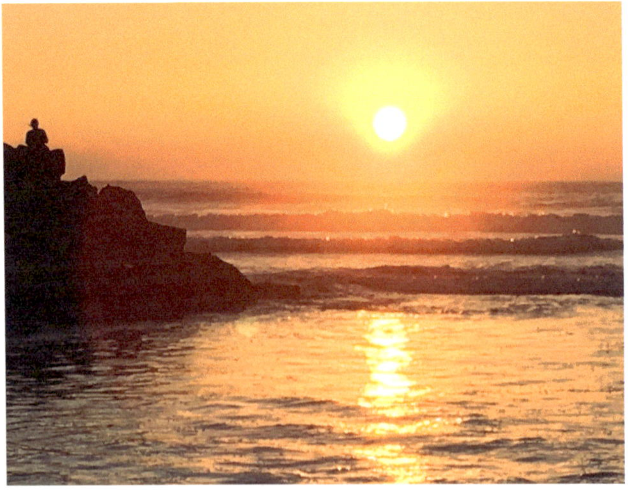

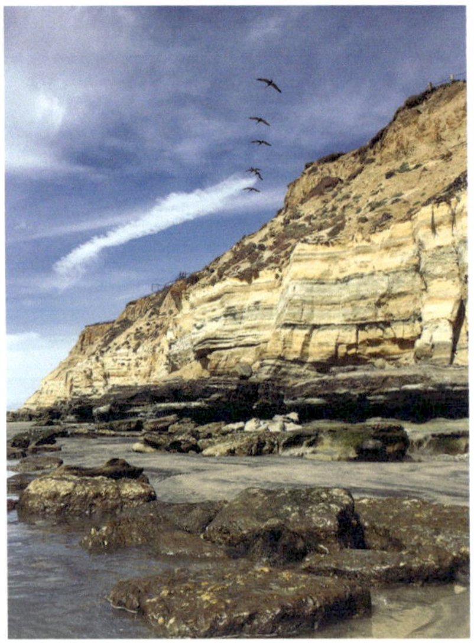

CREATING MY OWN SELF-CALMING SCENE

This is a picture I have found or a drawing I have made that helps me feel calm (I can imagine taking a trip here whenever I need to, so I can get calm and stay calm).

THIS IS HOW I LOOK
AFTER I USE A SELF-CALMING STRATEGY

This is a picture of me successfully
being with my team *after* I use my
self-calming strategy.

13.7 G.R.E.E.N. Scene #1

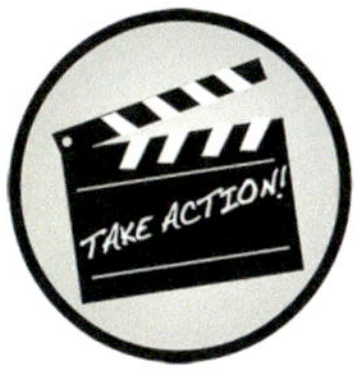

Reasons for Acting in This Scene

1. Acting in this scene can help you practice strategies to feel more calm and in control.
2. Acting in this scene can teach you to use strategies to feel calmer whenever that is useful for you.
3. Acting in this scene lets you practice asking for help when you need it.
4. Acting in this scene can help you successfully follow directions.

Directions for This Scene

1. The Scene Director and Acting Students review the appropriate pages from Section 12:
   - Making the Best G.R.E.E.N. Scenes (12.2)
   - Wise Action Tool: **Surveying the Scene before Taking Action** (12.2)
   - Rules for Acting in G.R.E.E.N. Scenes (12.3)
   - Using the G.R.E.E.N. Scene Review Form (12.4)—if others are watching the scene
   - G.R.E.E.N. Scene Warm-Ups (12.5)
2. The Director puts the Directions sheet in front of the student and makes sure that the acting student has a favorite calming scene to use. The Director also provides an example of an assignment that the student might need help completing.

3. The Director cues up "Brake to Take a 5 Break" to be played in the middle of this scene.

4. The Director gets the clapboard and says:

"Quiet on the set! Scene 1, Take 1. Action!"

If the scene gets repeated with the same set of actors, the Director will say:

"Quiet on the set! Scene 1, Take 2. Action!" etc.

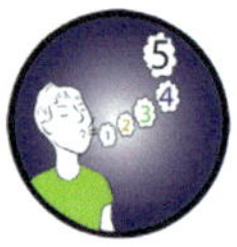

The Scene: I Take a 5 Break to Get Calm!

Narrator: You are frustrated and upset because you do not know what you are supposed to do for the class assignment in front of you. You feel that you cannot get calm. This keeps you from thinking of how to do your assignment. You do remember that you can raise your hand to let your teacher know that you feel frustrated.

Student raises hand and waits for the teacher to call on them.

Teacher: *Yes. What do you need?*

Student: *I am starting to feel frustrated.*

Teacher: *OK, This might be a good time to use some strategies that can help you get calm. Then you can tell me what is frustrating you. Can you use a calming strategy on your own, or would you like my help?*

Student: *I need your help, please.*

Teacher: *Great. Raise your hand after you get your calming picture. Wait for me and we can take a break together.*

Student gets calming picture and starts looking at it while waiting quietly for the teacher.

Teacher: *It looks like you are ready. Look at your calming picture while you listen to "Brake to Take a (5) Break." I'll go through the steps with you.*

Narrator: The teacher plays "Brake to Take a (5) Break" and takes all the steps with the student.

Teacher: *How do you feel now?*

Student: *I feel calmer.*

Teacher: *I feel calm, too. It looks like you are ready for me to help you with your assignment. Are you ready for me to help you?*

Student: *Yes, please.*

Teacher: *I'll be glad to help you. Show me which page or which question was frustrating you and we can work on it together.*

Student (points to the assignment the Director gave the student before the scene): *This part right here. Thanks for your help.*

Teacher: *You are welcome. Now let's see what the directions say.*

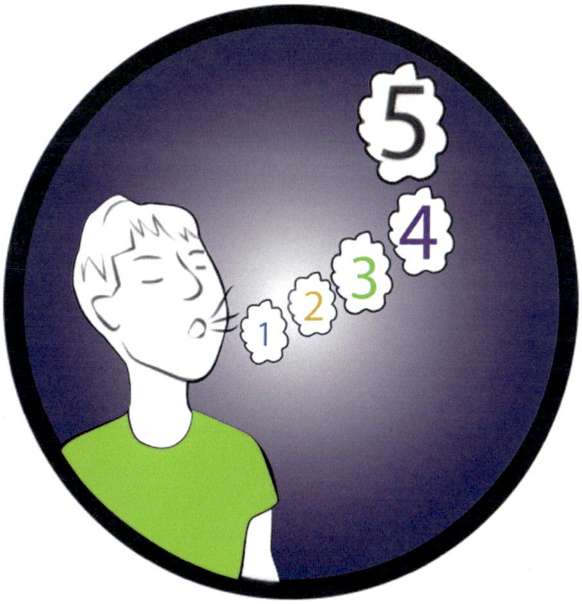

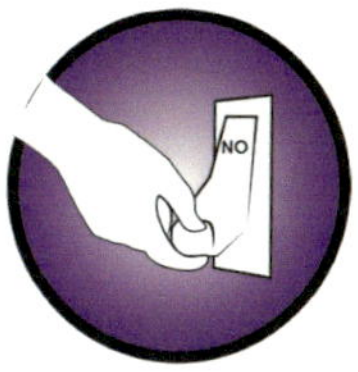

14 Flipping the Switch for Self-Control

14.1 Read and Discuss: Powerful Humans Have Self-Control to Act Safely

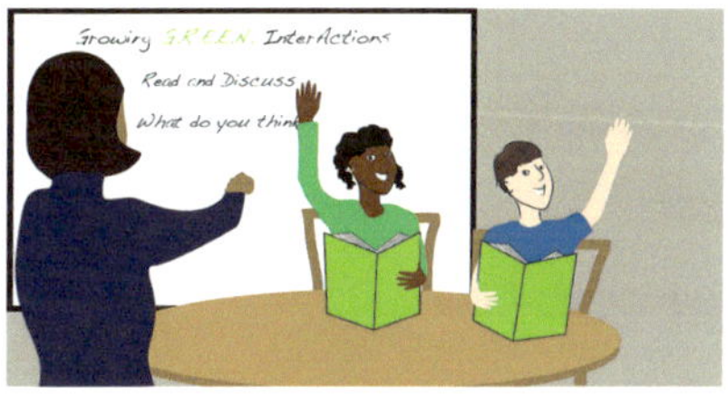

Because you have a **powerful** human brain that lets you Think First to choose your actions, you can have **self-control** to act safely. You can make action choices so you can stay safe and act **safely** with others around you.

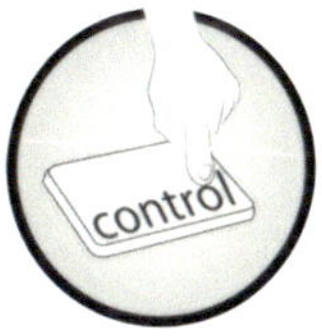

What does it mean to act **safely**?

Acting **safely** means your actions *don't* hurt you or the people or things around you.

You look around and **survey the scene to see who and what is around** you so you can move carefully to not hurt others or get hurt yourself.

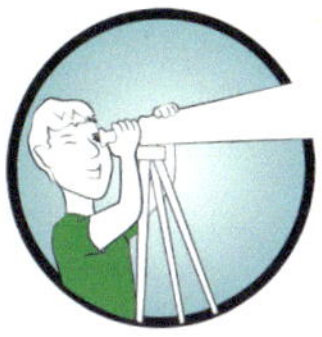

Can you act **safely** when you act quickly and impulsively *without* thinking of what you are doing? Unfortunately, the answer is no!

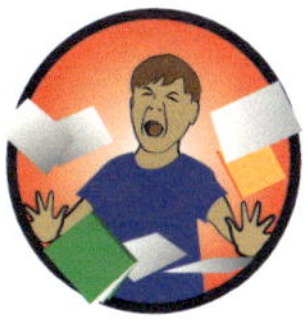

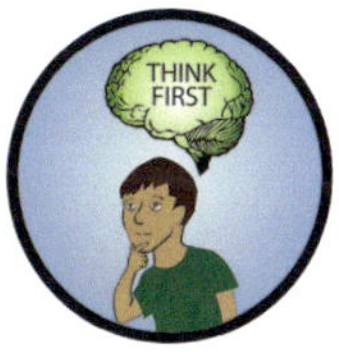

To act **safely**, you must take the time to Think First to make sure your actions *won't* hurt anyone or anything, so you and everyone else can continue moving **forward** to achieve **Personal Goals** and **Common Team Goals**.

When you try to be your best at being a human being with a **powerful** brain, you can work hard to find ways to achieve **self-control** so you can act **safely** and stay safe. With **self-control**, you can stop your actions if they will not be safe. **Self-control** comes from helping your brain put up its own stop light. You can listen to your

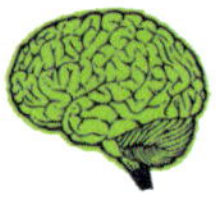

brain telling you to "Take a break to step on your brakes so you can **change** your direction!"

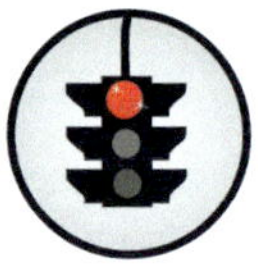

Discuss the following:

1. What does it mean to act **safely**?

2. What is a negative consequence when you do *not* act safely?

3. What is a **positive** consequence of having **self-control**?

4. When do *you* need to use **self-control** to act **safely**?

5. What do *you* think about to help you have **self-control**?

6. If someone tells you that you are not being safe, can you use a **self-control** strategy?

7. Can you step on your own brake and **flip the switch** quickly to **change** your actions to make them safer?

yes no sometimes

14.2 Step on the Brake and Flip the Switch!

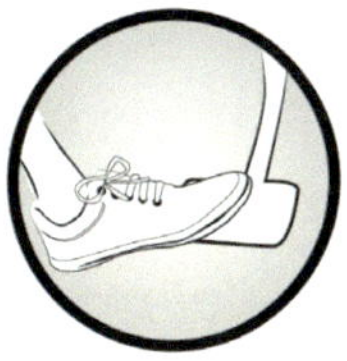

If you look carefully, you will notice when a red signal appears and tells you to step on the brake and **flip the switch.** This will help you stop so you can head in a better direction with your words and actions. This is an important skill to learn so you can **navigate** well with others. When you notice that you are heading in the wrong direction, you can use the strategy that helps you to stop going that way. Then you can feel proud of your **self-control**!

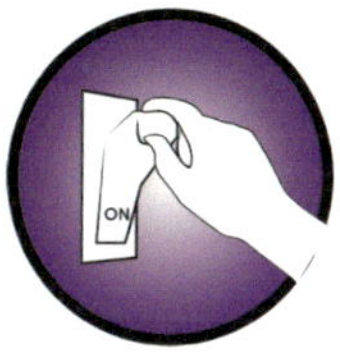

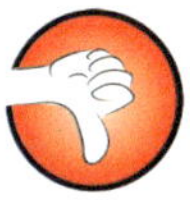

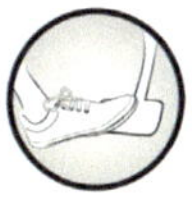

1. What is a negative action that you would like your brain to help you stop doing? ______________________________

____

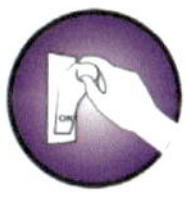

2. Can you think about **flipping the switch** so you could **change** your actions and make them **positive** instead?

yes no

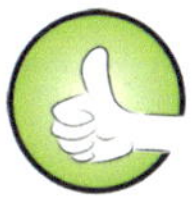

3. What **better** action can you do instead? ______________________________

____

14.3 Survey the Scene: Who Needs Their Switch Flipped for Self-Control?

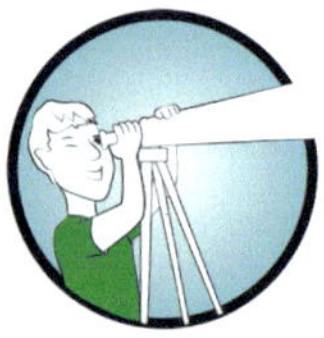

Directions: Circle the words that describe the action. Circle if the person is acting safely or not. If you decide the person is out of control and not acting safely, also circle the words to guide them to flip the switch to change the scene. Then the person can think of ways to use self-control. On the line, write what you think the person could do to make a better scene after flipping the switch.

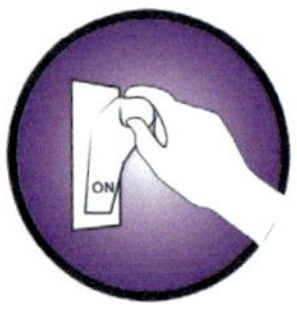

1. I move away from things when I am mad or upset so I don't throw anything or hurt anything.

   acting safely   *not* acting safely   flip the switch

   ____

2. I throw things when I am feeling mad at people.

   acting safely   *not* acting safely   flip the switch

   ____

3. I move at a speed that lets me look first to see where I am going.

   acting safely   *not* acting safely   flip the switch

   ____

4. I go as fast as I can without looking where I am going.

   acting safely   *not* acting safely   flip the switch

   ____

5. I am careful when I am around animals and others.

   acting safely   *not* acting safely   flip the switch

   ____

6. I kick and hit people and animals.

   acting safely   *not* acting safely   flip the switch

   ____

14.4 Guiding G.R.E.E.N. Thought: I Control My Own Body So No One Else Is Bothered

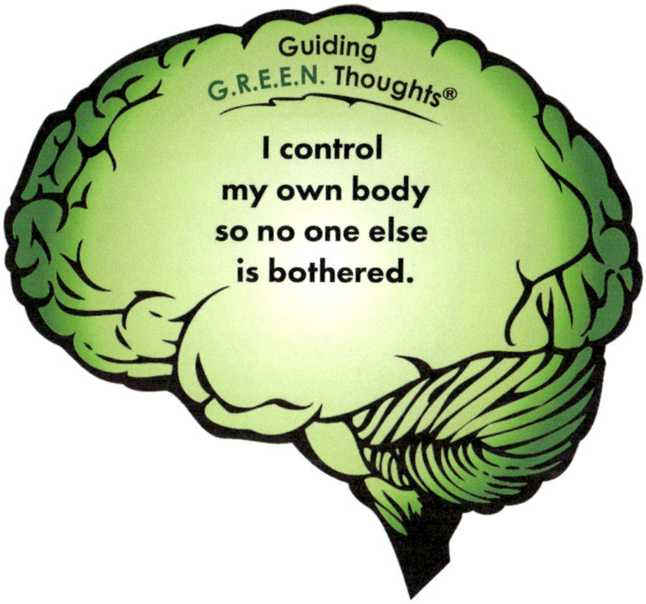

When you are in your real-life scenes with the people around you, It is important to be in control of your body. You may want to move to where you want to move, or touch the things you want to touch, or make any sound you want to make, but you will find that your actions might be bothering the people around you. If you don't stop, other people will think your action is **R.E.D.** because you are *not* showing that you care about the others on your Team.

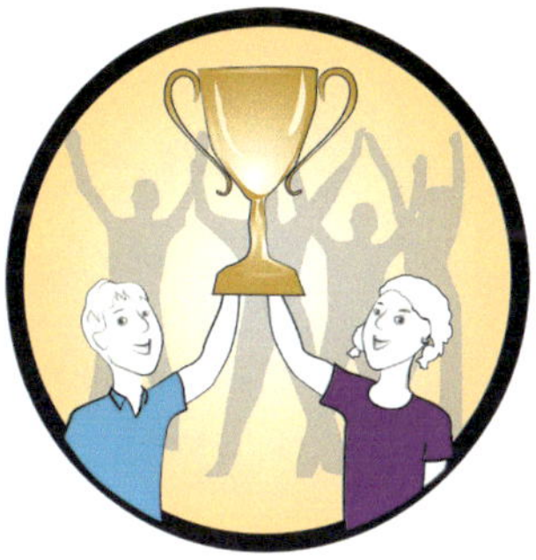

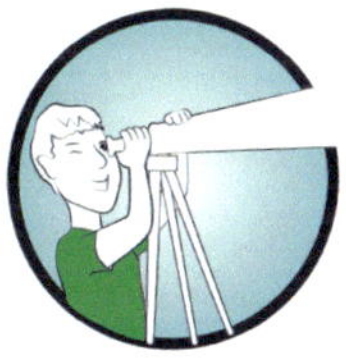

Survey the scene to get feedback from people on your Team. When you notice that you are bothering someone with your body actions, you can work hard to step on your brake to stop those actions.

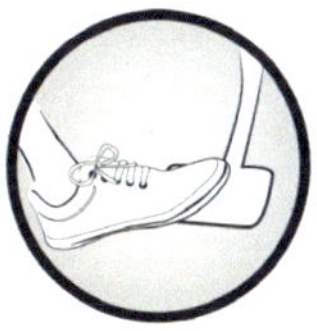

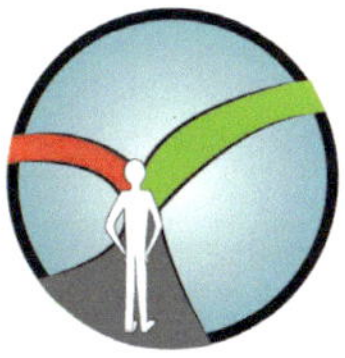

Instead of getting mad at the other person, or starting to bother the other person even more, you can make a **better** choice for the Team and make a **transformation** (see Making **Powerful Transformations**).

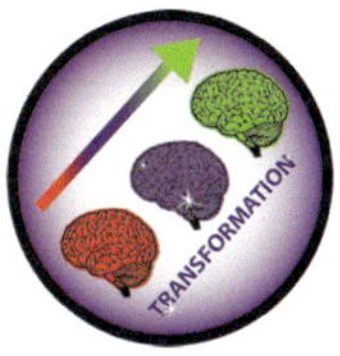

14.5 Bothering Someone or *Not*! What Are the Consequences?

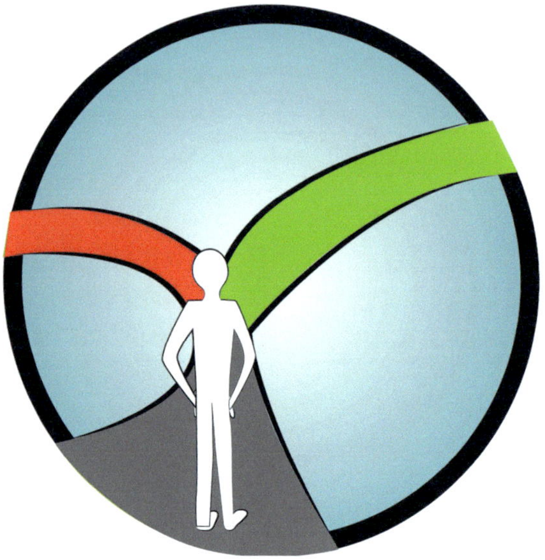

1. What is something you sometimes do with your body that bothers the people on your Teams? ____

____

2. What are the negative consequences of continuing to bother someone else when the person asked you to stop? ______________________________

____

3. What can you do to stop your actions if you find that you are bothering another person? ____

____

4. What are the **positive** consequences if you can stop bothering the other person? ____

____

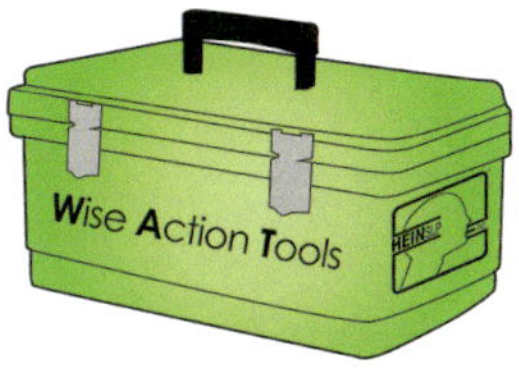

SELF-CALMING BY QUIETLY SQUEEZING A FIDGET

If you are feeling hyper, and have a lot of extra energy, you can quietly squeeze a calming fidget tool in one of your hands to release some of your energy. This will help you get out some energy in a way that does not bother other people on your Team.

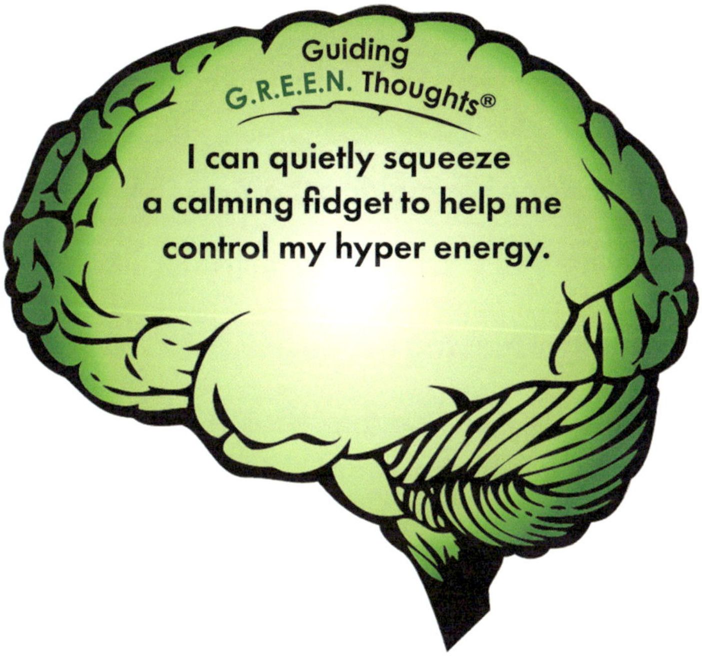

It takes practice to use a calming fidget tool quietly. It is easy to forget to get your body calmer and *not* to get acting *more* hyper! Quietly squeezing the fidget can calm your body to help you focus. But, you have to learn self-control so you don't bounce it, or throw it, or drop it and distract yourself and other people on your Team.

Practice using the fidget tool in the right way with your **powerful self-control**, so it can help you focus!

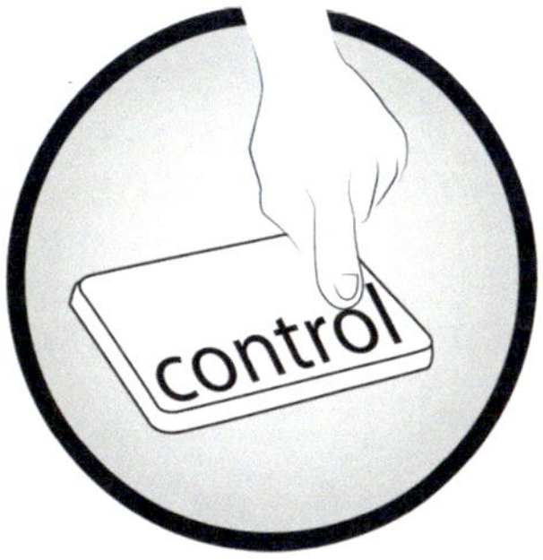

14.6 Things to Do before G.R.E.E.N. Scene #2

Reasons for acting out this scene

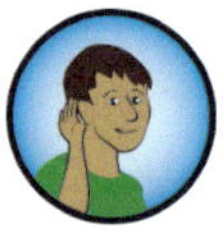

1. Acting in this scene is a way to practice accepting feedback from someone else when your actions are bothering others on the Team.

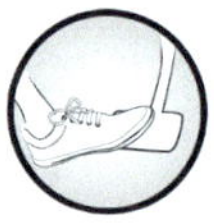

2. Acting in this scene is a way to practice stopping an action.

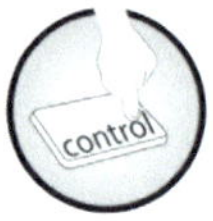

3. Acting in this scene is a way to practice controlling your own body.

Follow these Directions for Making the Best G.R.E.E.N. Scene:

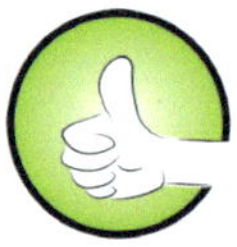

1. Read through this G.R.E.E.N. Scene with your Team.
2. Follow the steps for **Making the Best G.R.E.E.N. Scenes** (12.2).

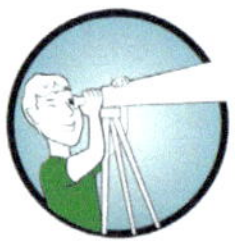

   A. Answer the questions on the **Wise Action Tool** called "**Surveying the Scene before Taking Action**" (12.2).

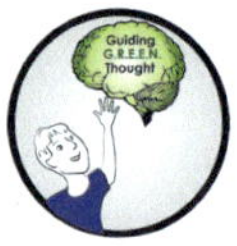

   B. Choose a useful **Guiding G.R.E.E.N. Thought** from the ones that are provided on the page following the script, or think of a **Guiding G.R.E.E.N. Thought** of your own that would be useful to make the best G.R.E.E.N. Scene.

   C. Choose observers to be Scene Reviewers to give honest reviews on the **G.R.E.E.N. Scene Review Form** (12.5).

3. Review the **Rules for Acting in G.R.E.E.N. Scenes** (12.3).
4. Check if your Acting Team is ready by reviewing the **G.R.E.E.N. Scene Warm-Ups** (12.5).
5. For this scene, the Scene Director gives Marco a pencil and asks him to start tapping only after the Director calls "Action!"

6. The Scene Director gets the clapboard and says, "Quiet on the set! G.R.E.E.N. Scene #2. Take one. Action!" (If the scene gets repeated with the same set of actors, the Director will say, "Quiet on the set. G.R.E.E.N. Scene #2. Take two. Action!")

G.R.E.E.N. *Scene #2: I Choose to Control My Own Body*

Marco starts tapping his pencil as if it is a fidget toy.

Narrator: It is not easy for Marco to stay calm in his classroom, and he has not liked getting feedback from others, but he is working hard to choose to be **helpful** for his Classroom Team.

Teacher: *Please stop tapping your pencil because you are disturbing your classmates.*

Narrator: Marco hears his teacher and **surveys the scene** in the classroom. He sees that his classmates are trying to concentrate on their seatwork.

Marco (stops tapping and says to his teacher): *I'm sorry. I'll be quiet, but I need to do something with my hyper energy right now. Can I hold a fidget quietly to help me control my body?*

Teacher: *Yes, you can get a fidget from the fidget box and quietly squeeze that. See if that will help you. If not, you can let me know, and we can figure out where you can quietly move around in the classroom. But first, do your best to use the fidget quietly.*

Marco quickly chooses a fidget, sits down, and starts using it quietly. He then raises his hand to say something to the teacher.

Marco's Teacher: *Yes, Marco?*

Marco: *This fidget should work for now. Thanks for your help. I will make sure to hold it quietly.*

Marco's Teacher: *Thanks for asking for what you need. I am glad you found a way to quietly deal with your hyper energy. I am sure the rest of the Classroom Team also* ***appreciates*** *it. Now we will continue with the lesson.*

14.7 Guiding G.R.E.E.N. Thought Choices for G.R.E.E.N. Scene #2

Help Marco **navigate G.R.E.E.N.** Scene #2 by circling one or more useful **Guiding G.R.E.E.N. Thoughts** from the ones below. Choose the most **helpful** one for guiding him to make the best choices. You may also write your own **Guiding G.R.E.E.N. Thought** if you can think of a different one that could be useful in this G.R.E.E.N. Scene.

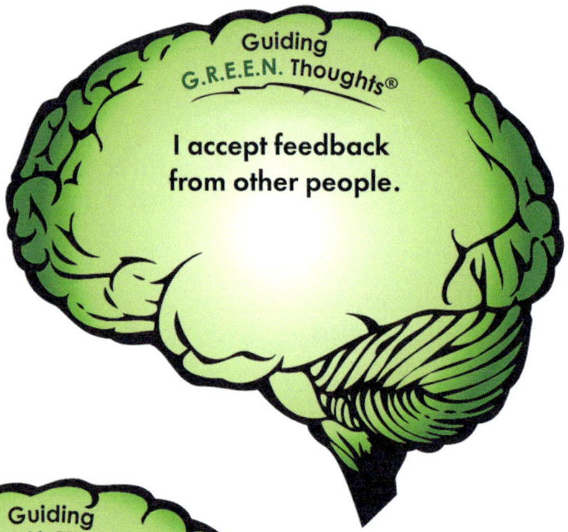

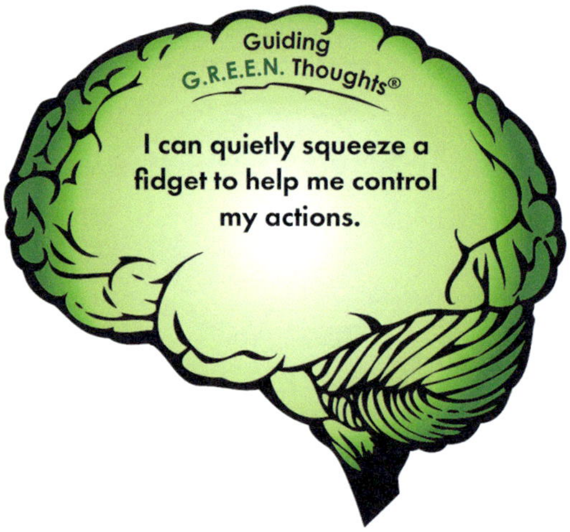

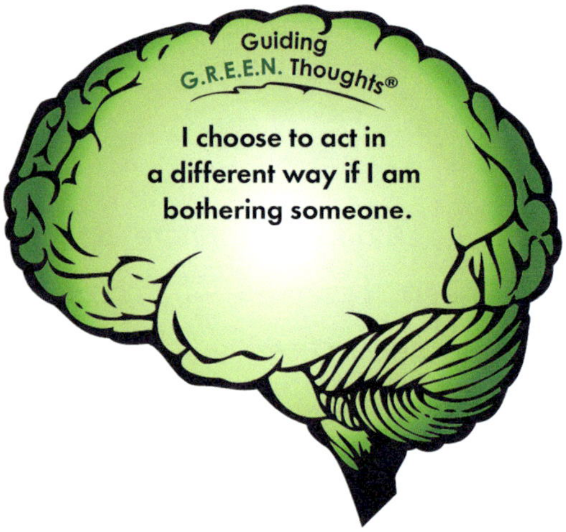

My own Guiding G.R.E.E.N. Thought for this scene:

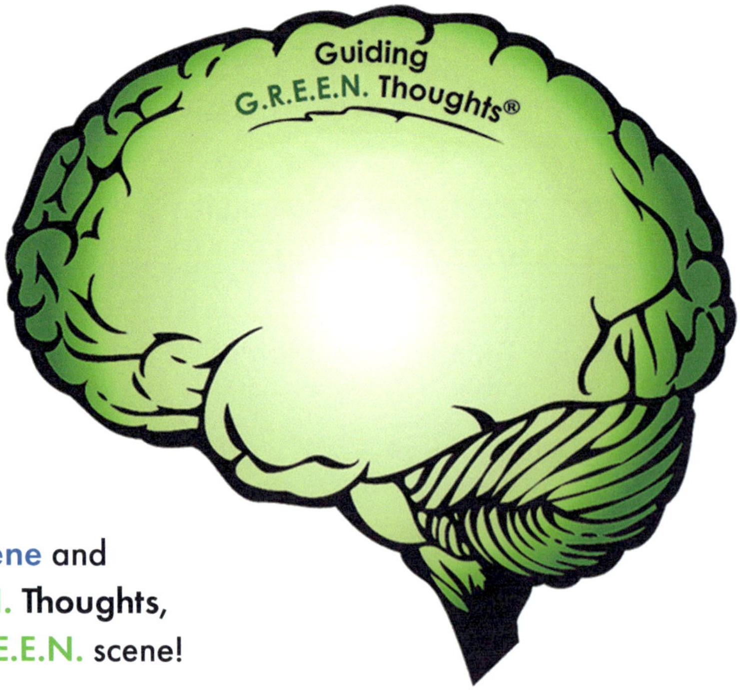

Once you have surveyed the scene and chosen useful **Guiding G.R.E.E.N. Thoughts**, you are ready to act out the G.R.E.E.N. scene!

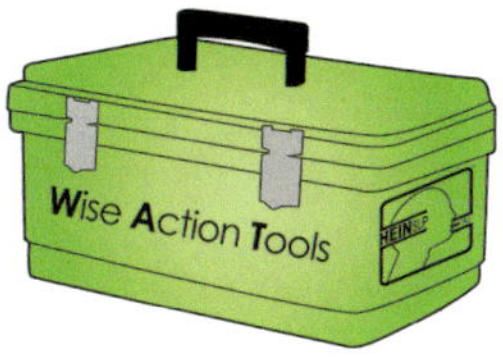

WRITING YOUR OWN GUIDING G.R.E.E.N. THOUGHT FOR SELF-CONTROL

You can write your own **Guiding G.R.E.E.N. Thought** that can help you control your body.

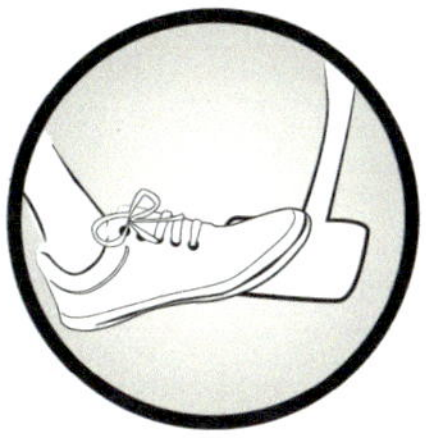

If you are making noises, saying words, or acting in ways that are bothering someone else, you can **step on the brakes** and use a **Wise Action Tool** instead. You can find a **Guiding G.R.E.E.N. Thought** and take your best action. Sometimes you will find that your best action is to stop an action!

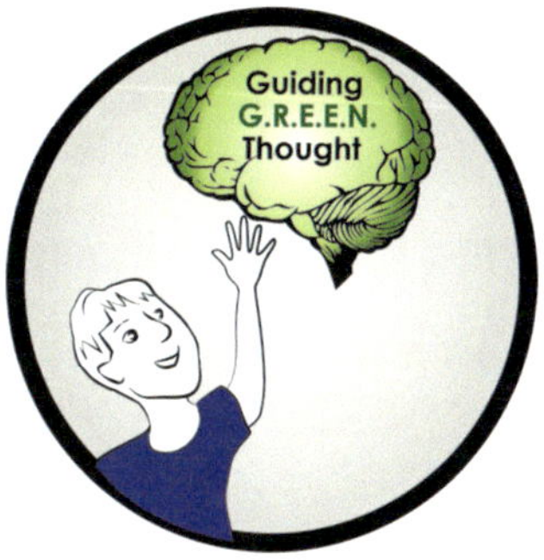

You can also write your own thought and tell why your **Guiding G.R.E.E.N. Thought** will help you and your Team. The most important step will be to actually do what the **Guiding G.R.E.E.N. Thought** says!

The more you practice controlling your body to stop action that is bothering other people, the more you realize that it really makes your scene better.

And the more you practice stopping any of your body's negative actions, the easier it will be to use **self-control** the next time you need it.

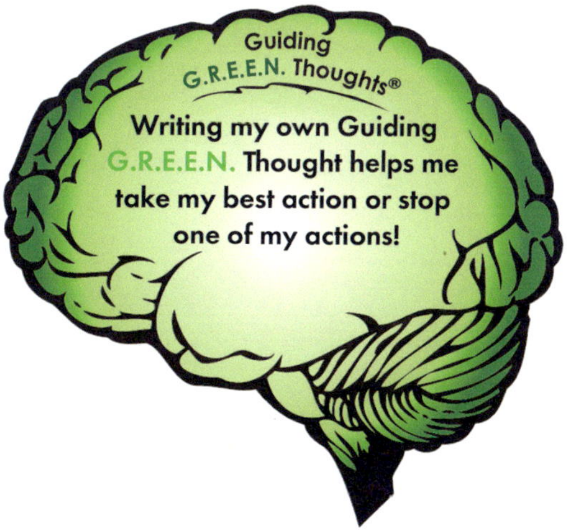

14.8 Things to Do before G.R.E.E.N. Scene #3:

After you act out G.R.E.E.N. Scene #2, you can write and act out your own G.R.E.E.N. Scene #3. Use a situation from your own life where someone asks you to stop doing something with your body because the action is bothering them or someone else. It should help you **navigate** successfully around the others on your Team if you can prove to yourself that you can accept feedback and be in control of your own body!

1. Think First to Help You Write Your Own Best G.R.E.E.N. Scene

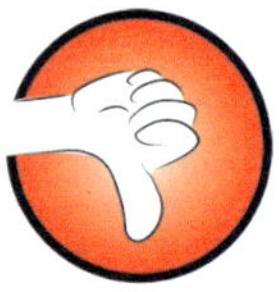

A. Think of something you do that might bother people on one of your Teams. In this scene you will show your **self-control** by stopping the action when asked to do so. On the first line of the script, write this bothersome action that you will be able to stop in this G.R.E.E.N. Scene.

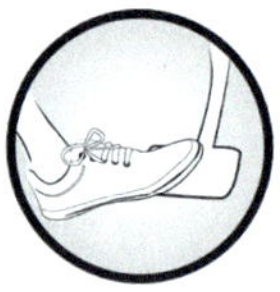

B. Think of a good reason why a Teammate would want you to stop your action. Write down this reason on the second blank line of G.R.E.E.N. Scene #3.

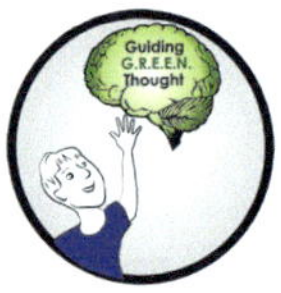

C. Write down a **Guiding G.R.E.E.N. Thought** (**G.G.T.**) that will help you have **self-control** so you can focus on doing whatever your team needs you to do. You can write on the page after the script or on one of the blank **G.G.T.** stickies. On your script, ask for a chance to write out a helpful **G.G.T.** or to read one that you know is helpful to you. Write this on the third blank line of script.

D. Think about what the other person might say after you show your **self-control**. Add this to the fourth blank line of the script. *Thank you for showing me that you can have self-control to stop . . .*

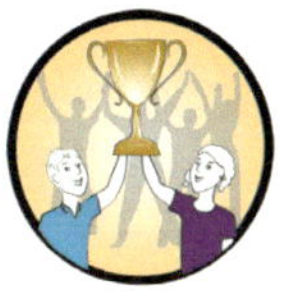

E. What could you say to show that you were **grateful** for your Teammate helping you use your **self-control** so you could then focus on helping the Team? Add this to the fifth line of the script.

2. **Make the Best** G.R.E.E.N. **Scene**: After you write out your script, and before you act it out, take all the steps for **Making the Best** G.R.E.E.N. **Scenes** found in Sections 12.2–12.5.

The Scene Director gets that clapboard and says, "Quiet on the set! **G.R.E.E.N.** Scene #3. Take one. Action!" (If the scene gets repeated with the same set of actors, the Scene Director will say, "Quiet on the set. **G.R.E.E.N.** Scene #3. Take two. Action!")

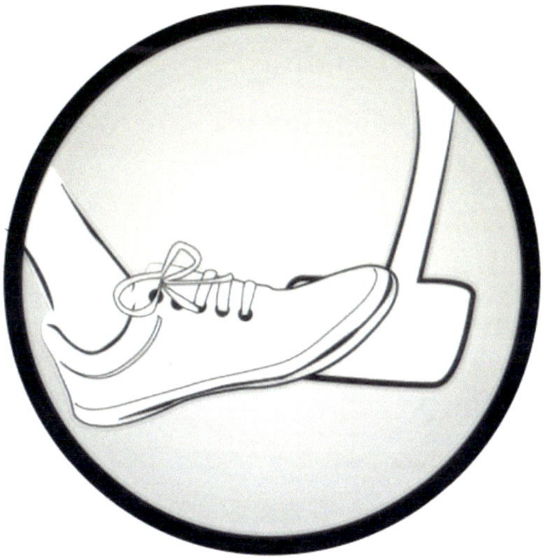

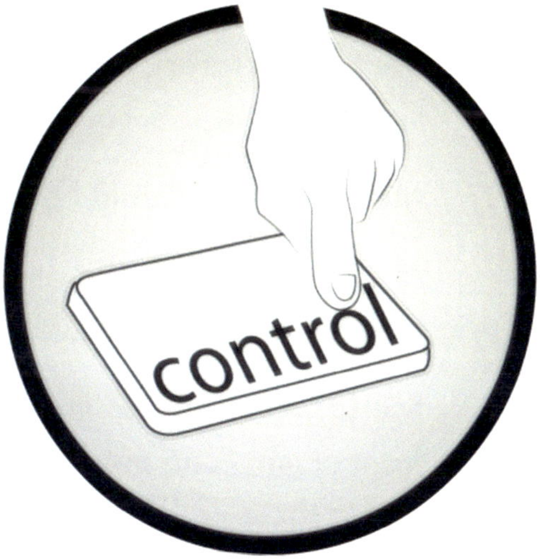

G.R.E.E.N. Scene #3: My Own Self-Control Scene

I can practice self-control in my own life scene! I can write it out and practice it now. I can then show self-control in my real-life scenes.

This is what I have been doing that is bothersome to others: ____________________

____

Me (as Narrator): This is me starting to do the bothersome action to someone else.

Me (as Actor): (briefly doing the bothersome action)

Other person on my Team: *Please stop!*

Me (as Actor): *Why should I stop?*

Other person on my Team (politely giving a good reason that makes sense):

____

____

Me (as Actor): *OK, I am sorry I bothered you. I will stop.*

Me (as Narrator): I ask for help in getting a **Guiding G.R.E.E.N. Thought** that will help me have **self-control** and successfully stop my bothersome action.

Me (as Actor): *Could I please* ____________________________________?

Me (as Narrator): The other person helps me get a **Guiding G.R.E.E.N. Thought** to help me so I can focus on doing whatever would be **helpful** to my Team and me.

Me (as Actor): *I can look at the* ***Guiding G.R.E.E.N. Thought*** *that I now have in front of me. I can now show the other person on my Team that I have the* ***self-control*** *to focus on doing whatever is asked of me. (I show* ***self-control*** *for a minute or longer depending upon the situation).*

Other person on my Team (after I show my **self-control**): *Thank you for showing me* ____________________________________

Me (as Actor): *Thank you for helping me* ____________________________

____

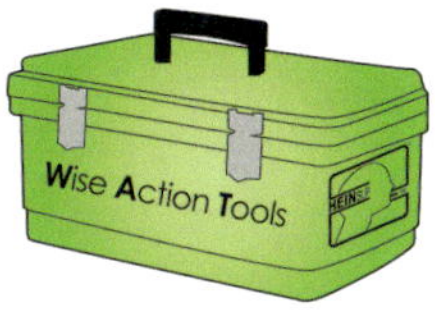

MY OWN GUIDING G.R.E.E.N. THOUGHT FOR HAVING SELF-CONTROL TO STOP HARMFUL ACTION

Here is my **Guiding G.R.E.E.N. Thought** to help me step on the brakes to stop any harmful actions I might be taking.

I have self-control to
stop taking harmful actions
so I can help my Team.

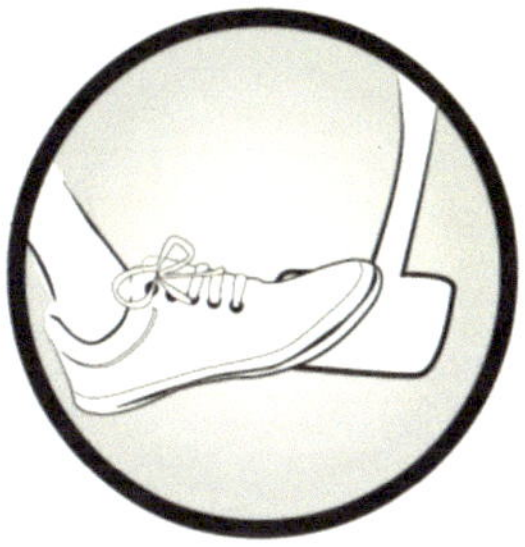

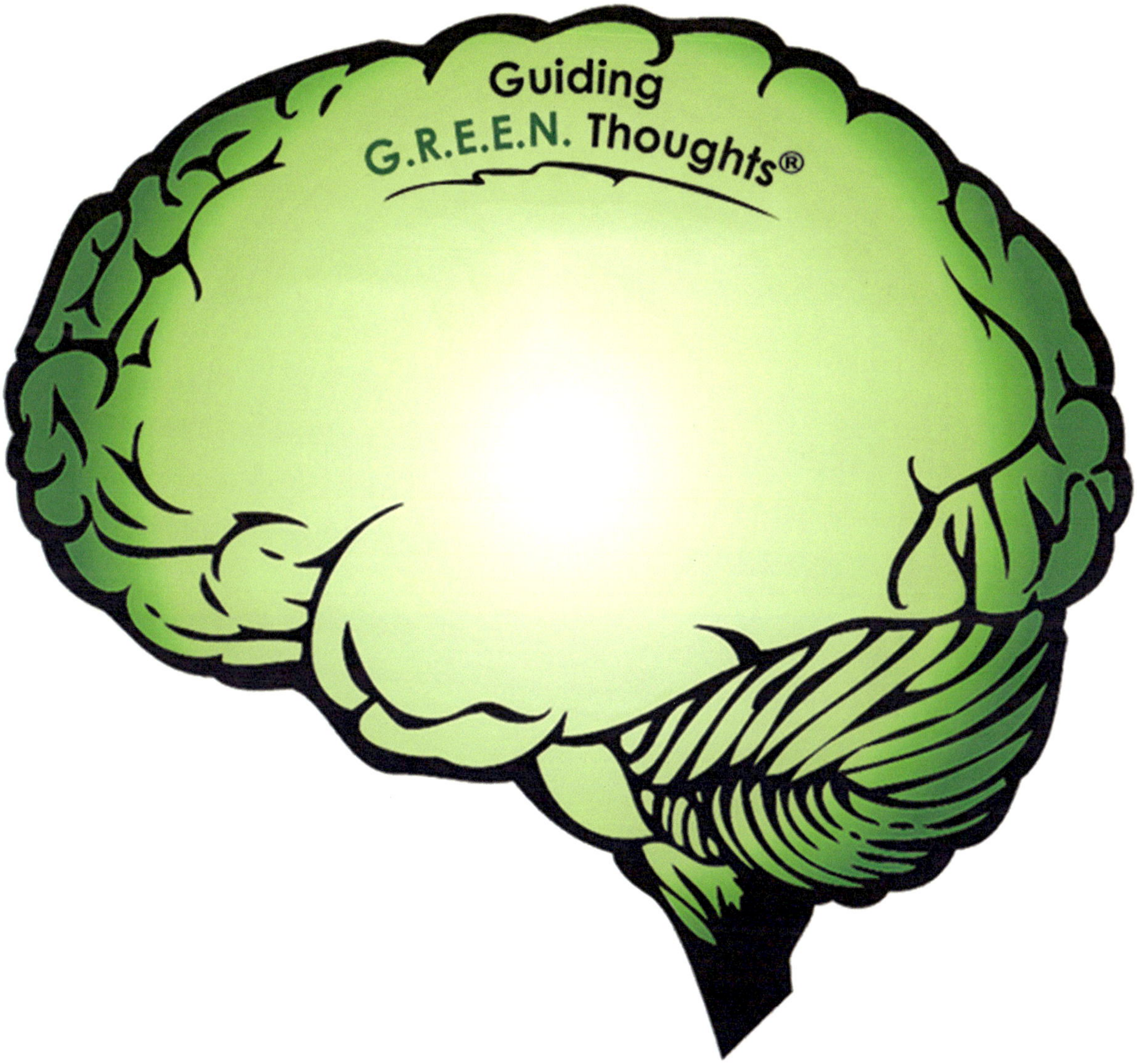

15 Making Powerful Transformations

15.1 Guiding G.R.E.E.N. Thought: I Make Transformations to Improve the Scene

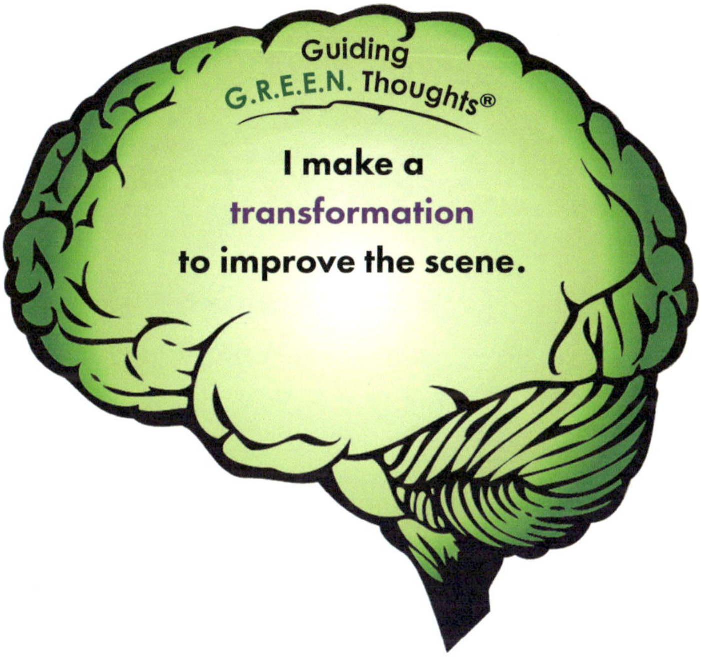

When you are **navigating** through the scenes of your life, things don't always go as you expect. Knowing what to do or say to the people on your Teams can be challenging.

Things can get complicated. To **navigate** through any complications, it is helpful to be **open-minded**.

You can be open to listening for any constructive feedback from people on your Team. You can ask yourself:

What is my Team telling me that I could do or say to make the scene ***better*** 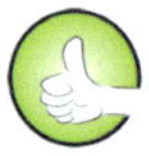 *right now?*

You can learn how acting differently could be **better**. If you can understand *why* you should **change** what you are doing, it can help you make the **change**.

Why Should I Change What I Am Doing?

You can use your own feedback from signals you get from your body. This also can help you **change** how you are doing something to make it **better**. The ability to be self-aware of your feelings, your needs and your actions is an important skill to learn.

I Want to Make Every Scene Better.

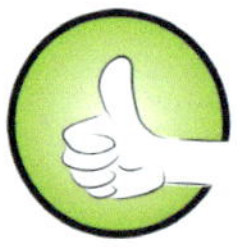

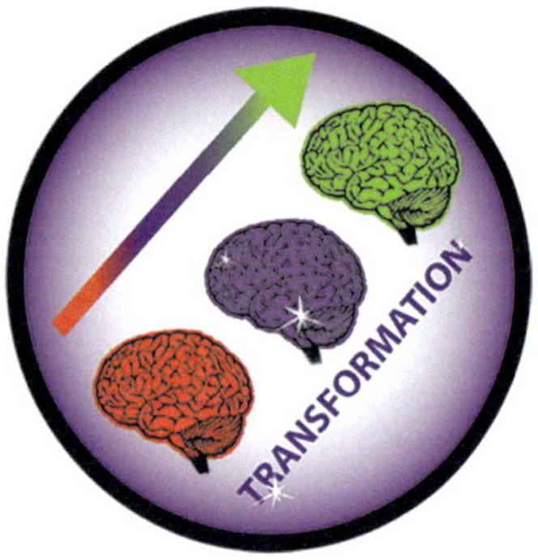

You can make a **transformation** on your own or with your Team in order to do whatever needs to be done to act **G.R.E.E.N.** in any life scene.

You can feel proud of yourself when you **transform** your feelings or actions and act more **G.R.E.E.N.** to meet your **goals**.

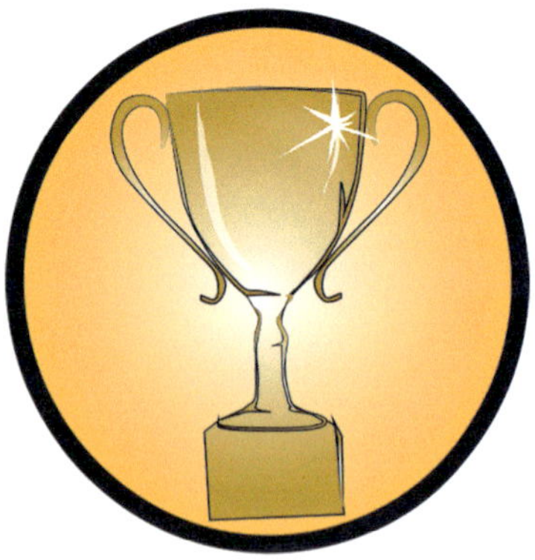
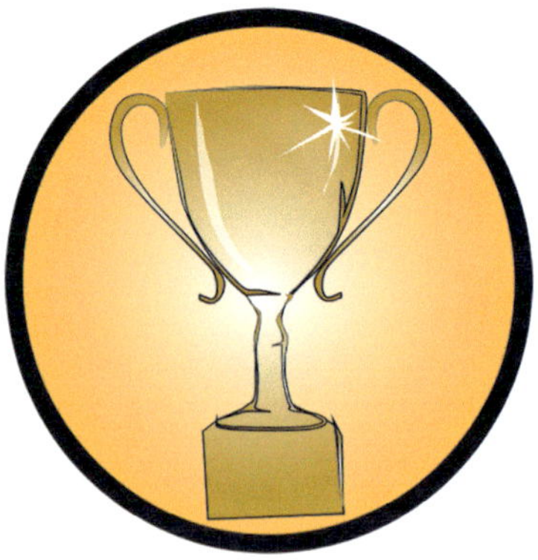
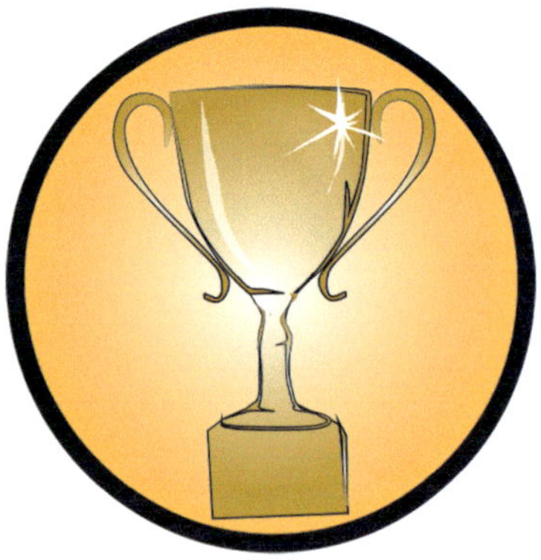

15.2 Transform Yourself to Reconnect with Others

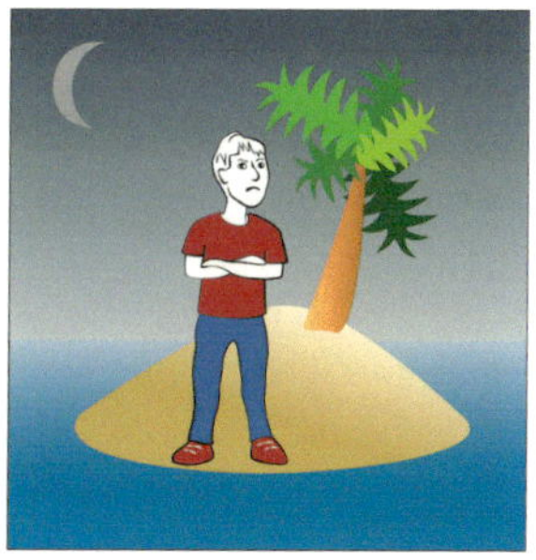

Sometimes you may think and act as if you are on your own separate island. It is as if you are in your own solitary **R.E.D.** bubble. You either don't notice the others on your Team or *don't* care about them. At these times, you might only be thinking about your own needs!

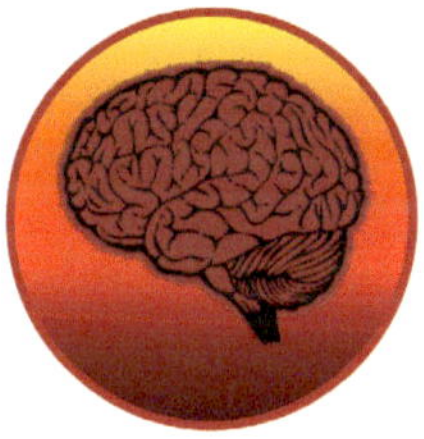

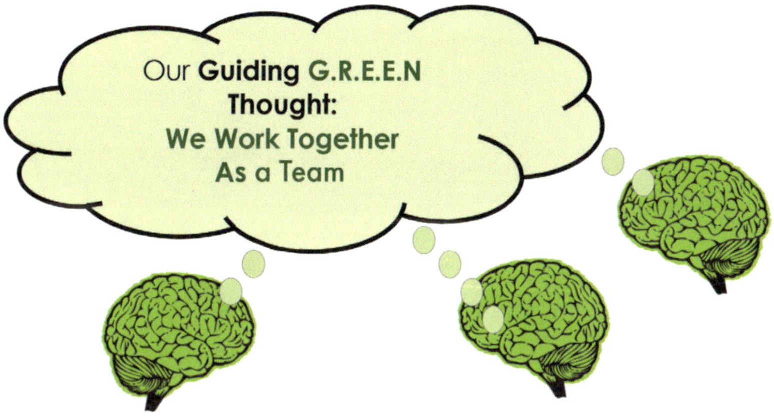

When you only think about yourself, you might be taking steps backward to disconnect from others. Instead, it is important to take steps **forward** and make civilized connections with people.

Take a step forward to connect →

I took steps to *disconnect* from other people.	-4	-3	-2	-1	0	+1	+2	+3	+4	I took steps to make positive civilized connections with other people.

← Take a step backward to disconnect

To get out of your own solitary **R.E.D.** bubble (or off your separate "island") and begin taking civilized steps toward your Teams, **pay attention to feedback** from others or from yourself to put on the brakes, take a break, and begin the **powerful** strategy of **transforming** yourself! You have the **power** to move yourself out of that solitary **R.E.D.** bubble.

When you understand that you *can* make a **transformation** and burst the solitary, **R.E.D.** bubble, you can return to thinking about others on your Teams.

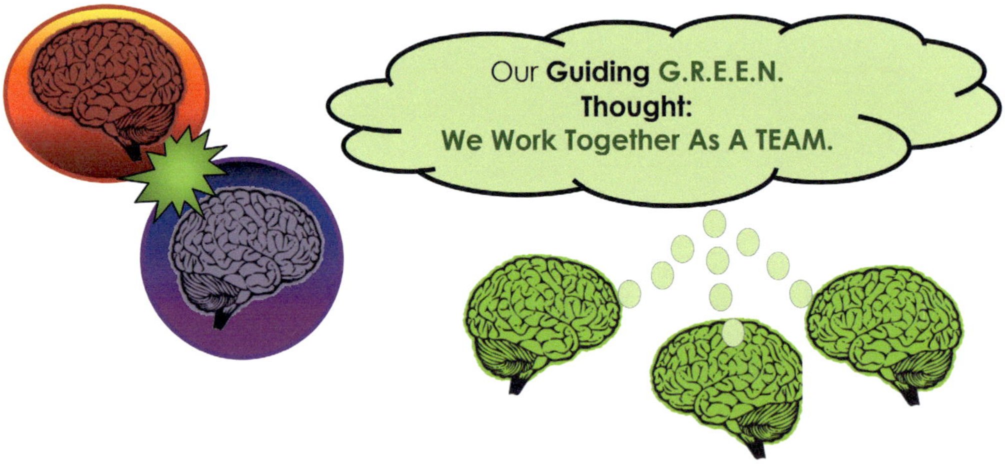

You can use **Guiding G.R.E.E.N. Thoughts** to remember **Common Team Goals**. You and your Team will work much **better** when everyone is working together.

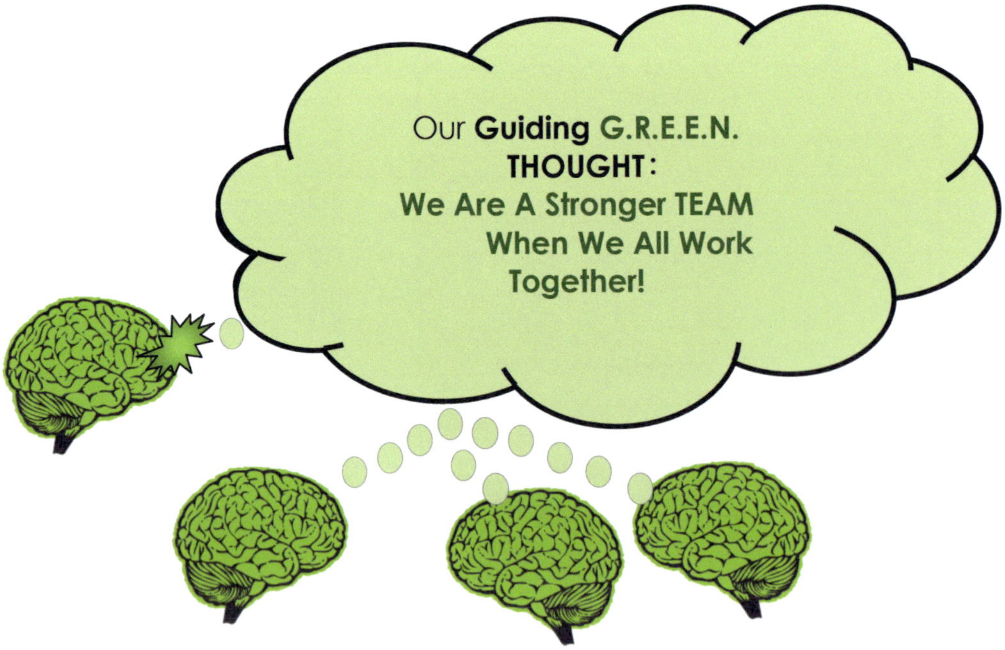

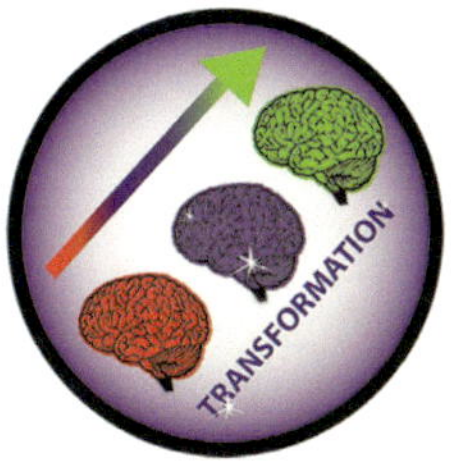

DON'T LISTEN TO THE MOON

A Song for Guiding **G.R.E.E.N. Thoughts**®

by Herb Hein

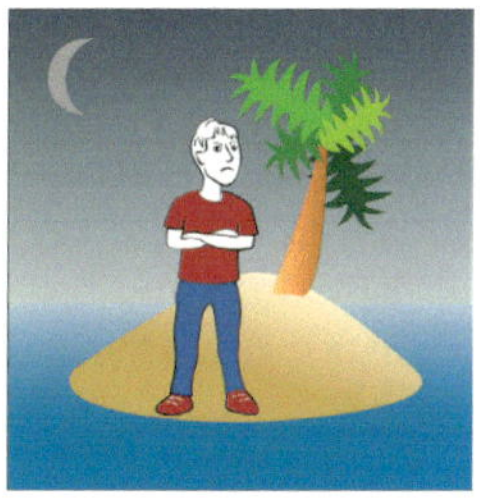

Liberate your island!
Become connected
and a part of what we can build together.
Free up your island!
Be connected
in a world where we live all right.

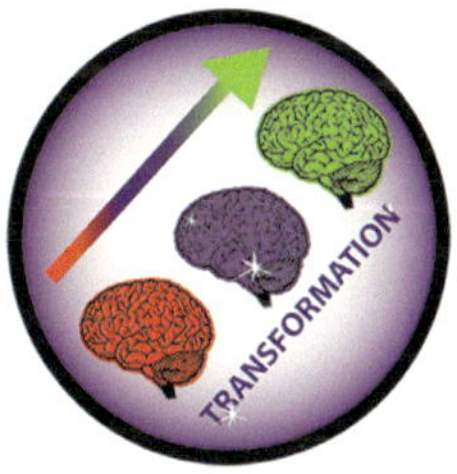

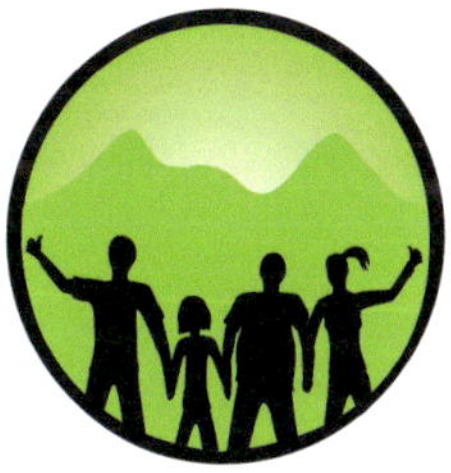

We can make it all right!
Don't listen to the moon at night.
Don't let it pull you to your darker side.
Take every chance to do what's right
to stand tall in the light

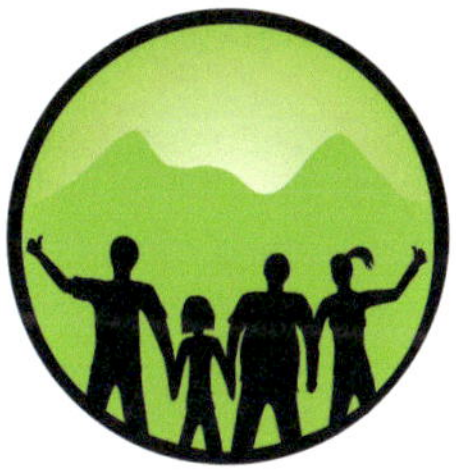

to stand tall in the light
in the light!
Reach out and give me your hand!
Don't make me work so hard!
Do your part, to reach the land
where we live all right.
We can make it all right!
Don't listen to the moon at night.
Don't let it pull you to your darker side.
Take every chance to do what's right
to stand tall in the light
to stand tall in the light...in the light...in the light!
Don't listen to the moon!

15.3 A Transformation Story: A Solitary R.E.D. Brain Is Transformed

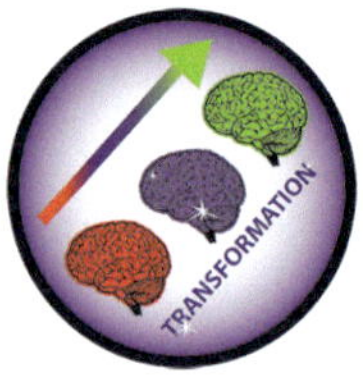

1. The solitary **R.E.D.** brain stands alone! It has a bubble around it keeping it alone and separated from everyone else.

2. The Team sends information to the solitary **R.E.D.** brain. The **R.E.D.** brain may resist the information, but the Team continues to send information to the solitary **R.E.D.** brain.

Attention! Attention! Feedback! Feedback!
We have a complication! We are *not* working together well!

3. The solitary **R.E.D.** brain begins to hear the feedback and *chooses* to make a **change** so it is not by itself anymore.

4. It decides it wants to be part of the Team, so it begins its **transformation!**

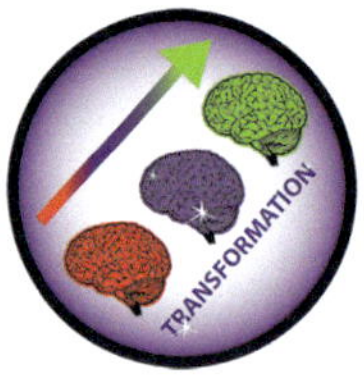

The transforming brain Flips The Switch to turn on self-regulation.

The **R.E.D.** bubble bursts, allowing **Guiding G.R.E.E.N. Thoughts** to enter.

5. The **transforming** brain becomes calm and focused and takes steps to start acting **G.R.E.E.N.** with the rest of the Team**.**

6. No one is acting in a solitary **R.E.D.** way anymore.

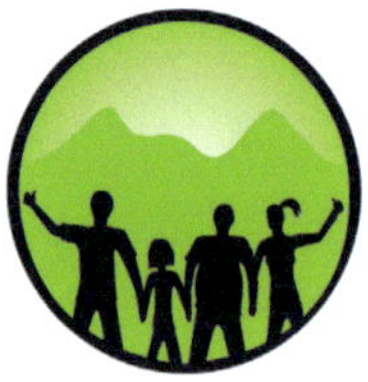

Everyone Is acting as if they are part of the Team.

The Team can now work **better** together to meet the **Common Team Goals**.

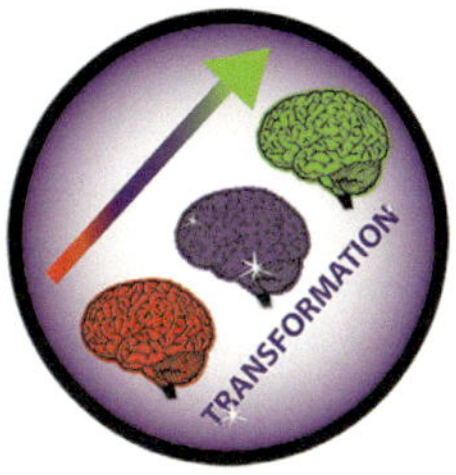

TRANSFORMATION SONG

A Song for Guiding G.R.E.E.N. Thoughts®

by Herb Hein

Receiving Information... 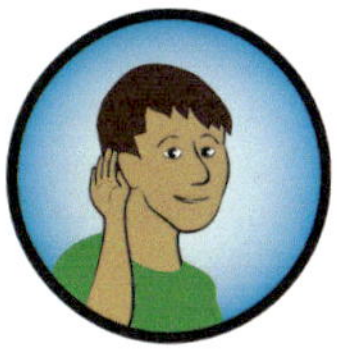

We have a complication! 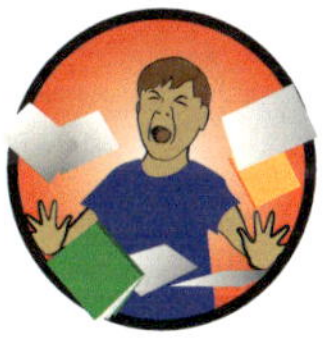

We need a transformation! 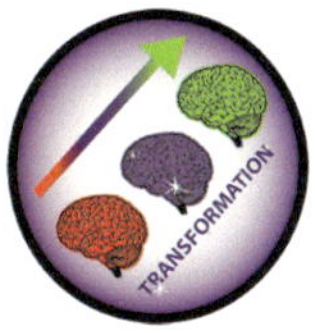

Turn on self-regulation 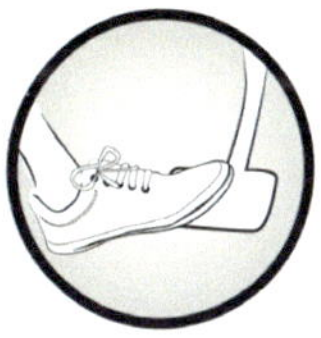 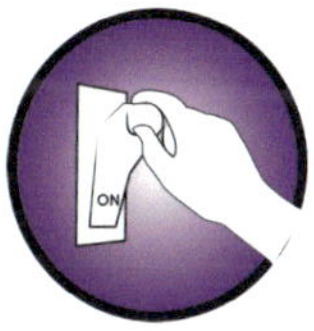

and self-calming installation 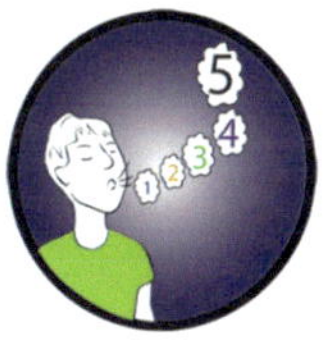

for G.R.E.E.N. Thought Liberation! 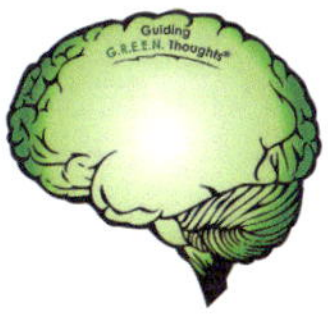

15.4 When to Use the Thought Transformation Scene Changer

You will find the **Thought Transformation Scene Changer** in the next section. This useful tool will help you make any scene **better** with your **powerful transforming** thoughts!

1. Use the **Thought Transformation Scene Changer** to show **transformations** that have already happened.

   Give yourself credit for having already made **positive changes** in your thinking and actions. Fill out this **Thought Transformation Scene Changer** to show the **changes** you made. This form will help you keep using your **powerful** brain to take steps **forward** toward **positive transformation**.

2. Use the **Thought Transformation Scene Changer** to show **transformations** you are making now. Or use it for **transformations** you are planning to make soon.

   Fill out the **Thought Transformation Scene Changer** for any new **transformations** you want to make in your life.

   Keep **transforming**!

   Keep making yourself **better**!

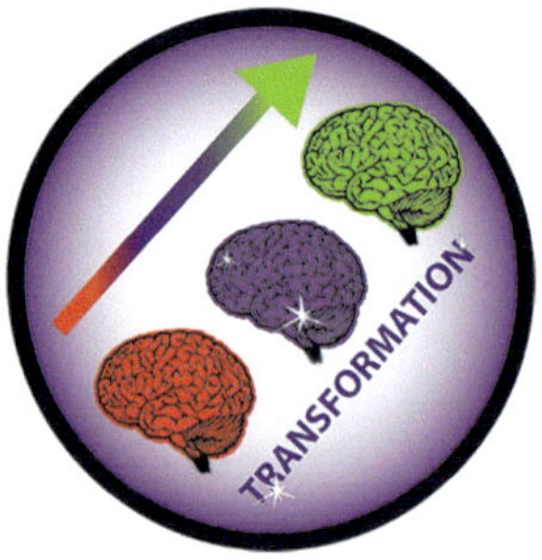

   Keep thinking of **Guiding G.R.E.E.N. Thoughts** that can help you make the **change**?

15.5 How to Use the Thought Transformation Scene Changer

Decide what kind of **change** you want to make in how you think and act in your life. This will be your **transformation**!

1. The scene at first—follow the directions for drawing and writing about the scene as it is *before* G.R.E.E.N. **Thought** Transformation.

2. Reach up to your brain for **Guiding** G.R.E.E.N. **Thoughts** to help you improve the scene. Write your **Guiding** G.R.E.E.N. **Thoughts** in the brains in the middle of the Transformation Scene Changer. Start at the bottom and work your way up. You will find many **Guiding** G.R.E.E.N. **Thoughts** in this program, or you may choose one or more of your own.

   To make a **transformation**, you need to remember these **Guiding** G.R.E.E.N. **Thoughts** during your day so that you can use them during challenging situations. The Thought Transformation **Scene** Changer can be looked at frequently during the day to help you remember the **changes** you are trying to make and what to think and do to make those **changes** occur.

3. Follow the directions to write and draw what happens *after* the **transformation**. Make sure to include how other people around you are acting and feeling because of your **transformation**.

4. Is the new scene **better**?

   Decide if the new scene is **better** and answer why you think so.

5. Find words to describe your transformation to make it even more **powerful** and to help you remember it!

My **transformation** is about changing from ________________________________

"old," negative thoughts/actions

to ____.

"new," positive thoughts/actions

Thought Transformation Scene Changer

Name ______________________ Date ______________

1. The Scene at first, *before* G.R.E.E.N. Thought Transformation.

a. Write or draw how I am acting with other people in this scene *before* the G.R.E.E.N. Thought Transformation.

b. What feedback am I getting from others about my actions? ____________________

____

c. How are all the people in this scene feeling, including me? ____________________

____

2. Get the Power!

Change the scene!

Be **open-minded** to make a **Transformation**.

Think of Guiding **G.R.E.E.N.** Thoughts to make it happen!

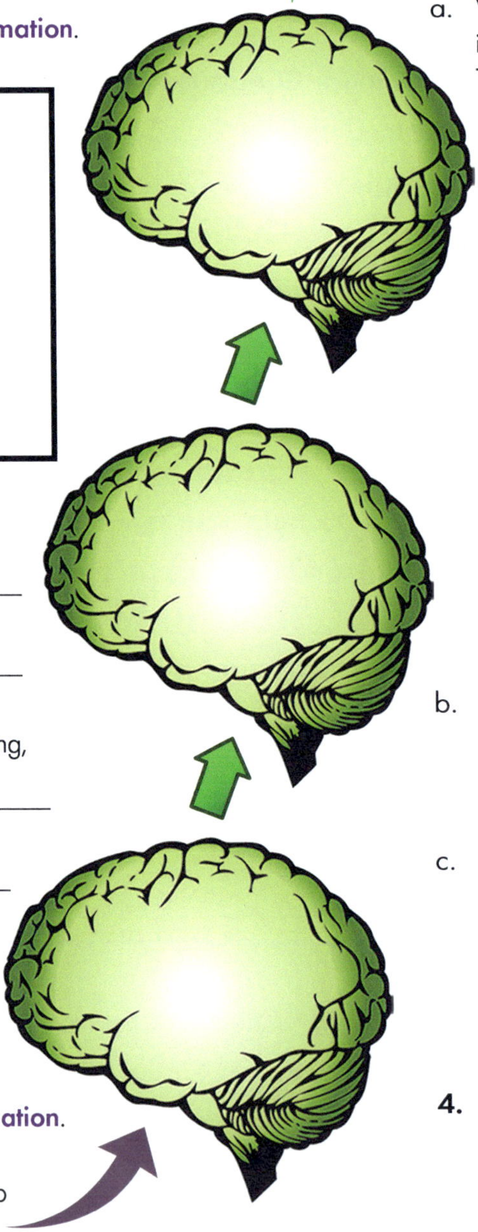

3. The new scene *after* G.R.E.E.N. Thought Transformation.

a. Write or draw what is happening in this scene *after* **G.R.E.E.N.** Thought **Transformation**.

b. What feedback am I getting from others about my actions? ____________________

____

c. How are all the people in this scene feeling now, including me?

____

____

4. Is this new scene better?

yes no

Why? ____________________

____

5. This page shows a powerful Transformation from ______________ to ______________.

15.6 Survey the Scene: What Changes Are Needed for G.R.E.E.N. Scene #4?

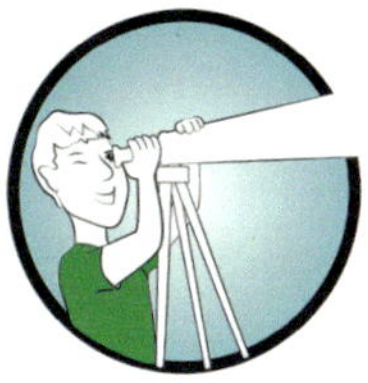

1. **Survey the scene** to locate any **R.E.D.** actions or words. With a red pencil, underline any words or action that you think are **R.E.D.** and could be **changed** to **G.R.E.E.N.**

Remember that **R.E.D.** stands for:

R = Rude

E = Egocentric

D = Disruptive

2. **Change the scene** to make it **G.R.E.E.N.** so it can be acted out.

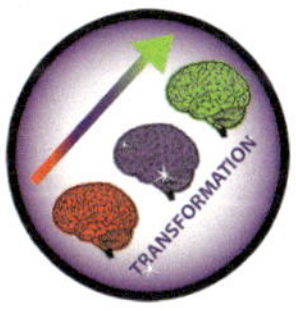

3. Take action in **G.R.E.E.N.** Scene #4

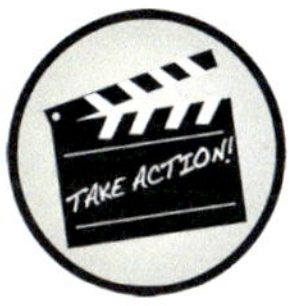

Travis likes to do math only in his head. He does not like to write out his math problems. This is OK when he is doing easy math, but when math got more complicated, he starts to skip steps and make mistakes. His teacher, Mrs. Patience, wants him to follow a step-by-step plan:

1. Take your time.
2. Write out the problem.
3. Do the problem and show how you are doing each step.
4. Check your work.

Travis gets frustrated and says, "I can't figure this out!"

Mrs. Patience comes over to him and says, "Let me help you. Let's write out the math problem instead of you only doing it in your head. That way we can see the details in the problem and track them."

Travis resists the new idea and says, "I never do it that way. I only do it in my head!"

His teacher takes a deep breath to stay patient and calm and says, "Why don't you try it out?"

Travis continues to resist his teacher's suggestion and says, "No! It takes too long to write it out. That's a terrible idea!"

Mrs. Patience takes a deep breath and then says, "Well, I see you are getting frustrated that you cannot figure out the problem. From my point of view, it is taking you a longer time to do it in your head. The rest of the class is ready to go to P.E., and you are not finished with your math."

15.7 Change the Scene to Make It G.R.E.E.N.: Help Travis Make a Transformation

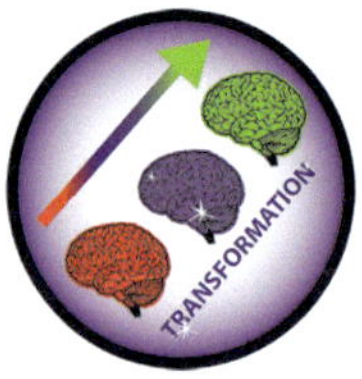

1. What should be the **Common Team Goal** 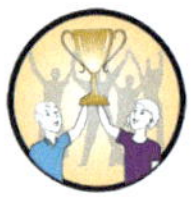 in this scene? ______

   ____

2. What will be a negative consequence if Travis continues to act **R.E.D.** 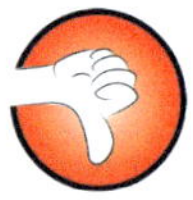 in this scene?

   ____

3. What will the **positive** 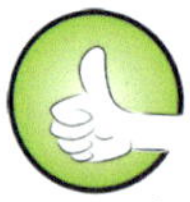 consequence be if Travis **rewinds** the scene, makes a **transformation**, and takes his best actions for himself and his Classroom Team? ____________________________

   ____

15.8 Help Travis Choose Guiding G.R.E.E.N. Thoughts for His Transformation

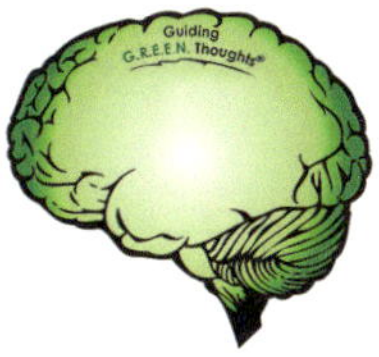

Choose **Guiding G.R.E.E.N. Thoughts** that might help Travis make a **transformation** and **change the scene** to **G.R.E.E.N.** for himself and the Classroom Team.

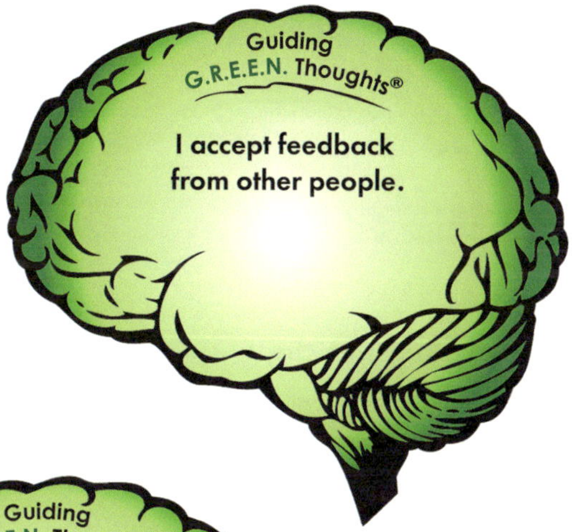

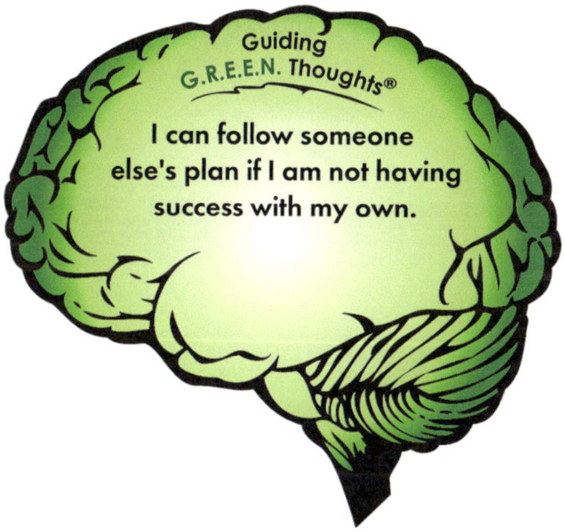

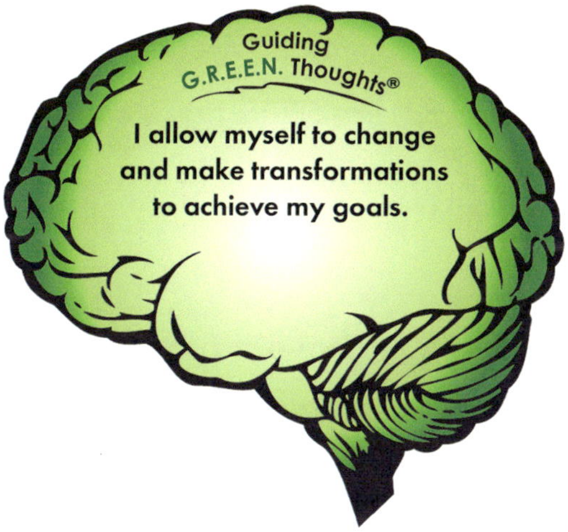

My own **Guiding G.R.E.E.N. Thought** for this scene:

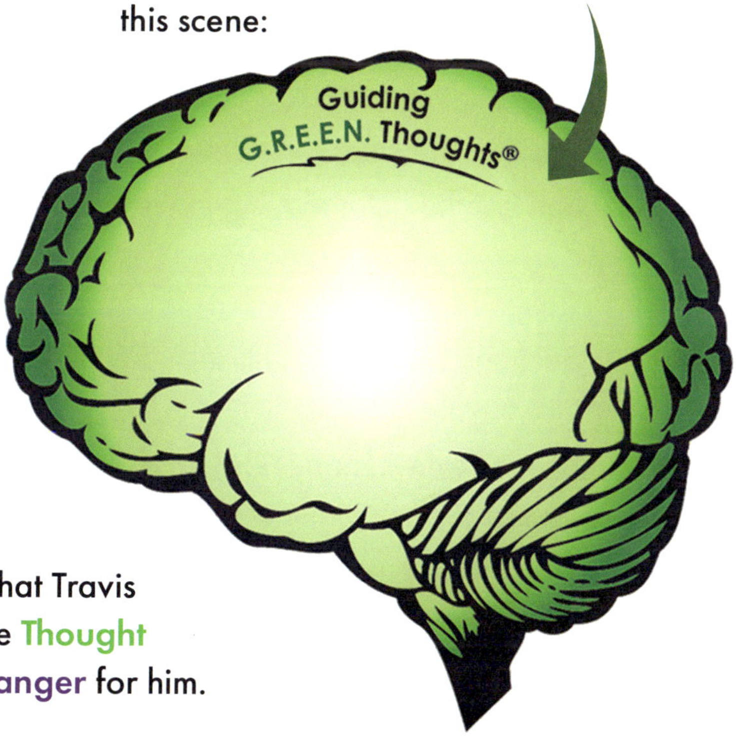

Show the **transformation** that Travis could make by filling out the **Thought Transformation Scene Changer** for him.

15.9 G.R.E.E.N. Scene #4: I Can Follow Your Plan

Reasons for Acting in This Scene

1. Acting in this scene is a way to practice making a **transformation**.

2. Acting in this scene helps you choose to listen to someone else's advice so you can be more successful and achieve your **goals**.

Things to Do before G.R.E.E.N. Scene #4

1. The Scene Director has the actor playing the role of Travis fill out the **Transformation** Scene **Change**r before acting in the scene to help Travis see the **powerful transformation** he has made to make the scene **G.R.E.E.N.**

2. The Director gives the actor playing the role of Travis the **Guiding G.R.E.E.N. Thoughts** that have already been chosen and written out to help Travis think about them when he needs them.

3. The Director also gives Travis a two- or three-step math word problem to do and has the actor playing the role of the teacher sit next to Travis.

4. Take all the necessary steps for **Making the Best G.R.E.E.N. Scenes** found in Sections 12.2–12.5. This includes Surveying the **G.R.E.E.N.** Scene (12.2), reviewing the Rules for Acting in **G.R.E.E.N.** Scenes (12.3), using the **G.R.E.E.N.** Scene Review Form (12.4), and **G.R.E.E.N.** Scene Warm-Ups (12.5).

5. The Director gets the clapboard and says, "Quiet on the set! **G.R.E.E.N.** Scene #4, Take 1! Action!" (If the scene gets repeated with the same set of actors, the Director will say, "Quiet on the set! **G.R.E.E.N.** Scene #4, Take 2! Action!")

G.R.E.E.N. *Scene #4: I Can Follow Your Plan* (We Help Travis Rewind the Scene to Make It G.R.E.E.N.!)

Narrator: *Travis only likes to do math in his head. He does not like to write out his math problems. This is OK when he is doing easy math, but when math got more complicated, he starts to skip steps and make mistakes. His teacher, Mr. (or Mrs.) Patience, tries to get him to follow a step-by-step plan:*

1. Take your time.
2. Write out the problem.
3. Do the problem and show how you are doing each step.
4. Check your work.

Travis (speaking in a slightly frustrated tone of voice): *I can't figure this out!*

Teacher: *Let me help you. Let's write out the math problem instead of only doing it in your head. That way we can see the details in the problem and track them.*

Travis: *I never do it that way. I only do it in my head!*

Teacher: *Why don't you try it out? Try the step-by-step plan once to see if it works. I'll go through it with you.*

Narrator: Travis tells himself the **Guiding G.R.E.E.N. Thoughts** he needs in order to make a **transformation** so he can work **better** with his Team.

Travis: *OK, I'll give it a try.*

Teacher: *Thanks, Travis, for being so **open-minded.***

Travis (writes out the steps to the math problem and gets an answer): *I think writing it out helped me track what I was doing.*

Teacher: *I think you are right, Travis. Now check your work to see whether you made any mistakes.*

Travis (checks his work): *I don't think I made any mistakes.*

Teacher: *Yes, you got the right answer! Maybe you can write out the step-by-step plan next time, too, so you won't get as frustrated.*

Travis: *I think that's a good idea when the problem has many steps that need to be tracked.*

15.10 A Word Problem for Travis to Use in G.R.E.E.N. Scene #4

A Multi-step Math Word Problem for Travis:

Mr. Rossini is busy in his bakery. His next job this morning is to make two dozen of his famous raisin cookies for the principal of the Twin Oaks Middle School. Then he will bake six dozen more for today's window display. He needs to put six raisins in each cookie. How many raisins does he need?

Step One: Circle the key words in the problem.

Step Two: Add up how many dozen.

→ Write the answer here ____________________

Step Three: Multiply by 12.

→ Write the answer here ____________________

Step Four: Multiply by 6.

→ Write the answer here ____________________

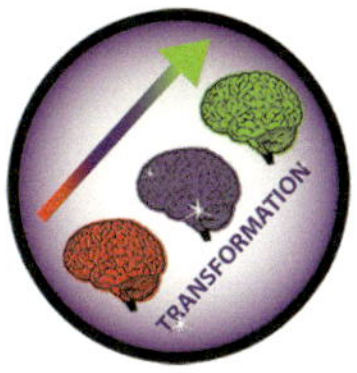

16 T.O.P. Ideas Help You Make Transformations

Think First!

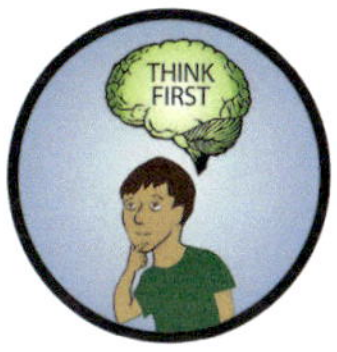

Be Open-Minded!

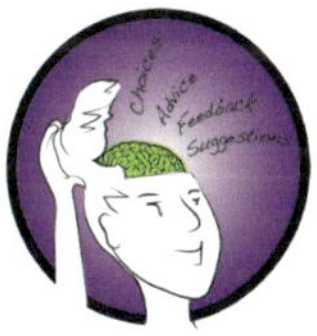

Be Positive!

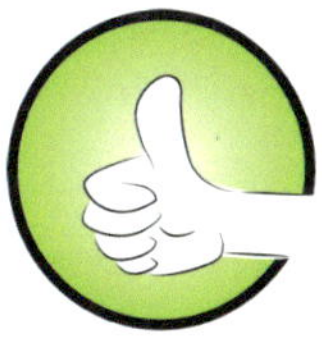

16.1 T.O.P. Ideas: Think First, Be Open-Minded, and Be Positive

The next **G.R.E.E.N.** Scenes will help you focus on three ideas that can be at the TOP of your head when you are with your Teams. They help you make **transformations** that make things **better** for yourself and your Teams.

Think First!

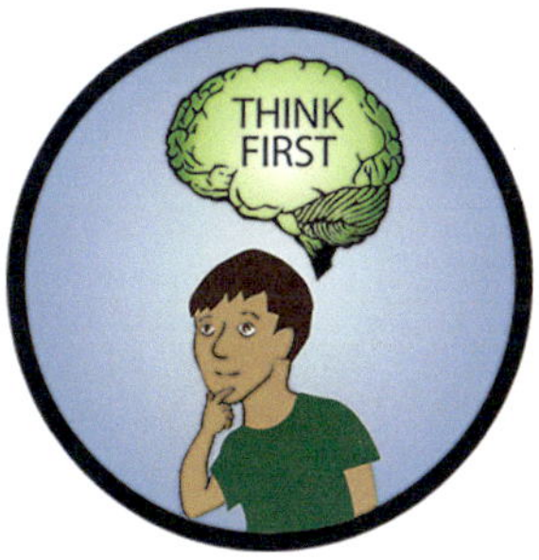

You have already learned how important it is to Think First so you can act **positively**. When you Think First, you understand how your actions affect others. Because you Think First about the consequences of your actions, you can make the best choices.

Be Open-Minded!

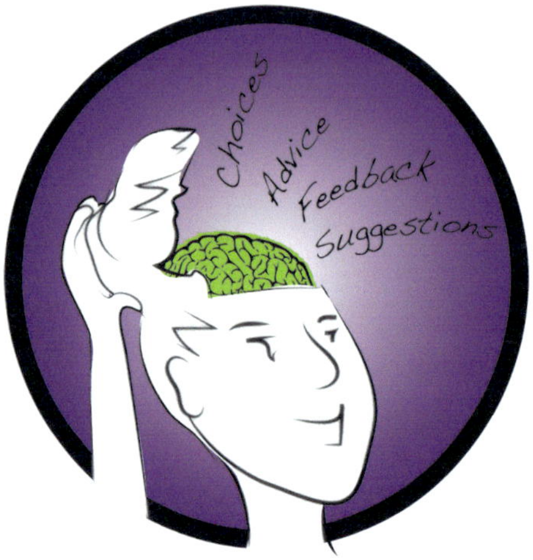

When you are **open-minded**, you are open to new ideas that might be different or better than your first idea. Being **open-minded** helps you to avoid getting stuck with only one idea that might not be the best. It lets you be open to ideas from people on your Team.

It helps you **change** how you are thinking about something if you get feedback that another idea might be **better** for the Team.

Be Positive!

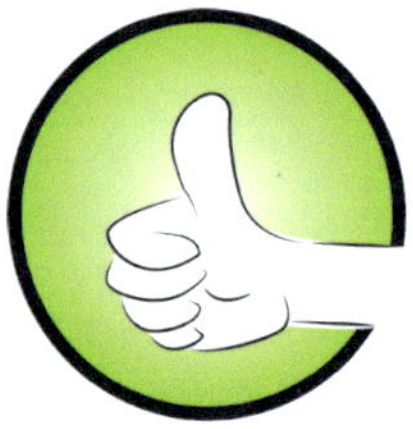

Being **positive** means you can think about making things **better** for yourself *and* the people and things around you. Being **positive** helps you strive to do your best to work with others.

16.2 G.R.E.E.N. Scene #5: Thirsty but Still Thinking First (Remember Team Rules *before* You Act)

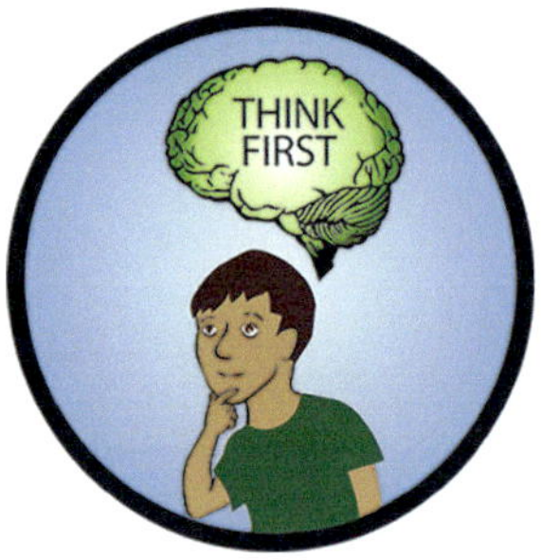

Reasons for Acting in this Scene:

See if you are ready to Think First to act **G.R.E.E.N.**! This **G.R.E.E.N.** Scene will give you a chance to Think First so you can follow some basic rules.

Sometimes people do not want to think about rules. Sometimes people do not want to follow rules because they think the rules might stop them from doing what they want to do. But when we are on a Team, we help out when we Think First to remember the Team rules and follow them. This lets the Team reach its **Common Team Goals** together. Since you and your Teammates have **powerful** human brains, you can Think First before you take action. This will help you reach your **Personal Goals** while helping the Team reach its **Common Team Goals**.

Things to do before G.R.E.E.N. Scene #5:

Take all the necessary steps for **Making the Best G.R.E.E.N. Scenes** found in sections 12.2–12-5. This includes **Surveying the G.R.E.E.N. Scene** (12.2), choosing the best **Guiding G.R.E.E.N. Thought** for this scene (16.4), reviewing the **Rules for Acting in G.R.E.E.N. Scenes** (12.3), using the **G.R.E.E.N. Scene Review Form** (12.4), and engaging in the **G.R.E.E.N. Scene Warm-Ups** (12.5).

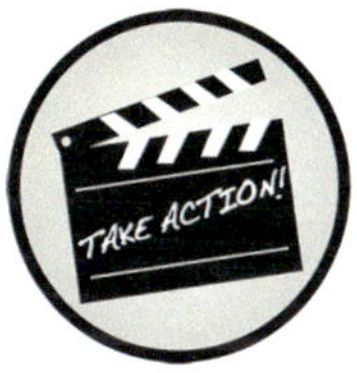

The Director gets the clapboard and says, "Quiet on the set. G.R.E.E.N. Scene #5. Take one! Action!" If the scene gets repeated with the same set of actors, the Director will say, "Quiet on the set. G.R.E.E.N. Scene #5. Take two! Action!"

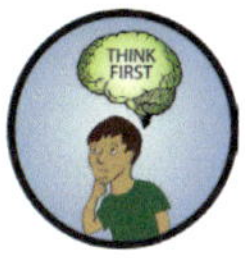

16.3 G.R.E.E.N. Scene #5: Thirsty but Still Thinking First!

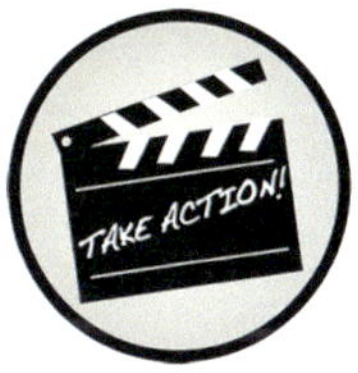

Narrator: You are thirsty during class, so you want to go to the water fountain. You could get up and get a drink, but you Think First. You remember the rule in this class. You must raise your hand and ask the teacher for permission before you get up.

Thirsty student: (While sitting in your seat, you raise your hand.)

Teacher (calling on you after seeing your hand raised): *Yes? What do you need?*

Thirsty student: *Could I please get a drink of water?*

Teacher: *Yes, certainly.*

Thirsty student: *Thank you.*

Teacher: *Thank you for raising your hand and asking first.*

Thirsty student: *You're welcome.*

16.4 Choosing Guiding G.R.E.E.N. Thoughts for G.R.E.E.N. Scene #5

Here are some **Guiding G.R.E.E.N. Thoughts** to help our characters Think First. Help the Thirsty Student in G.R.E.E.N. Scene #5 by circling a **helpful Guiding G.R.E.E.N. Thought** from the choices below. You also may write your own **Guiding G.R.E.E.N. Thought** if you can think of a different one that could be useful in this G.R.E.E.N. Scene.

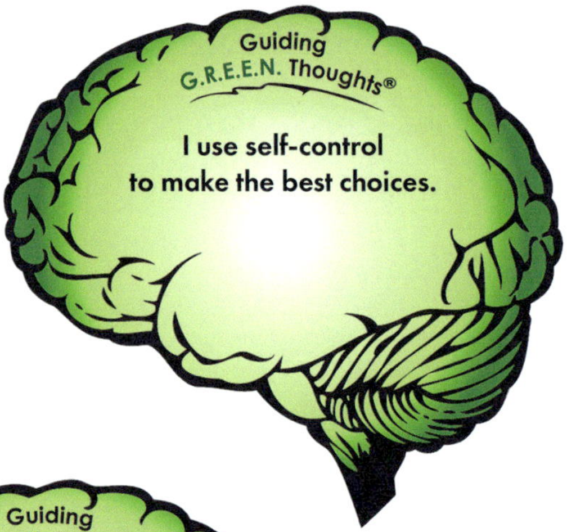

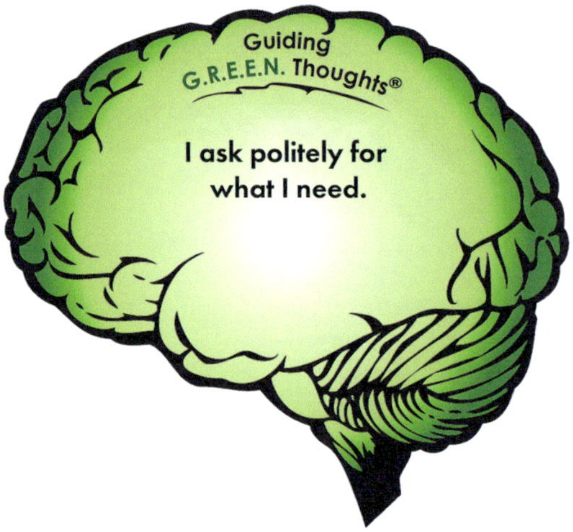

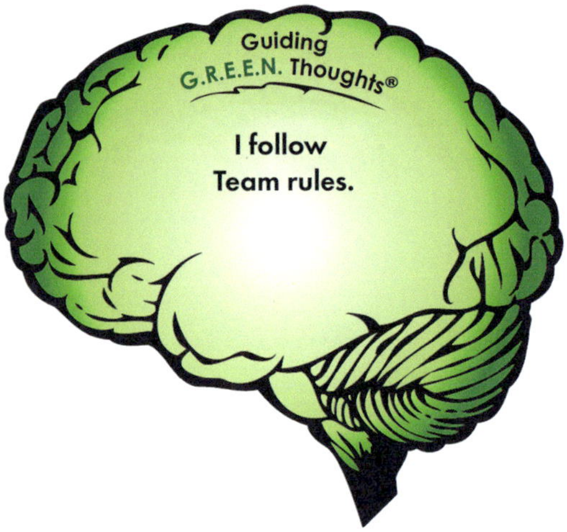

My own Guiding G.R.E.E.N. Thought for this scene:

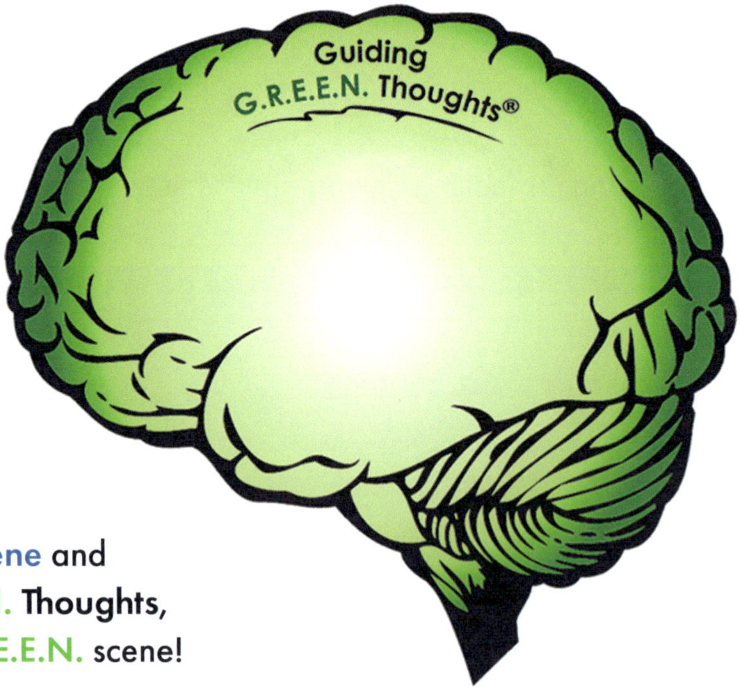

Once you have surveyed the scene and chosen useful **Guiding G.R.E.E.N. Thoughts**, you are ready to act out the G.R.E.E.N. scene!

16.5 Be Open-Minded to New Ideas

When you have an **open mind**, you are ready to think about new and different choices. With an **open mind**, you can listen to ideas that other people share with you. You might even **change** your own thoughts and actions when you hear about these other ideas.

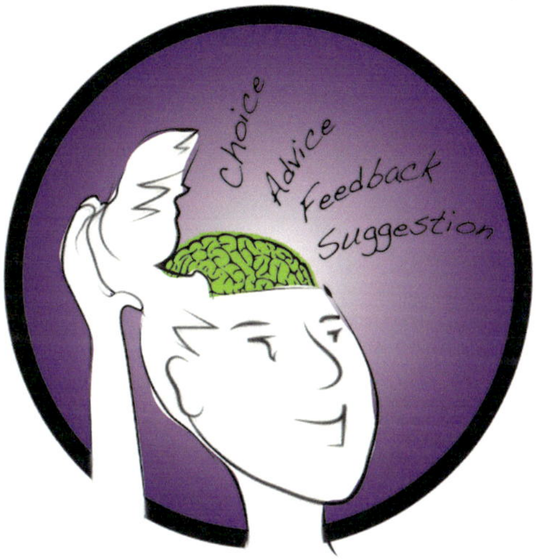

With an **open mind**, you listen to advice and constructive feedback from people on your Teams. This might help you improve your thoughts and your actions.

Are you ready to have an **open mind** to act **G.R.E.E.N.**? Here is a **G.R.E.E.N.** Scene to help you act **G.R.E.E.N.** with an **open mind**!

Things to Do before G.R.E.E.N. Scene #6

Take all the necessary steps for **Making the Best G.R.E.E.N. Scenes** found in sections 12.2–12-5. This includes **Surveying the G.R.E.E.N. Scene** (12.2), choosing the best **Guiding G.R.E.E.N. Thought** for this scene (16.7), reviewing the **Rules for Acting in G.R.E.E.N. Scenes** (12.3), using the **G.R.E.E.N. Scene Review Form** (12.4), and engaging in the **G.R.E.E.N. Scene Warm-Ups** (12.5).

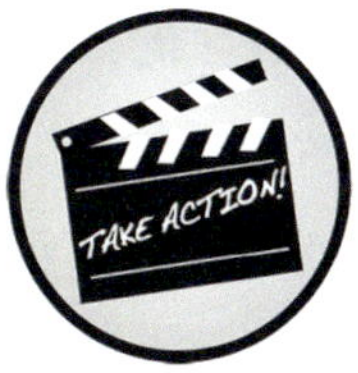

The Director gets the clapboard and says, "Quiet on the set. **G.R.E.E.N.** Scene #6. Take one! Action!" If the scene gets repeated with the same set of actors, the Director will say, "Quiet on the set. **G.R.E.E.N.** Scene #6. Take two! Action!"

16.6 G.R.E.E.N. Scene #6: Open-Minded Like Oscar!

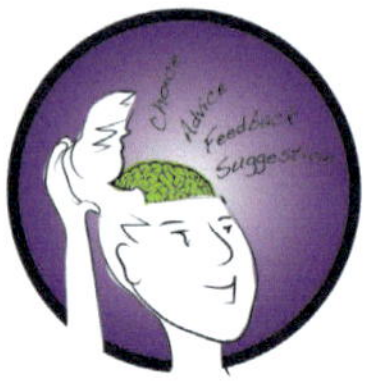

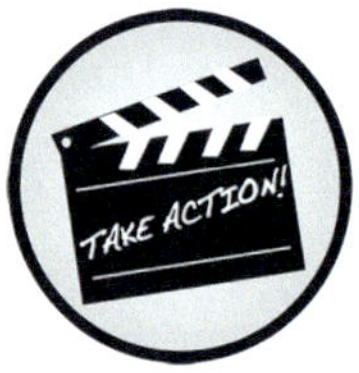

Narrator: Oscar does not really like getting new ideas from other people. He likes to do things his own way. But he is learning to be **open-minded** to new ideas. He is learning to listen to new ideas and try them out because they sometimes make his life better. New ideas also sometimes make life **better** for other people on his Team.

Right now, he is doing his homework at the kitchen table. He likes doing his homework there because the kitchen table is where he always has done his homework. His brother, Marco, is making loud sounds while playing in the family room, next to the kitchen. His mother, Mrs. Gomez, is getting dinner ready and talking on the phone. Oscar is having trouble concentrating on his homework.

Oscar: *Can everyone please be quiet? I'm trying to do my homework.*

Mrs. Gomez: *I must go now and talk with Oscar. I'll talk to you later (ends phone call and walks to Oscar). Are you having trouble concentrating here?*

Oscar: *Yes, I am. I am supposed to read this and answer the questions, but it is hard to do my work with Marco making noises and you talking on the phone.*

Mrs. Gomez: *I have an idea that might make it easier for you to concentrate. Would you like to hear it?*

Oscar: *Yes. What is your idea?*

Mrs. Gomez: *Your father and I bought you the desk in your room, but you have not used it to do your homework. Why don't you go work there? Your room is quieter and you should be able to concentrate better.*

Oscar: *But I always do my homework here in the kitchen.*

Mrs. Gomez: *Well maybe it's time to try a new idea. Why don't you try working in your room today and see if it is easier to concentrate? You might really like it. And that way your brother and I can still talk and make some noise out here without it bothering you. You can still come out to ask me if you have a question about your work. What do you think? Can you go try it out?*

Oscar: *OK, I'll give it a try.*

Mrs. Gomez: *Great. I'll help you move your books.*

16.7 Choosing Guiding G.R.E.E.N. Thoughts for G.R.E.E.N. Scene #6

Help Oscar in G.R.E.E.N. Scene #6 by circling a useful **Guiding G.R.E.E.N. Thought** from the choices below. You also may write your own **Guiding G.R.E.E.N. Thought** if you can think of a different one that fits this G.R.E.E.N. Scene.

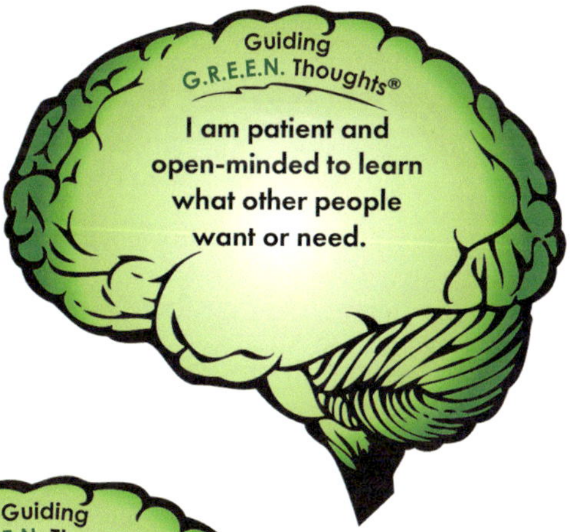

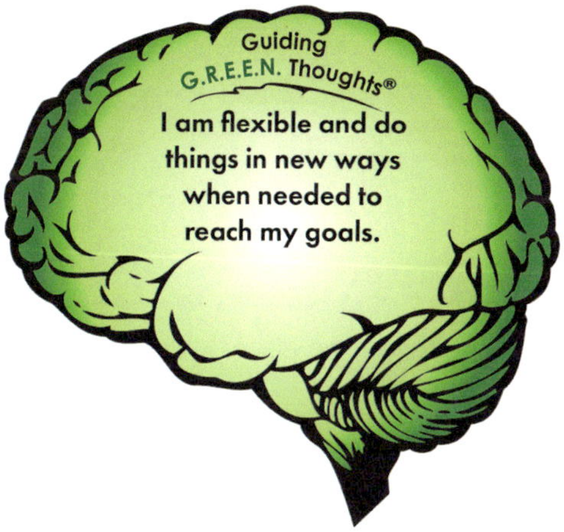

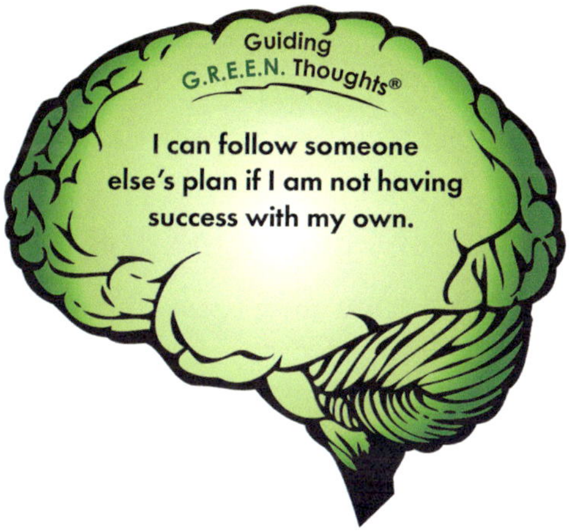

My own **Guiding G.R.E.E.N. Thought** for this scene:

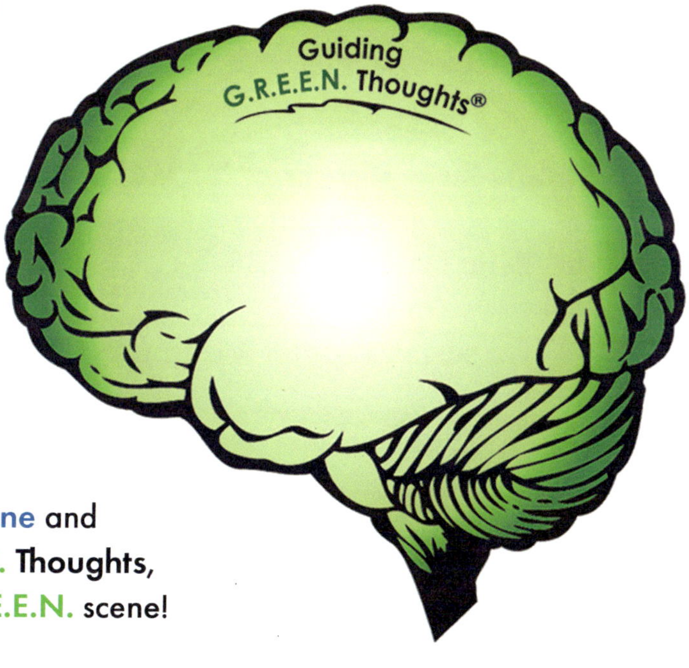

Once you have surveyed the scene and chosen useful **Guiding G.R.E.E.N. Thoughts**, you are ready to act out the G.R.E.E.N. scene!

16.8 Be Positive; Things Will Get Better!

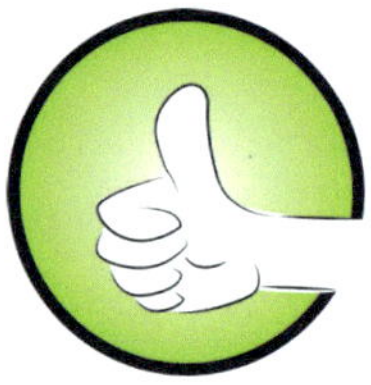

Being **positive** means having a good attitude to help you move **forward**. When you are **positive**, you can think about things getting **better** in any scene you are in for yourself and your Team. If you do not have a **positive** attitude, you might feel stuck. Without a **positive** attitude, you might have difficulty moving **forward** toward your **goal**.

The **G.R.E.E.N.** Scene that follows will help you act with a **positive** attitude!

16.9 G.R.E.E.N. Scene #7: Acting Positive Makes It Better

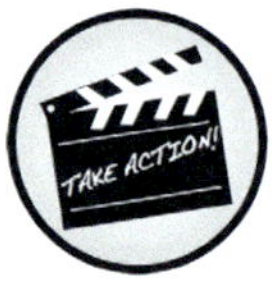

Reasons for Acting in this Scene:

1. Acting in this scene helps you see how you can benefit from making a **change** from having a negative attitude to having a **positive** attitude.

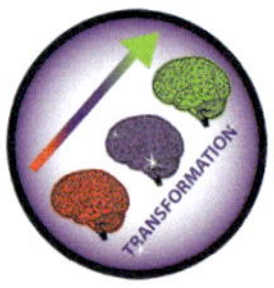

2. Acting in this scene is a way to practice taking useful feedback from someone on your Team who can help you achieve a **Personal Goal**.

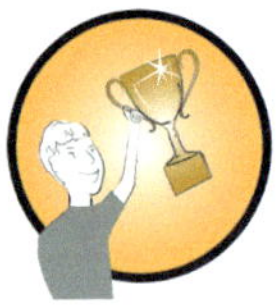

3. Acting in this scene helps you see how it is useful to take the time to look over your own work before having someone else look at it.

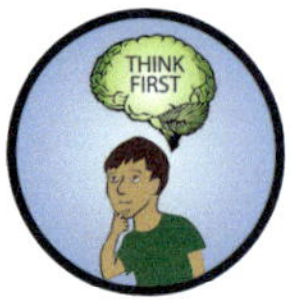

Follow these Directions for Making the Best G.R.E.E.N. Scene:

1. Read through this **G.R.E.E.N.** Scene with your Team.

2. Follow the steps for **Making the Best G.R.E.E.N. Scene (12.2-12-5)**

3. For this scene, you can also fill out a **Thought Transformation Scene Changer** to show Pat's **transformation**. (15.5)

4. For this scene, the Teacher gives Pat a copy of some work that Pat has previously written so Pat can agree to make a couple of **editing changes.**

5. The Director gets the clapboard and says, "Quiet on the set! **G.R.E.E.N.** Scene #7. Take one. Action!" (If the scene gets repeated with the same set of actors, the Scene Director will say, "Quiet on the set. **G.R.E.E.N.** Scene #7. Take two. Action!")

16.10 G.R.E.E.N. Scene #7: Acting Positive Makes It Better

Narrator: Pat did not like checking her work. She thought it was boring and got mad if someone asked her to look over her work again. She did not like spending time going over any work she had already done and had a negative attitude about editing. One day, her teacher handed-back her project. It had many red editing marks on it. Her teacher told her to rewrite the whole project. Pat felt terrible.

On the next assignment, her teacher asked her to Think First and keep an **open mind** about checking over her work. Pat remembered the red marks and bad grade, so she started editing her work without complaining! This started a **transformation**. Pat began to **change** her attitude about checking her work. After following her teacher's suggestion and reviewing her work, she found one or two mistakes. She made the **changes** and got a **better** grade! Pat tried this again and again, and her grades kept improving! She now has a **positive** attitude about checking her work and keeps getting **better** grades.

Teacher: *Pat, I think it would be a good idea for you to check your work to see if you can find any errors before your turn it in to me.*

Pat: *OK, I'll check it. If I find my own mistakes, there will be fewer mistakes for you to find.*

Teacher: *That's right. I **appreciate** your **positive** attitude. I'll look forward to seeing your best work when you turn it in.*

Pat: *Thanks for helping me do my best.*

Teacher: *You're welcome.*

16.11 Choosing G.R.E.E.N. Thoughts for G.R.E.E.N. Scene #7

Help Pat in G.R.E.E.N. Scene #7 by circling a useful **Guiding G.R.E.E.N. Thought** from the choices below. You also may write your own **Guiding G.R.E.E.N. Thought** if you can think of a different one that fits this G.R.E.E.N. Scene:

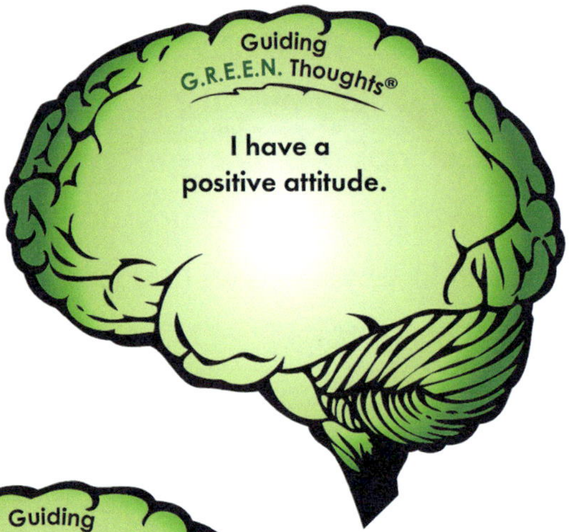

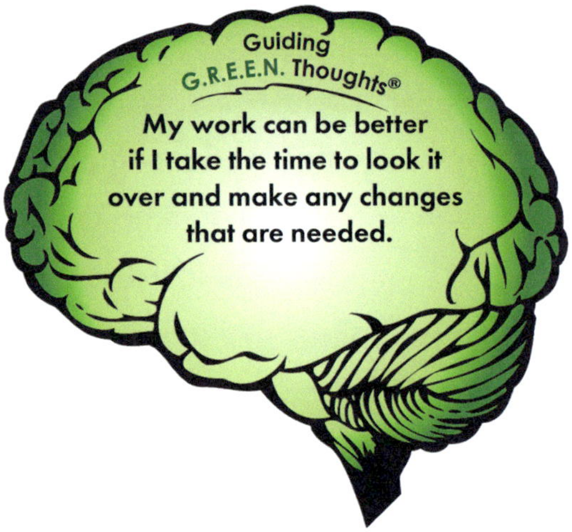

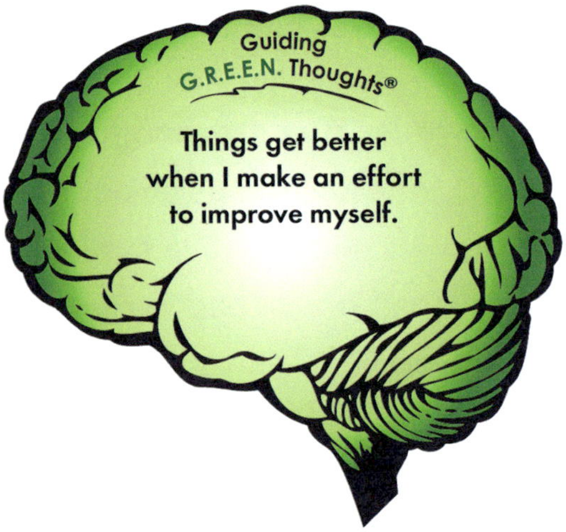

My own **Guiding G.R.E.E.N. Thought** for this scene:

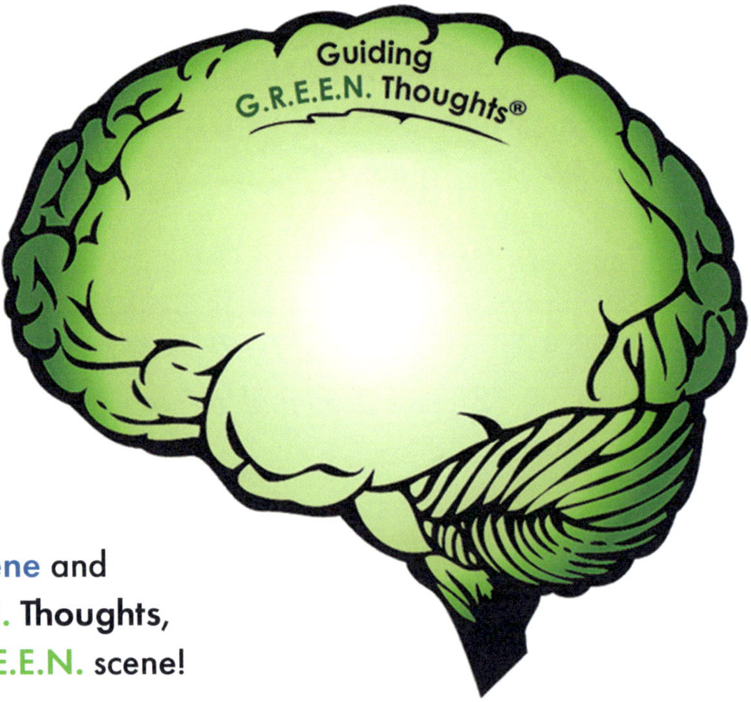

Once you have surveyed the scene and chosen useful **Guiding G.R.E.E.N. Thoughts**, you are ready to act out the G.R.E.E.N. scene!

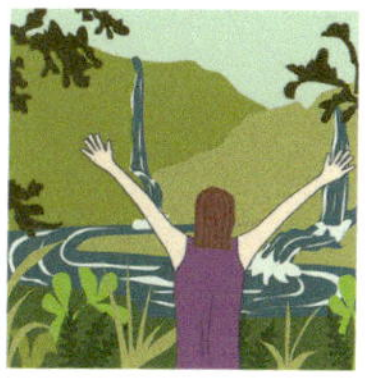

17 Being Grateful

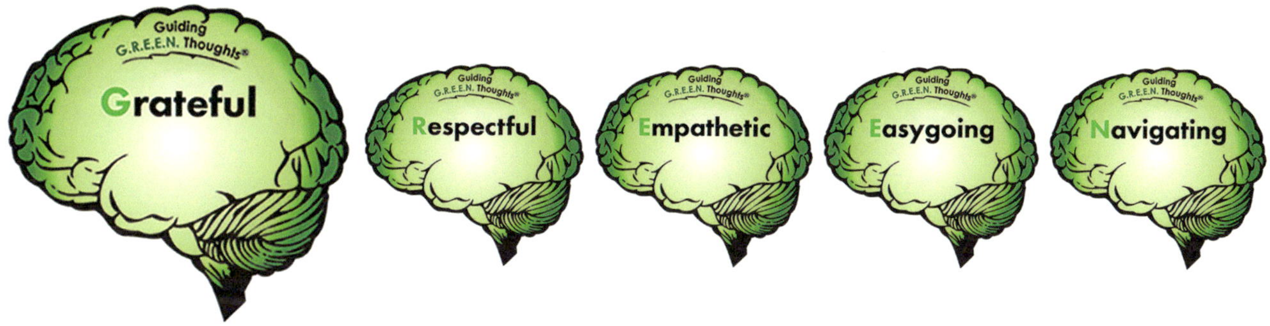

17.1 Acting in a Grateful Way

Being **grateful** means being **thankful** for what you have. When you are **grateful**, you show people that you **appreciate** what you already have in your life. You take time to think about how lucky you are to have people and things in your life. Then you show your **appreciation**.

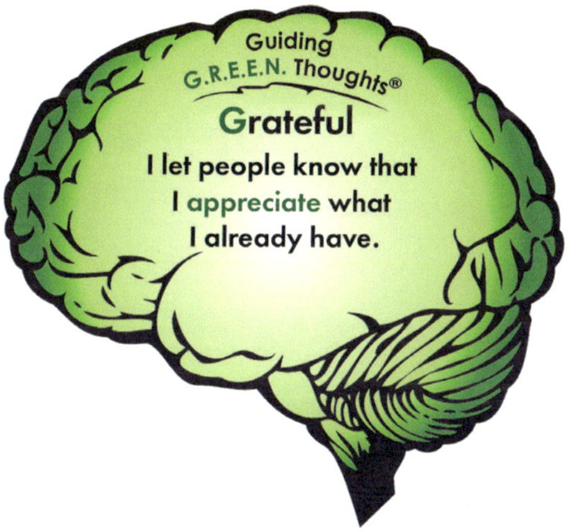

When you act **gratefully**, you let people know that for right now, you are glad to have the things you have. When you are **grateful**, you do not need to be greedy by asking for more than you have right now.

You can show your **gratitude** by using words to show your **appreciation**. You can also show you are **grateful** by doing **helpful, thoughtful** things for other people on your Home, School, and Friendship Teams.

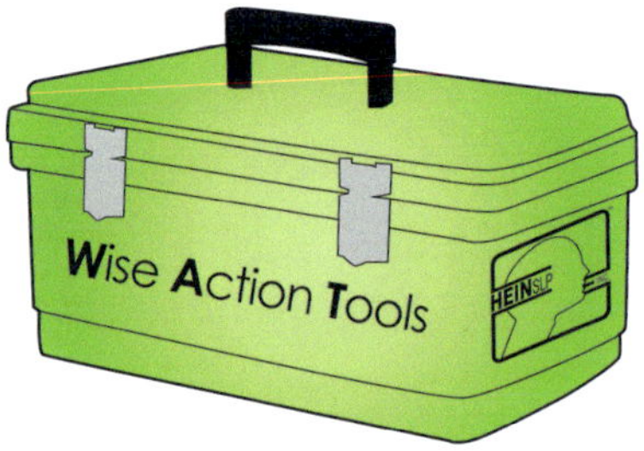

APPRECIATION BOX

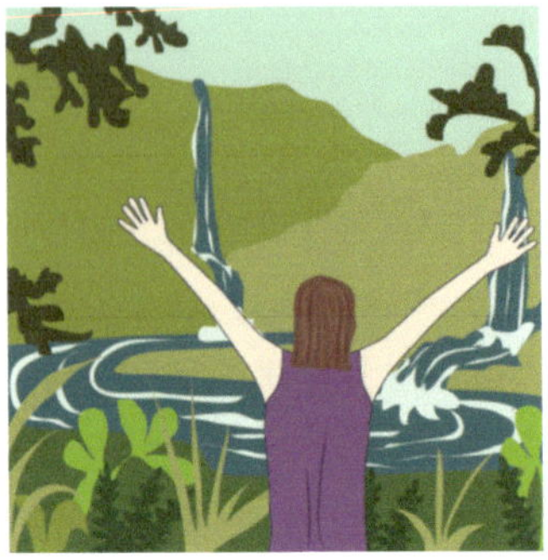

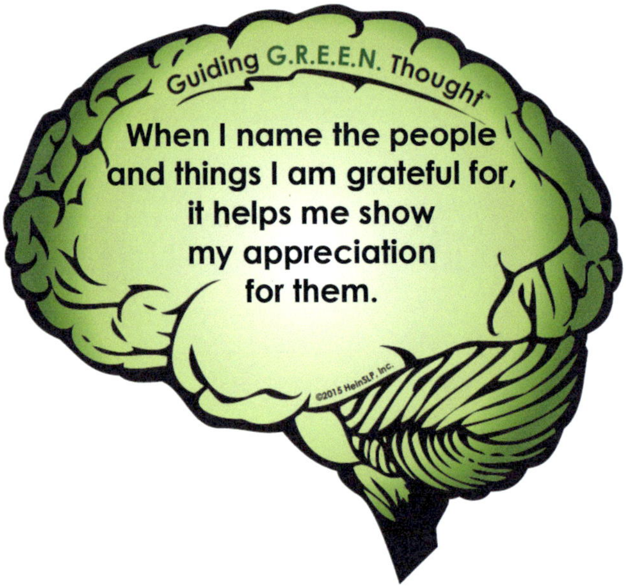

MY APPRECIATION BOX

This is a picture of me with the people and things that I am **grateful** for having in my life. I fill this box with everyone and everything I **appreciate.** I am in this scene too, because I **appreciate** being alive!

17.2 Guiding G.R.E.E.N. Thoughts for Acting Grateful

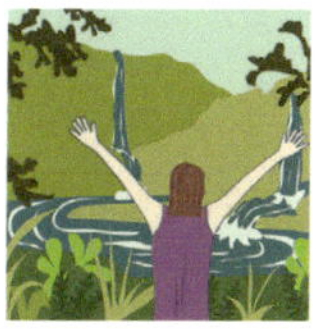

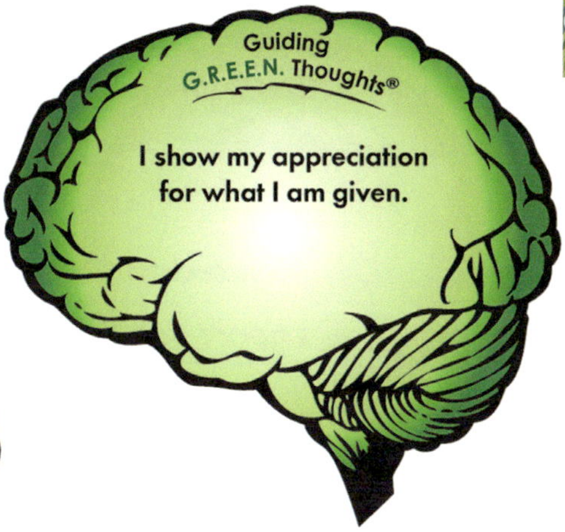

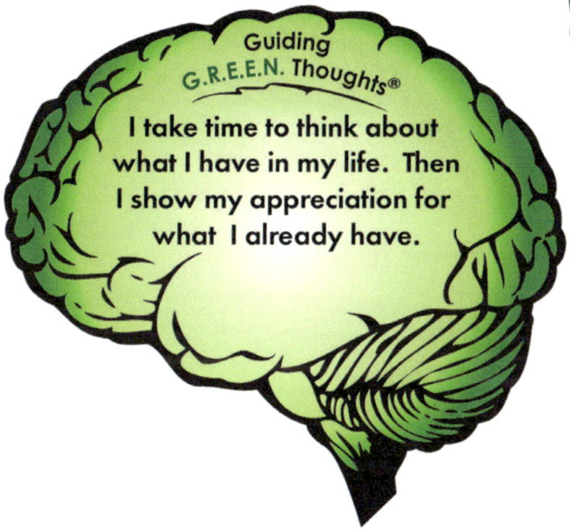

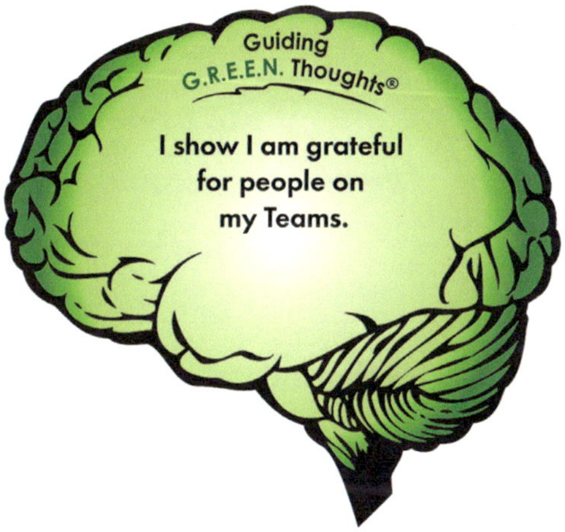

17.3 Telling What We Are Grateful for Is Powerful

The first step in showing **gratitude** is saying "thank you." An even more **powerful** way to show **gratitude** is to talk about what you are **grateful** for. This shows that you have taken the time to notice the good things in your life.

If someone has been **kind** and **thoughtful** and has given you things that you want or need, that person can feel appreciated when you talk with them about exactly what they gave you. If someone has helped you or taught you something, that person will feel appreciated when you tell them how they helped you.

Besides using your **grateful** words, you can show your **appreciation** even more by taking action to make the other person's life better, too.

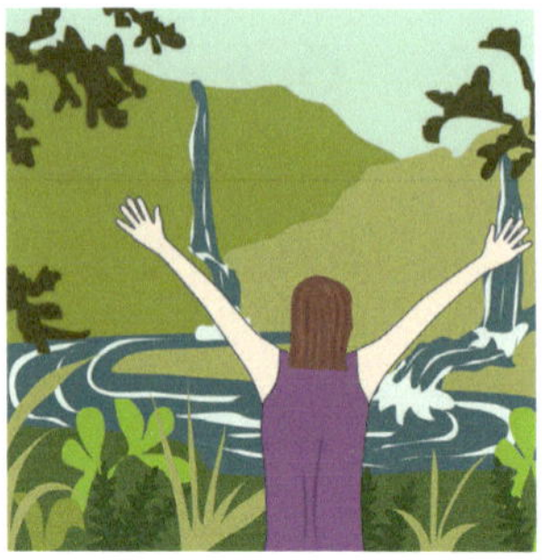

I APPRECIATE

A Song for **Guiding G.R.E.E.N. Thoughts**®

by Herb Hein

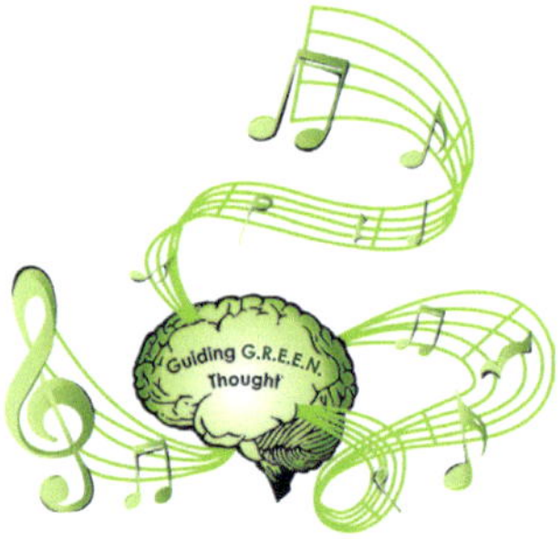

I appreciate I have shoes on my feet.
I appreciate I have something to eat.
I appreciate I have you so I don't have to feel lonely.
I appreciate I have somewhere to live.
I appreciate I have something to give.
I appreciate every day that I am alive.
And I know there's always something more.
We're meant to get up off the floor.
We have our brains and arms for reaching higher.
But for now, I am Grateful
and for now, I am satisfied
with everyone and everything that's around me.
I appreciate every breath that I take.
I appreciate every day I awake.
I appreciate when you give me a reason to smile.
'Cuz I know I'll be seeing something more
next time I rise up off the floor,
and I'll be ready...for reaching higher.
So for now...I am Grateful
and for now I am satisfied
with everyone and everything that's around me.
I say thank you! I say thank you! I say thank you!

17.4 Survey the Scene: Using Grateful Words and Actions for Getting Help with Math

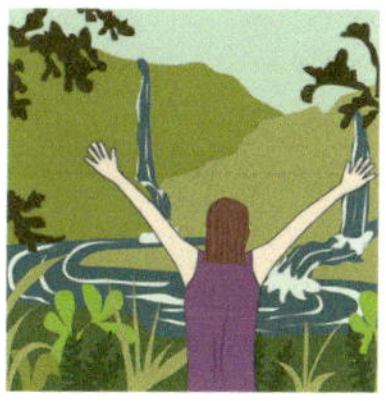

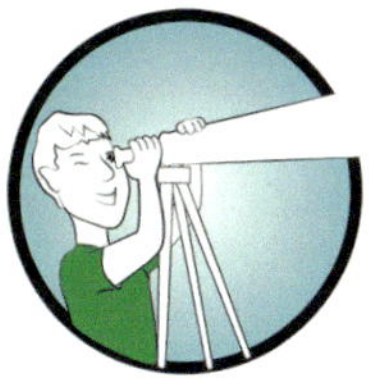

Jose's older brother, Carlos, helps him figure out how to do his math homework.

1. What can Jose say to show he is **grateful** for Carlos's help?

   Thank you, Carlos, for ____

   ____

2. What is something Jose can do for Carlos that day or the next day to show he really is **grateful**? ____________________________________

   ____

   (Some possible ideas are shown to help you think of a **grateful** action.)

   A. Help Carlos do one of his chores.

   B. Give Carlos a gift.

   C. Write a note to Carlos.

   D. Tell his parents how **helpful** Carlos was to him.

   E. ____

   ____

Thank you!

17.5 Survey the Scene: Using Grateful Words and Actions to Get Help during a Sad Time

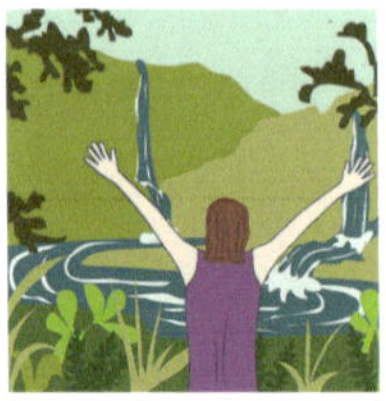

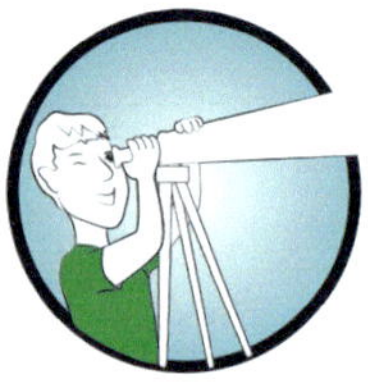

Kim's mother was sick and had to go to the hospital. The next day, when Kim went to school, she was looking sad and worried. Her teacher, Mrs. Liner, asked Kim if there was anything she wanted to talk about. During lunch, Kim shared about how she was feeling with Mrs. Liner. Mrs. Liner said some things to help Kim feel **better**.

1. What can Kim say to show she is **grateful** for Mrs. Liner's help?

   Thank you, Mrs. Liner, for ____

   ____

2. What is something Kim can do for Mrs. Liner that day or the next day to show she really is **grateful** for Mrs. Liner's help? ______________________

   ____

   ____

   (Some possible ideas are below to help you think of a **grateful** action.)

   A. Ask if she can help Mrs. Liner with something in the classroom.

   B. Make or buy Mrs. Liner a small gift.

   C. Write a note to Mrs. Liner.

   D. Draw a picture for Mrs. Liner.

   E. ____

Thank you!

17.6 Survey the Scene: Using Grateful Words and Actions for Getting Help Playing Basketball

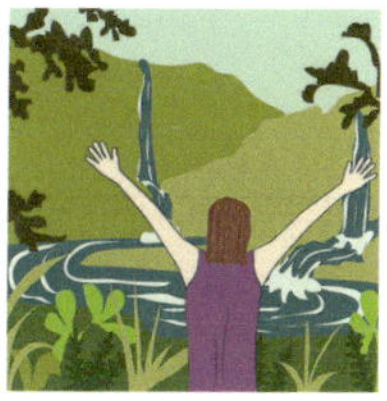

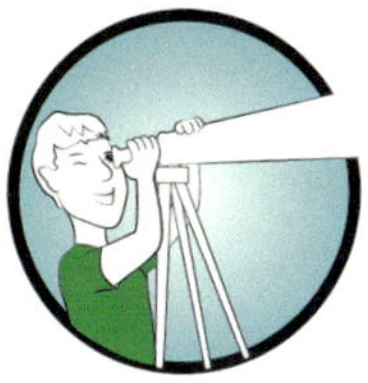

During lunch, Angela was telling her classmates that she wanted to try out for the basketball team. She thought she could get on the Team if she could shoot baskets a little bit better. Angela's classmate Anthony said he would be willing to give her some helpful tips during recess. He took the time to show Angela how to hold her hand a little bit differently so she could make shots into the hoop more consistently. That afternoon, Angela went to the basketball tryouts and made the Team!

1. What is something Angela could say to Anthony the next day at school to show she is grateful for Anthony's help.

   Thank you, Anthony, for ____

   ____

2. What is something Angela can do for Anthony the next day or in the next week to show she really is grateful for his help? __________________________

   ____

   (Some possible ideas are shown to help you think of a grateful action.)

   A. She can bring a special treat to share during lunch.

   B. She can write a note to Anthony.

   C. She can get or make Anthony a small gift.

   D. She can ask Anthony if there is anything she can help him do better.

   E. ____

Thank you!

17.7 Change the Scene to Make It G.R.E.E.N.: Help Lily Get Help

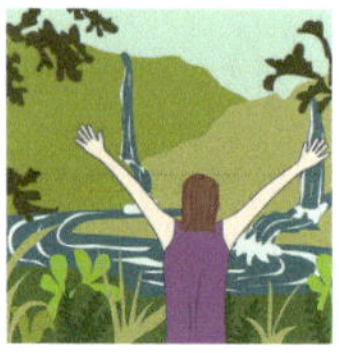

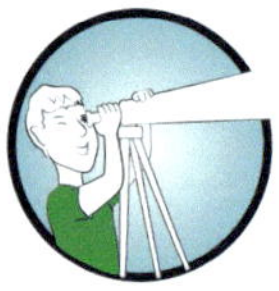

Survey the scene to see if Lily is thinking of the Team by acting **grateful** for her teacher' s help.

Lily was frustrated about a math problem that she had to solve. She put her head down on her desk. Lily's teacher, Mr. Garcia, came over to help her because Lily was looking upset. He said, "You look like you can use my help, Lily. Is there something I can help you with?"

Lily lifted her head and said, "I hate this class. I can't ever solve these math problems, and nobody is ever going to have enough time to really help me with them!"

1. Is Lily acting in a **grateful** way?

    yes   no

2. Is Lily using words that show that she is glad that her teacher came over to try to help?

    yes   no

3. What do you think a negative consequence might be for Lily acting in this way?

    ____

4. Help Lily **change the scene** to make it more **G.R.E.E.N.** What can she say or do to show Mr. Garcia she is **grateful** that he has offered to help her? _____

    ____

    ____

5. What do you think a **positive** consequence might be if Lily acted more **grateful** for her teacher being there to help her? ____________________________

    ____

17.8 G.R.E.E.N. Scene #8: Help Lily Say,"I Am Grateful for Your Help!"

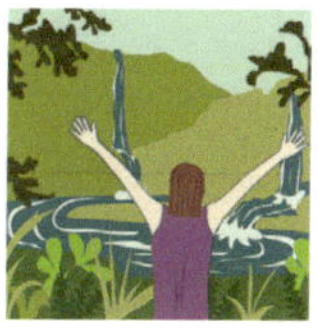

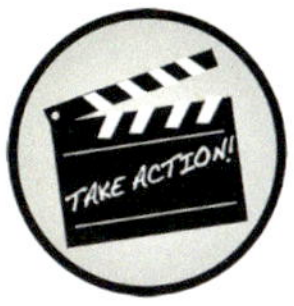

You have the **power** to **change** 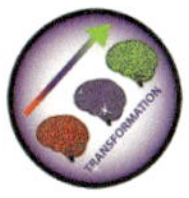 **the scene** to make it **better** for Lily and her Team. Take action and make it a **G.R.E.E.N.** Scene!

Narrator: Lily was frustrated about a math problem that she had to solve in class.

Lily (starts to quietly cry and puts her head on her desk).

Narrator: Lily's teacher sees Lily put her head on her desk. He thinks that Lily must be upset about something so he walks over to her.

Lily's Teacher: *You look upset, Lily. Is there something I can help you with?*

Narrator: Lily lifts her head and says:

Lily: ____

____

Teacher: ____

____

Lily: ____

____

After writing this **better G.R.E.E.N. Scene**, you can fill out the **Thought Transformation Scene Changer** (15.5) to show Lily's successful **transformation**.

Once you have written out **G.R.E.E.N. Scene #8** showing Lily's **transformation**, you can act it out. Take all the necessary steps for **Making the Best G.R.E.E.N. Scenes** found in sections 12.2–12-5. This includes **Surveying the G.R.E.E.N. Scene** (12.2), choosing a **Guiding G.R.E.E.N. Thought** for this scene, reviewing the **Rules for Acting in G.R.E.E.N. Scenes** (12.3), using the **G.R.E.E.N. Scene Review Form** (12.4), and engaging in the **G.R.E.E.N. Scene Warm-Ups** (12.5).

The Director gets the clapboard and says, "Quiet on the set. G.R.E.E.N. Scene #8. Take one! Action!" If the scene gets repeated with the same set of actors, the Director will say, "Quiet on the set. G.R.E.E.N. Scene #8. Take two! Action!"

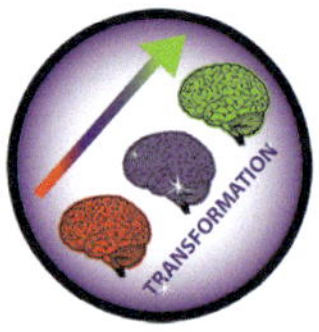

17.9 Change the Scene to Make It G.R.E.E.N.: Greedy or Grateful for Ice Cream?

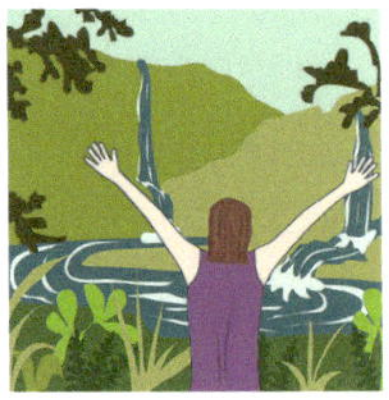

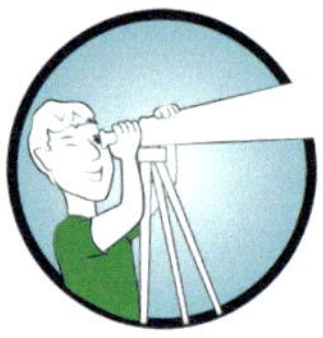

Survey the scene to see if Peter is thinking of the Team by acting **grateful** for having a bowl of ice cream for dessert.

Peter: *We were eating dinner last night. My mother made my favorite pasta with meatballs. She let me have seconds because she knew it was my favorite. Then we were having dessert. She gave me a bowl of ice cream, but I wanted to have seconds of that, too! She said it was too much sugar for me, and I should be satisfied with one bowl. I told her I really, really needed a second bowl of ice cream and that it was stupid to worry about the sugar. I also told her she was being mean by not letting me have seconds for dessert. She left the room crying and my Dad said I was not going to have any dessert for a week. My parents are so unfair!*

1. Is Peter acting in a **grateful** way?

yes no

2. Was his mother being mean to him, or was she helping him make wise choices in what he was eating?

   A. being mean

   B. helping him make wise choices

3. What is the negative consequence of Peter acting greedy during dinner?

____

____

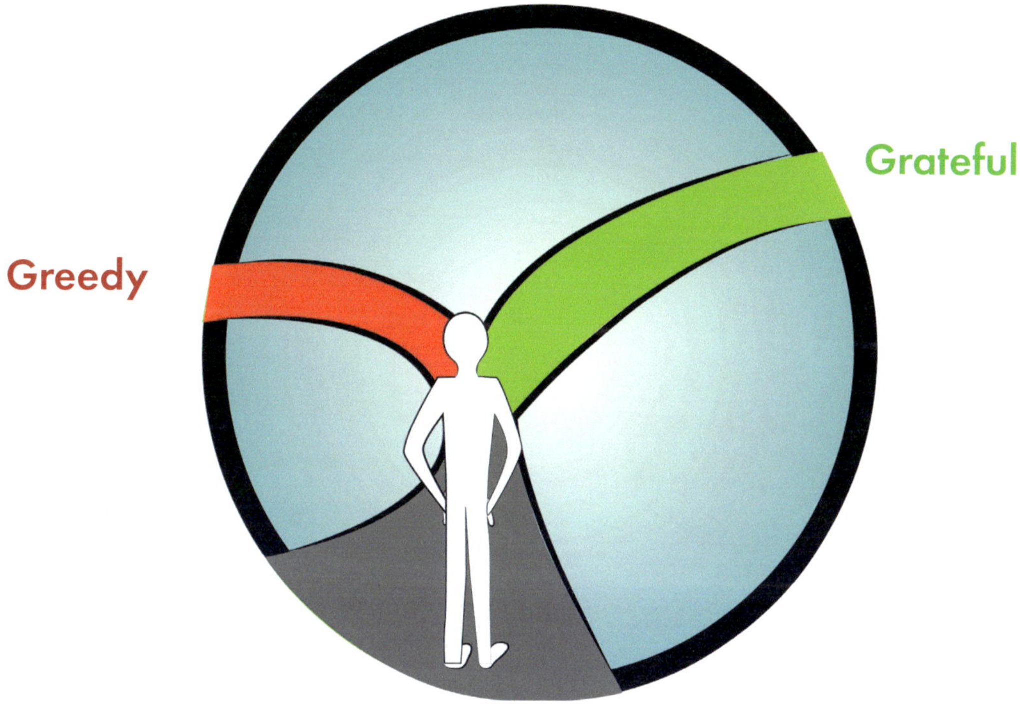

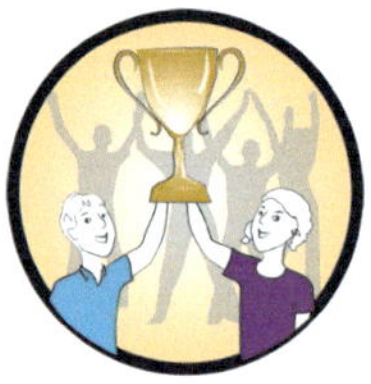

4. What are some **Guiding G.R.E.E.N. Thoughts** that Peter could think about to help him show that he knows the **Common Team Goals** during dinner?

Circle the **Guiding G.R.E.E.N. Thoughts** that fit the scene from the ones given below. If you would like, you can add your own thought that you think might help Peter in this scene as well.

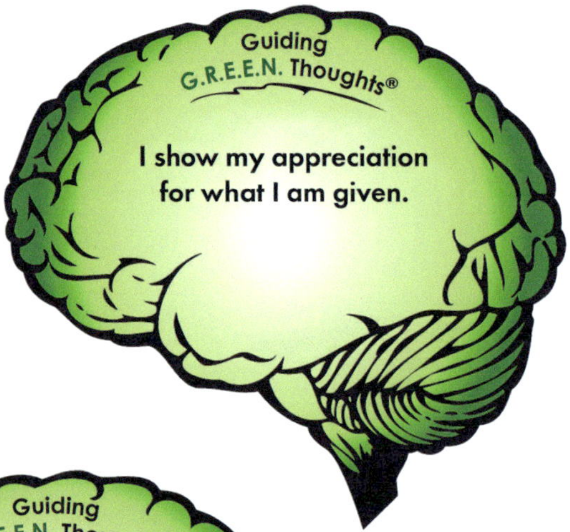

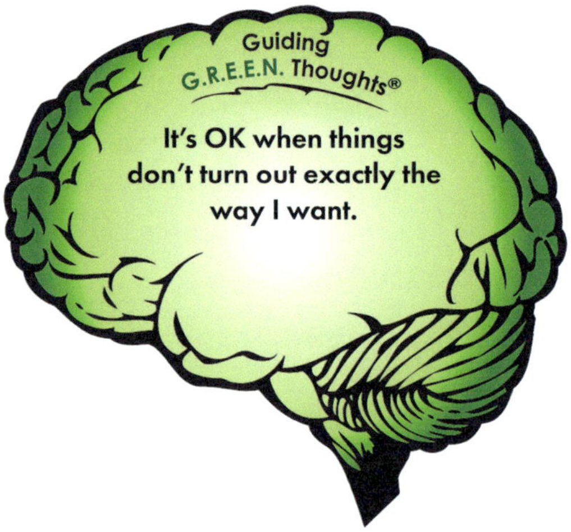

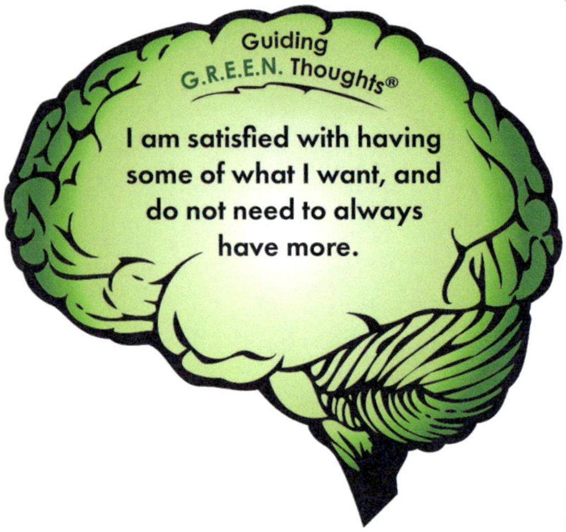

My own **Guiding G.R.E.E.N. Thought** for this scene:

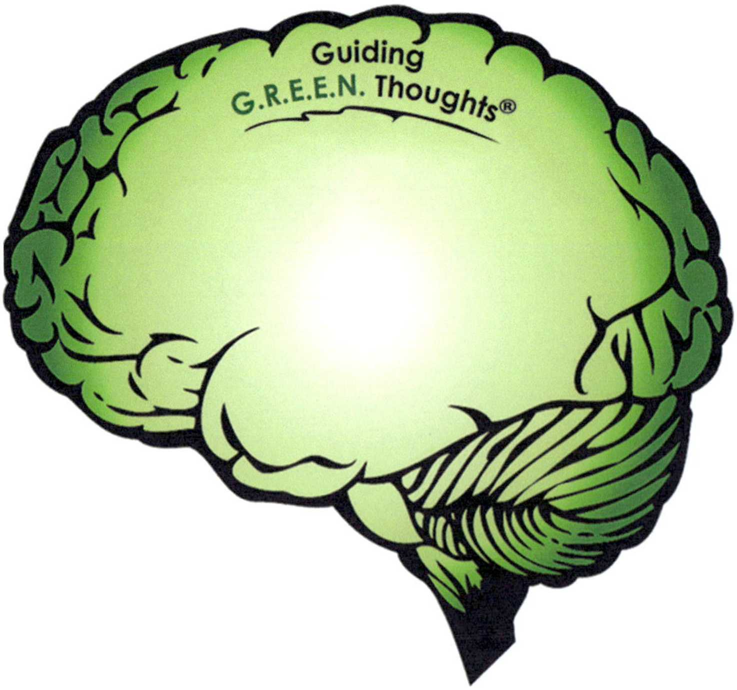

5. Help Peter **change the scene** to make it more **G.R.E.E.N.** What can he say or do to show his mother he is **grateful** to have her on his Home Team?

____

____

Thanks for making a great dinner.

Thanks for giving me seconds of pasta and meatballs.

Thanks for the ice cream.

Thank you for ______________________________________

____

I **appreciate** ______________________________________

6. What do you think could be a **positive** consequence if Peter acted more **grateful** for the food his mother gave him to eat? ______________________

____

7. Fill out the **Thought Transformation Scene Changer** to show Peter's **transformation**. (15.5)

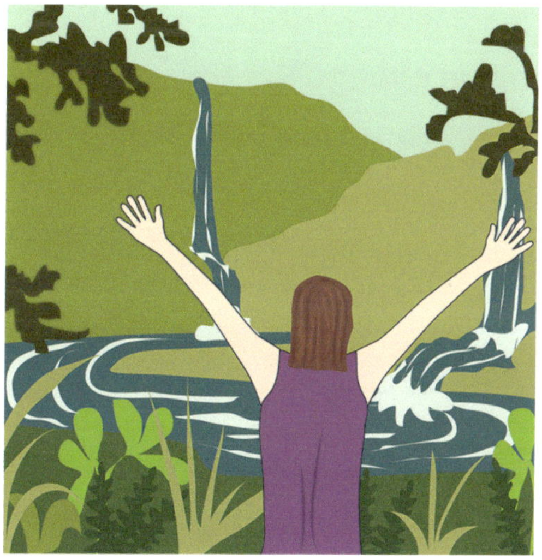

I appreciate what you gave me!

Thank you!

17.10 Change the Scene to Make It G.R.E.E.N.: Is One Enough?

Is this person thinking of the Team by acting **grateful**?

After a lesson, Robbie's teacher said, "Because it is the last day before vacation, I am going to give each of you an ice pop." When it was Robbie's turn, the teacher handed him one. Robbie didn't say anything except, "Is this little pop all we're getting? And don't you have any cherry ones?"

1. Is Robbie acting in a **grateful** way?

   yes no

2. Is Robbie showing he **cares** about the feelings of others on his Class Team?

   yes no

What do you think a negative consequence might be if Robbie acts in this way? ______________________________

____

3. Help Robbie **change the scene** to make it more **G.R.E.E.N.** What can he say when his teacher offers him an ice pop? ______________________________

   ____

4. What do you think a **positive** consequence might be if Robbie acted more **grateful**? ______________________________

   ____

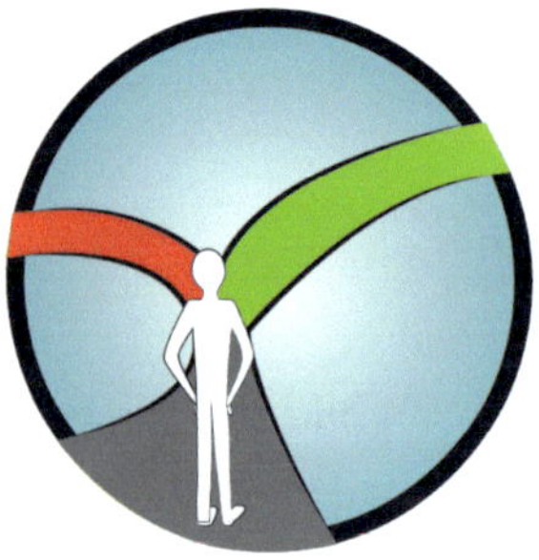

17.11 G.R.E.E.N. Scene #9: Thank You! One Is Enough for Me

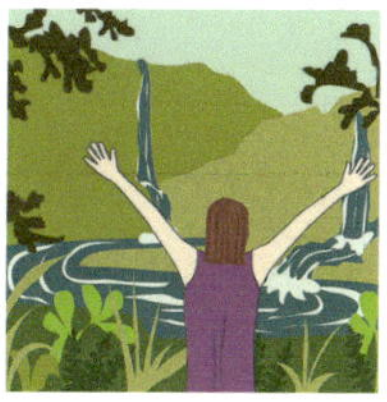

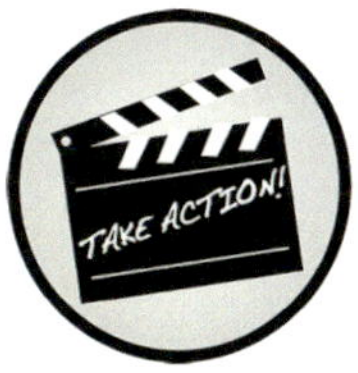

You have the **power** to **change the scene** to make it better for Robbie and his Team. Take action and make it a **G.R.E.E.N.** Scene!

Narrator: After the last lesson on the last day of school before vacation, Robbie's teacher decided to give out a treat for her class.

Teacher: *Because it is the last day before vacation, I am going to give each of you an ice pop.*

Narrator: When it was Robbie's turn, the teacher handed him one.

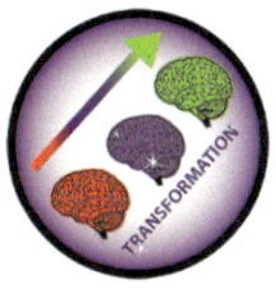

Robbie: ____

____

Teacher: ____

What **Guiding G.R.E.E.N. Thought** would help Robbie in this scene?

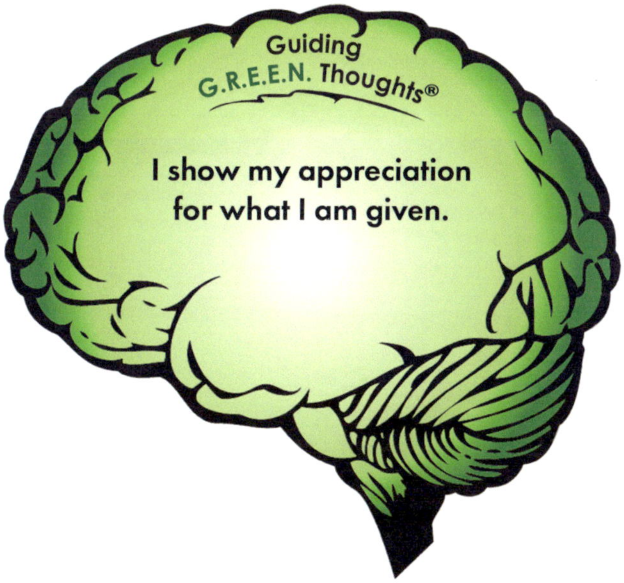

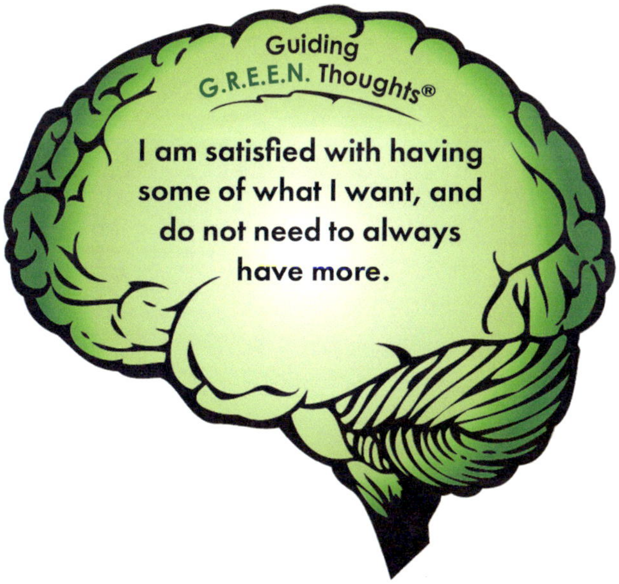

After writing this **better G.R.E.E.N. Scene**, you can fill out the **Thought Transformation Scene Changer** (15.5) to show Robbie's successful **transformation**

Once you have written out **G.R.E.E.N. Scene #9** showing Robbie **transformation**, you can act it out. Take all the necessary steps for **Making the Best G.R.E.E.N. Scenes** found in sections 12.2–12-5. This includes **Surveying the G.R.E.E.N. Scene** (12.2), choosing a **Guiding G.R.E.E.N. Thought** for this scene, reviewing the **Rules for Acting in G.R.E.E.N. Scenes** (12.3), using the **G.R.E.E.N. Scene Review Form** (12.4), and engaging in the **G.R.E.E.N. Scene Warm-Ups** (12.5).

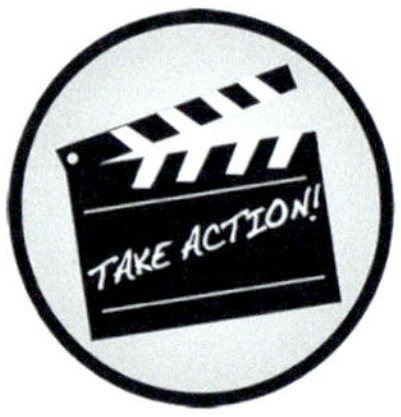

The Director gets the clapboard and says, "Quiet on the set. G.R.E.E.N. Scene #9. Take one! Action!" If the scene gets repeated with the same set of actors, the Director will say, "Quiet on the set. G.R.E.E.N. Scene #9. Take two! Action!"

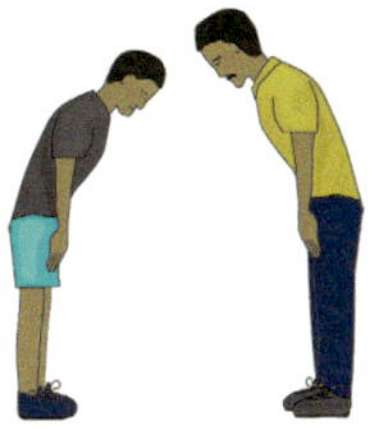

18 Learning to Respectfully Respond to Others

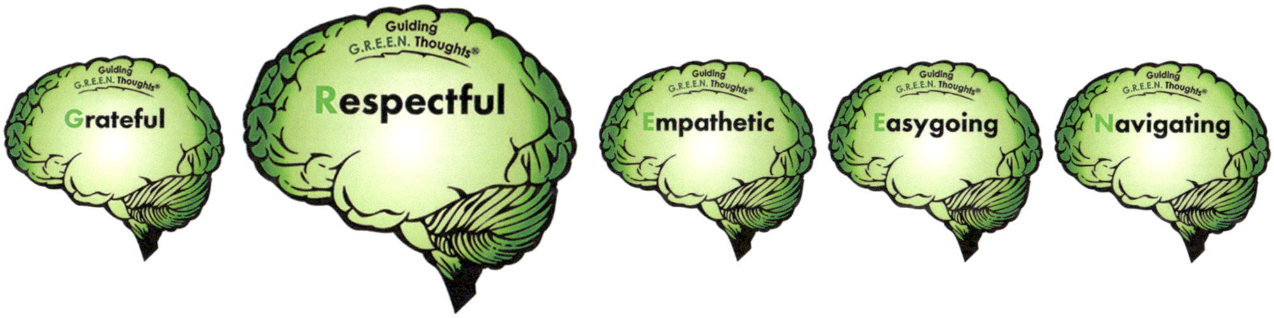

18.1 Add Respect to Your Interactions!

You have learned to be **grateful** for what you have and to know how to show this to others on your Teams. Now you can focus on learning how to act **respectfully** when people on your Teams are talking to you.

18.2 What Does It Mean to Be Respectful?

Respectful: Acting **respectful** means you notice the people and things in your life and treat them with **care**. We all have heard the phrase, "Respect your elders," so we know that we should be **kind** and **polite** to older people. We also get along **better** on our Teams when we show we **care** about people of all ages and the toys, animals, and other things around us. When you act **respectfully**, you are making choices with your words and actions so the people with you feel comfortable and safe.

When you are **respectful**, you **pay attention to people** when they are talking to you. When you are **respectful**, you choose **considerate** and **polite** words. When you are **respectful**, other people will feel that their needs are as important as yours. With your **polite words**, **tone of voice** and **positive attitude**, you let people on your Teams know you consider it important that they are spending time to be with you.

18.3 Guiding G.R.E.E.N. Thoughts for Being Respectful

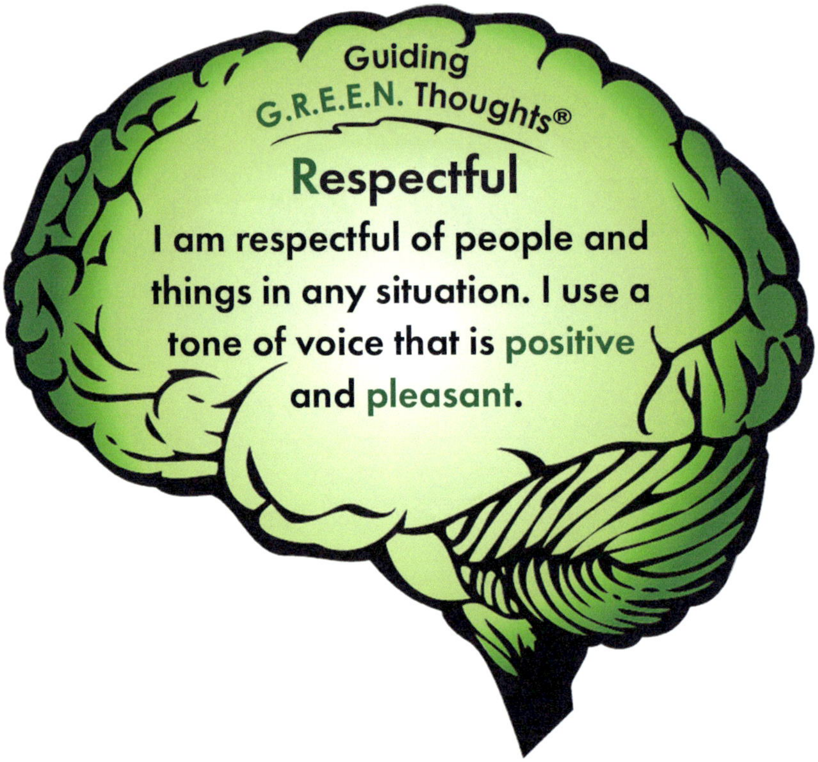

- I show respect to the people and things in my life.
- I use a positive and pleasant tone of voice.
- I look at you when you are talking to me.
- I answer you right away with a positive tone of voice.
- I use a tone of voice that shows I am interested in what you are saying.
- I pay attention to choose appropriate topics of conversation.
- I tell the truth when I am talking with other people on my Teams.

18.4 Ways to Act Respectfully

There are things to think about so you can talk with other people in a **respectful** way:

1. Have eye contact. Look at other people when they are talking to you.
2. Answer right away if someone asks you a question.
3. Use a **positive** and **pleasant** tone of voice and a speaking volume that matches the situation.
4. Take turns in order to have a **cooperative conversation**. You can be **respectful** and **easygoing** by taking turns listening and talking. All members of the Conversation Team are respected for sharing their ideas.
5. Stay focused on the topic and choose words that keep the conversation **positive**.

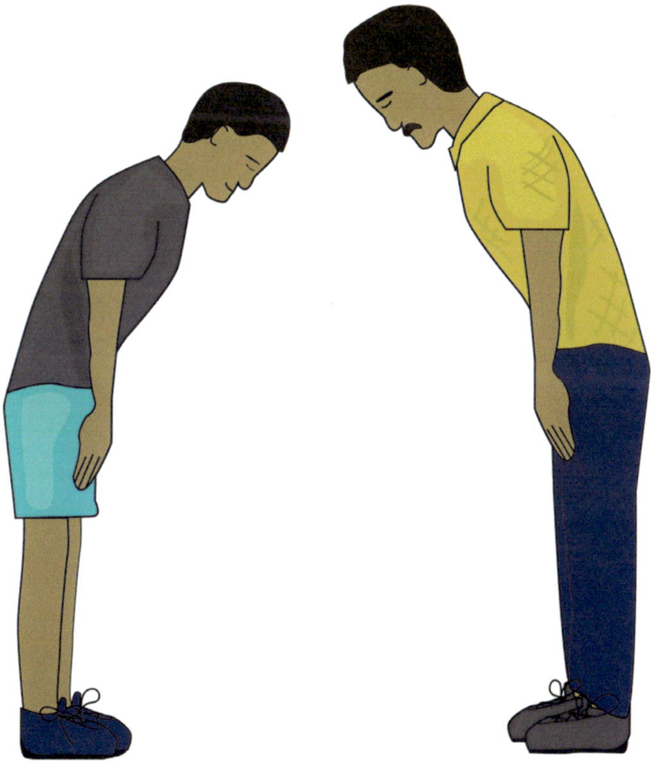

18.5 Survey the Scene: Choose to Act Respectfully

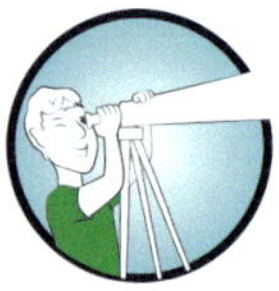

Help these people make the best choice to act **respectfully** to **connect** with the people on their Teams. Choose **G.R.E.E.N.** action to help the Team move **forward**!

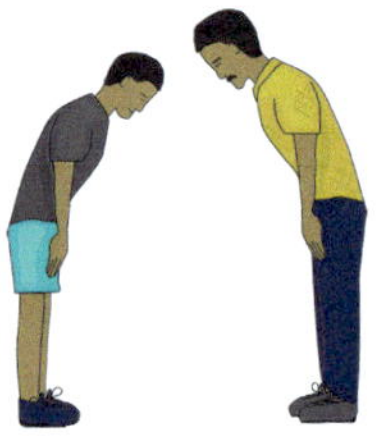

Directions: Do your best to determine which action is respectful. Circle your answer.

1. Max

   A. Max doesn't look at the person he is talking to.

   B. Max looks at the person he is talking to.

2. Jessica

   A. Jessica answers the person who asked her a question.

   B. Jessica ignores the person who asked her a question.

3. Paul

   A. Paul uses words that upset his conversation partner.

   B. Paul uses words that make his conversation partner feel comfortable talking with him.

4. Carla

   A. Carla uses a **positive**, interested tone of voice.

   B. Carla uses a sarcastic and negative tone of voice.

5. Aaron

   A. Aaron interrupts the other person who was sharing an idea and switches to his favorite topic.

   B. Aaron tells himself to stay focused on the Team topic and waits to take his turn to share his idea about that topic!

I DON'T IGNORE YOU

A Song for **Guiding** G.R.E.E.N. **Thoughts**®

By Herb Hein

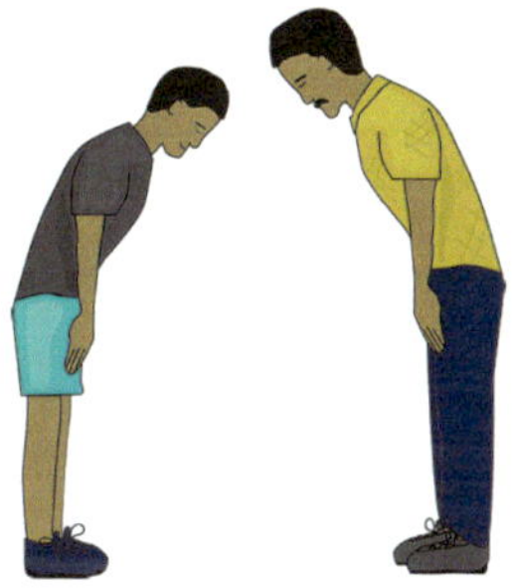

If you say something to me, I don't ignore you.

If you say something to me, I don't ignore you.

When you ask me a question, I answer right away.

When you ask me a question, I answer right away.

If you say something to me, I don't ignore you.

If you say something to me, I don't ignore you.

18.6 Quick G.R.E.E.N. Scenes for Eye Contact and Quick Responses

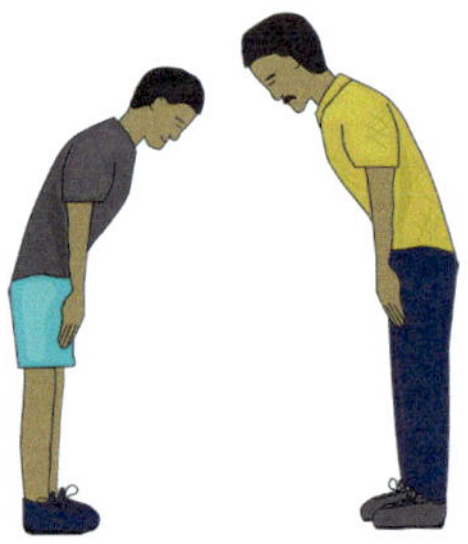

Here are some Quick **G.R.E.E.N.** Scenes to help you do two very important things when someone talks to you:

1. Look at the person talking to you. (Person B)
2. Answer the person (Person A) right after you are greeted or asked a question. This shows you heard them and **respect** them.

Date _______ Person A ________________ Person B ________________

Scene #1

Person A: *Hello! Good morning!/Good afternoon!*

Person B: ⟶ **Hello! Good morning!/Good afternoon!**

1. You looked at the person   yes   no
2. You answered right away: # of seconds _______

Scene #2

Person A: *How are you today?!*

Person B: ⟶ **Fine. How are you?!**

1. You looked at the person   yes   no
2. You answered right away: # of seconds _______

18.7 Change the Scene to Make It G.R.E.E.N.!: Help Matthew Respectfully Answer

At lunchtime, Matthew sat down at a table with some classmates. One of his classmates asked Matthew, "How are you doing today?" Matthew did not use any words to answer. He just burped loudly and laughed.

1. What did Matthew do that was rude, **R.E.D.**, friendship-disconnecting behavior? Underline it in red.

Let's **rewind** the scene and help Matthew reach up for a **Guiding G.R.E.E.N. Thought** so he can act in a more **respectful**, **G.R.E.E.N.**, **friendship-connecting** way.

These are some **Guiding G.R.E.E.N. Thoughts** that Matthew can reach for to help him make a better choice of actions:

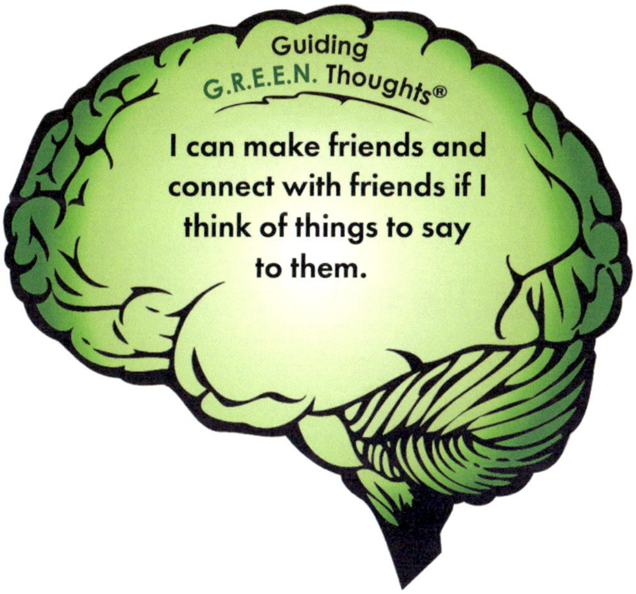

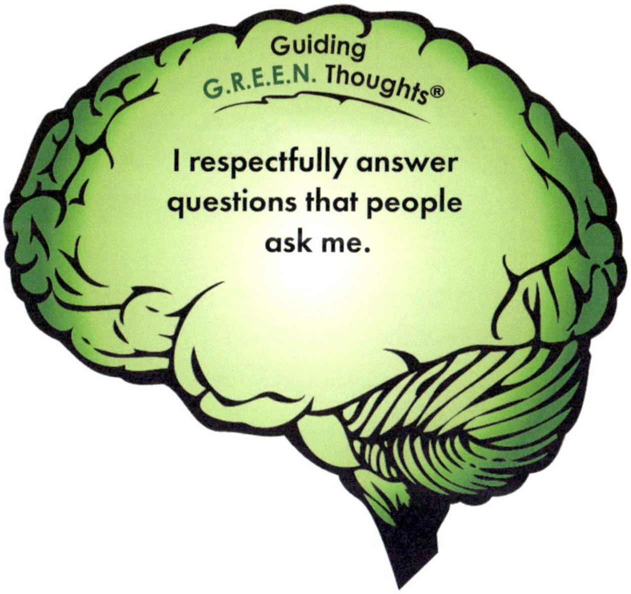

2. Answer the question as **respectfully** as you can, showing Matthew a **better** way to respond to the question.

Question: *How are you doing today?*

Answer: ____

PLEASE TELL ME SOMETHING RIGHT AWAY WHEN I ASK YOU A QUESTION!

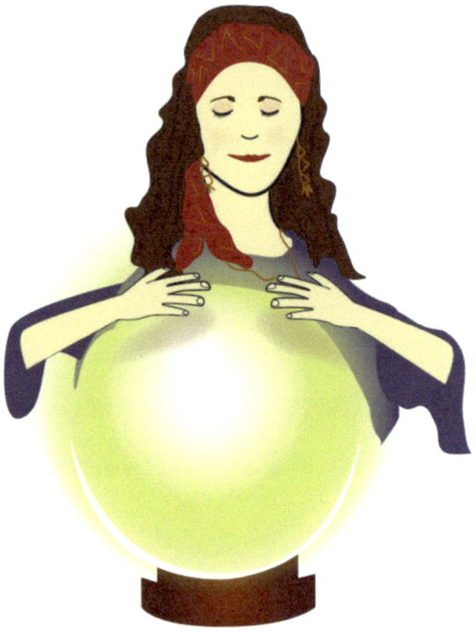

"Let me look into my crystal ball...
I try really hard, but I cannot read
your mind."

Help me help you. Please do one of the following after I ask you a question:

1. Quickly tell me the answer if you know it. **The answer is . . .**

or

2. Say, "**Wait a minute, please. I'm thinking**" if you need more time to think.

or

3. Say, "**Please tell me again**" if you did not hear what I said.

or

4. Say, "**I don't know. I need some help answering the question**" if you don't know how to answer the question correctly.

18.8 Change the Scene to Make It G.R.E.E.N. at School: Please Answer My Question

Survey the scene below. See what the problem is. Then **change the scene** to make it **G.R.E.E.N.**

1. Circle or highlight what the teacher thought was **R.E.D.** behavior in Stacey's situation.

   Stacey: *I got into trouble with my teacher because I didn't answer her questions. She said I just sat there and did not tell her anything. She got so mad at me.*

   Stacey's brother, Bill: *Why didn't you talk to her when she asked you questions?*

   Stacey: *Well...I didn't feel like it.*

   Stacey's brother, Bill: *Did you know the answer to the question?*

   Stacey: *Yeah...I just wasn't in the mood to answer.*

2. What could Stacey do in class the next time the teacher asks her a question that she knows how to answer? (#1) ______________________________

   ____

3. What **Guiding G.R.E.E.N. Thought** could Stacey use to be more **respectful** with her teacher? Finish writing the **Guiding G.R.E.E.N. Thought** below (see the Wise Action Tool at end of Section 18.7 for help choosing what to write):

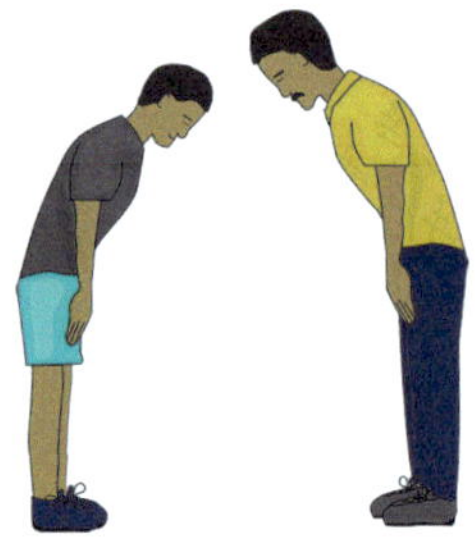

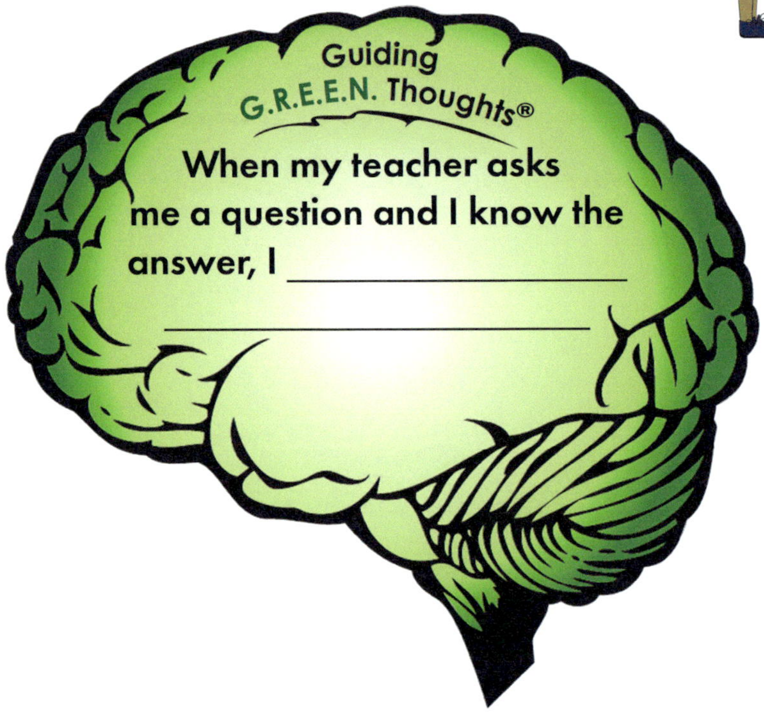

4. 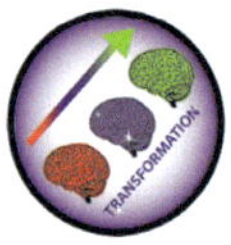 **Change the scene** and make it **G.R.E.E.N.**: Draw Stacey answering the question.

You have the **power** to help everyone in the scene act **G.R.E.E.N.!**

Draw Stacey acting **respectfully** toward her teacher.

A. Draw Stacey's teacher asking her a question.

B. Use a word bubble to write a question the teacher could be asking.

C. Use a word bubble to write what Stacey says to answer her teacher's question.

D. In the box on the right, show how you think the teacher feels when Stacey is **respectfully** answering her.

Here is Stacey's teacher asking her a question and Stacey answering right away!	This shows how Stacey's teacher feels after Stacey **respectfully** answers her.

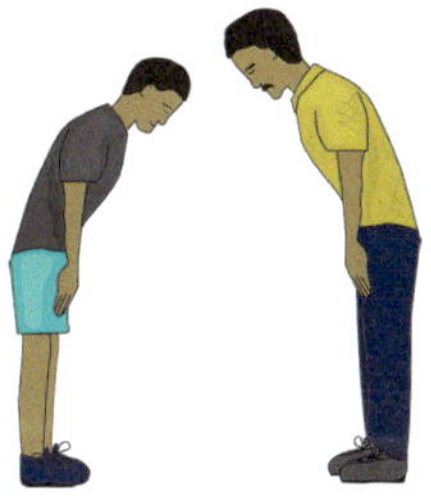

18.9 Change the Scene to Make It G.R.E.E.N. at School: Tell Me You Need More Time

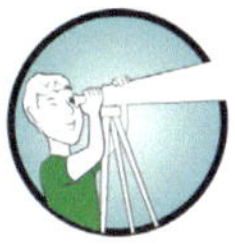

Survey the scene below to see what the problem is. Then **change the scene** to make it **G.R.E.E.N.**

1. Mark what the teacher thought was **R.E.D.** behavior in Marco's situation.

Marco: *I got into trouble with my teacher because I didn't answer her questions. She said I just sat there and did not tell her anything. She got so mad at me.*

Marco's Brother, Carlos: *Why didn't you talk to her when she asked you questions?*

Marco: *Well...I was taking my time thinking of what to say. She was asking a lot of questions and I didn't have enough time to think about all the answers.*

Marco's Brother, Carlos: *Didn't you tell her you were thinking of what to say?*

Marco: *No! I didn't know what to say. She just kept asking me more questions and wanting me to answer right away.*

2. What could Marco say to his teacher the next time he needed more time to think? (#2) ____

____

3. What **Guiding G.R.E.E.N. Thought** could Marco use to help him act more **respectfully** toward his teacher if he needs more time to think? Finish writing the **Guiding G.R.E.E.N. Thought** below (see the Wise Action Tool at the end of Section 18.7 for help with this): ________________________________

____

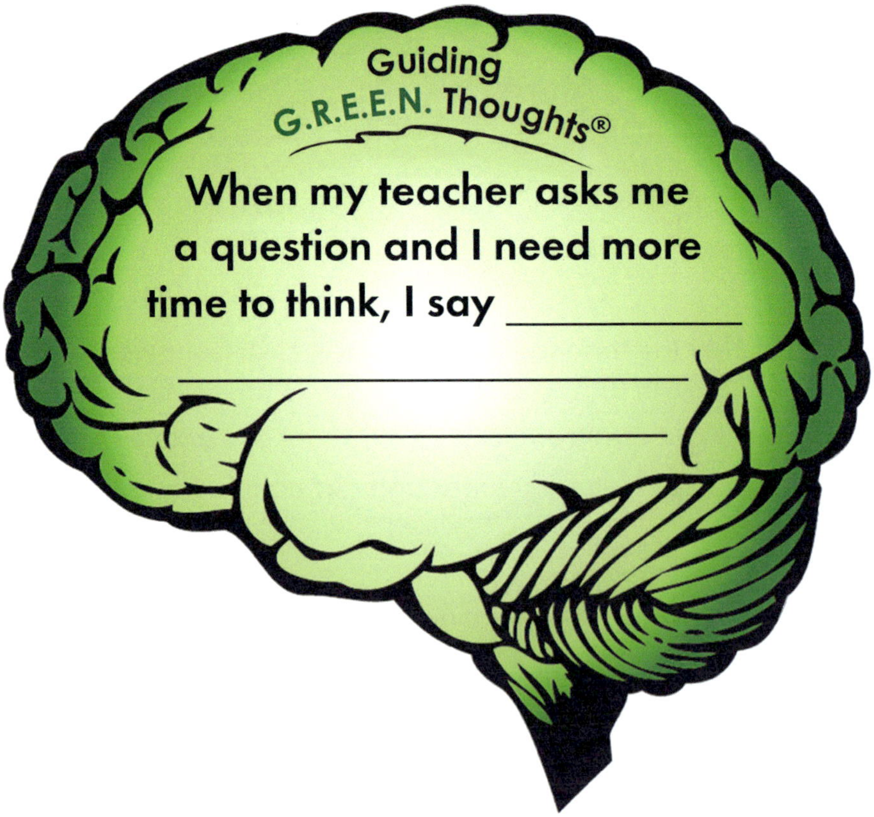

4. **Change the Scene** *and* make it **G.R.E.E.N.:** Draw Marco asking for more time to answer. You have the **power** to help everyone in the scene act **G.R.E.E.N.** Draw how Marco can act more **respectfully** toward his teacher and ask for what he needs.

   A. Draw Marco's teacher asking him questions.

   B. Use a word bubble to write what he could say to his teacher so she gives him time to think of an answer.

   C. Use a word bubble to write what his teacher could **respectfully** say back to him when he asks for what he needs. (*OK. I'll give you time to think.*)

   D. In the box on the right, show how Marco and his teacher feel when he answers the question after having time to think.

Here is Marco's teacher asking him a question and Marco **respectfully** asking for more time to think of an answer:	This shows how Marco and his teacher feel when Marco answers her question after having had time to think of his answer.

18.10 Change the Scene to Make It G.R.E.E.N. at School: Please Tell Me You Didn't Hear Me

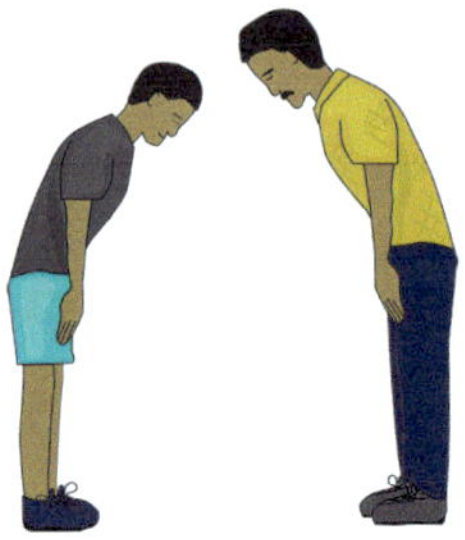

Survey the scene below to see what the problem is. Then change the scene to make it G.R.E.E.N.

1. Mark what the teacher thought was R.E.D. behavior in Albert's situation.

   Albert: *I got into trouble with my teacher because I didn't answer his questions. He said I just sat there and did not tell him anything. He got so frustrated with me!*

   Albert's friend John: *Why didn't you talk to him when he asked you questions?*

   Albert: *Well...I didn't hear the question he was asking me. I got distracted by something.*

   Albert's friend John: *Why did you just sit there and not say anything?*

   Albert: *I don't know. I thought he'd get mad at me if he found out I didn't hear him.*

2. What could Albert say to his teacher the next time he loses his attention when the teacher asks him a question? (#3) ______________________________

   ____

3. After asking a question, what do you think a teacher would find more rude?

   A. The student did not say anything.

   B. The student asked for the question to be repeated.

4. What **Guiding G.R.E.E.N. Thought** could Albert use to help him act more **respectfully** toward his teacher if he needs a question repeated? Finish writing the **Guiding G.R.E.E.N. Thought** below. (See Wise Action Tool at the end of Section 18.7)

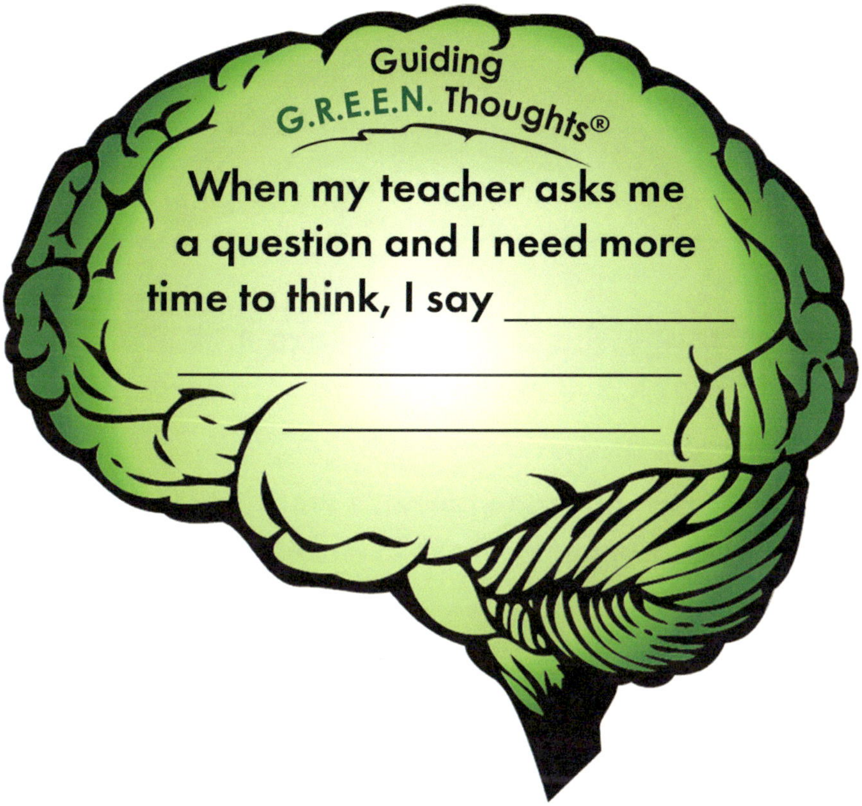

5. **Change the Scene** *and* make it **G.R.E.E.N.**: Draw Albert asking for a repeat.

   You have the **power** to help everyone in the scene act **G.R.E.E.N.** Draw how Albert can act more **respectfully** toward his teacher when he needs something repeated.

   A. Draw Albert's teacher asking him a question.

   B. Use a word bubble to write what Albert could **respectfully** say to his teacher when he needs the teacher to repeat the question.

   C. In the box on the right, use a word bubble to write what his teacher could **respectfully** say back to him after Albert **politely** asks for what he needs.

Here is Albert's teacher asking him a question and Albert **respectfully** asking for the question to be repeated:	This shows Albert's teacher **respectfully** responding to Albert's request while Albert listens carefully:

18.11 Change the Scene to Make It G.R.E.E.N. at School: Ask Me to Help You Understand

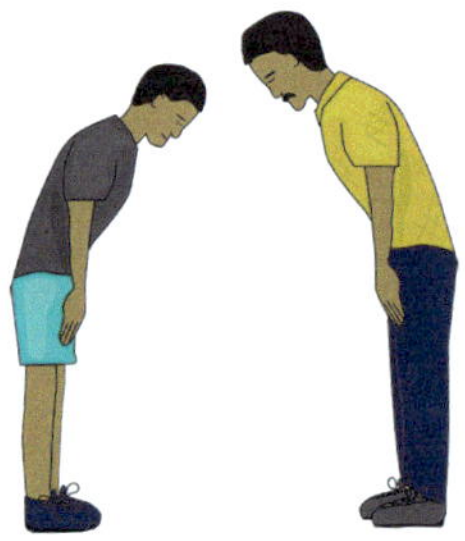

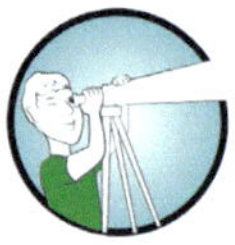

Survey the scene below to see what the problem is. Then **change the scene** to make it **G.R.E.E.N.**

1. Mark what the teacher thought was **R.E.D.** behavior in Jessica's situation?

   Jessica: *I got into trouble with my teacher because I didn't answer her questions. She said I just sat there and did not tell her anything. She got so frustrated with me.*

   Jessica's friend Taylor: *Why didn't you talk to her when she asked you a question?*

   Jessica: *Well...I didn't really understand what she was asking me because I also didn't really understand what was happening in that part of the story. She was asking me about the "motive" for the action of one character. Since I didn't know what she meant, I couldn't think of an answer!*

2. What could Jessica say to her teacher the next time she doesn't understand something the teacher is saying? ______________________________

   ____

3. After asking a question, what action do you think a teacher would think was more rude?

   A. a student asking for help understanding so they can know how to answer

   B. a student not saying anything

4. What **Guiding G.R.E.E.N. Thought** could Jessica use to help her act more respectfully toward her teacher when she needs help in understanding what is being said? Finish writing the **Guiding G.R.E.E.N. Thought** below (refer to the Wise Action Tool at the end of Section 18.7):

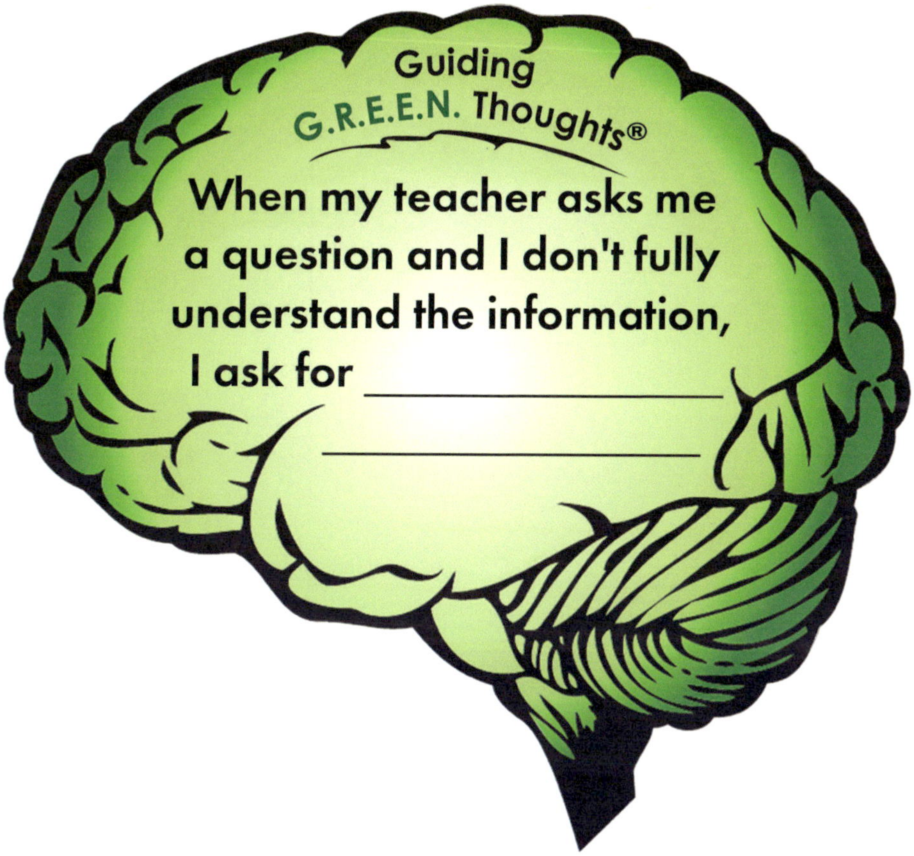

5. **Change the scene** *and* make it **G.R.E.E.N.**: Draw Jessica asking for help understanding her teacher's question.

You have the **power** to help everyone in the scene act **G.R.E.E.N.** Draw how Jessica can act more **respectfully** toward her teacher and get the help she needs.

A. Draw Jessica's teacher asking her a question.

B. Use a word bubble to write what Jessica could say to her teacher when her teacher asks her a question that she does not know how to answer.

C. In the box on the right, use a word bubble to write what her teacher could **respectfully** say back to her when Jessica **politely** asks for what she needs.

Here is Jessica's teacher asking her a question that she does not understand about the "motive" for a character's action, and Jessica **respectfully** asking for help in understanding the question.	This shows Jessica's teacher starting to help Jessica understand the question by **respectfully** asking if she understands the word "motive."

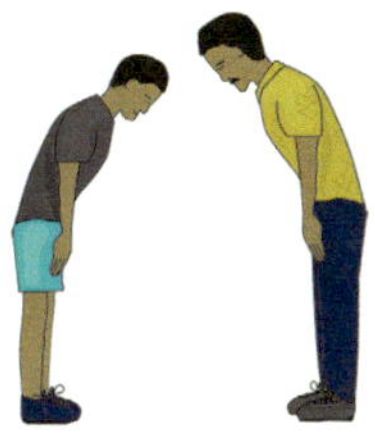

19 Respectfully Choosing Topic, Volume, and Tone of Voice

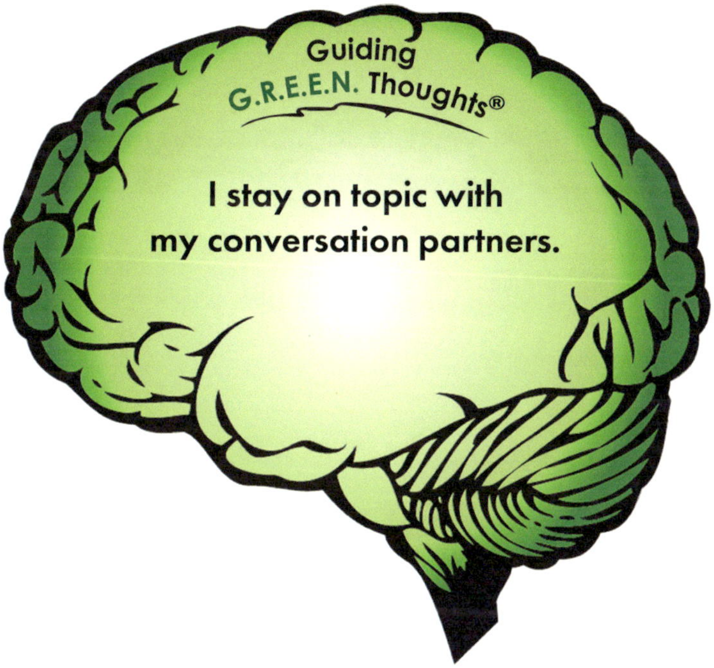

19.1 Being Respectful by Staying On-Topic

You may have a lot of things that you want to say. If you are talking to yourself, you can say all kinds of things whenever you want. But if you are talking with other people, you are on a Conversation Team with them. Your **goal** is to have a successful conversation. Everyone in the conversation takes the time to listen to one another and do their best to stay on the same topic and share ideas about that topic.

You might talk about a few topics in the same conversation. However, you and the others on your Conversation Team can work to stay on one topic together before switching to another topic together. You **take turns** talking about one topic and finish talking about that topic before moving on to a new one.

19.2 Using the On-Topic Tracker for a Respectful Conversation

You can use the **On-Topic** Tracker to help track the Conversation Team topic. This should help keep you from bouncing from one unrelated topic to another. You and your Teammates can help one another keep conversation topics related. When you ask questions and make comments about a common topic, you are acting **respectfully** toward others. If you keep getting off-topic, people may think you are not taking the conversation seriously. They might think you are acting rude.

1. Write out each topic you are talking about together with your Conversation Team.

2. If you stay on the topic when you make a comment or ask a question, you can circle that you were **on-topic**.

3. If you fall off the topic, circle off-topic.

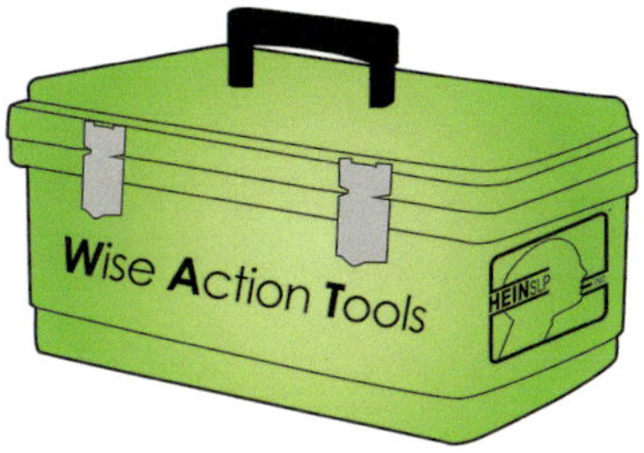

ON-TOPIC TRACKER

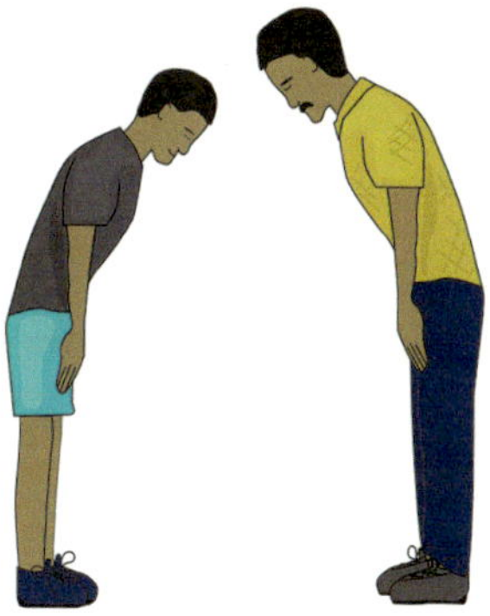

1. What is this Conversation Team Topic? ______________________________

____

2. Fill in the names of the conversation partners and check when each partner asks a question or makes a comment that relates to the Team topic. Check on the bottom if each partner stayed **on-topic** or went off-topic during this conversation.

______________________ CONVERSATION PARTNER #1	______________________ CONVERSATION PARTNER #2
____ question(s) asked about the Team topic __ __ __ __ __	____ question(s) asked about the Team topic __ __ __ __ __
____ comments made about the Team topic __ __ __ __ __	____ comments made about the Team topic __ __ __ __ __
ON-TOPIC OFF-TOPIC	ON-TOPIC OFF-TOPIC

3. Did both conversation partners stay **on-topic**? yes no

4. After both conversation partners have stayed **on-topic** about one topic, they can start to have another **on-topic** conversation about a different topic.

19.3 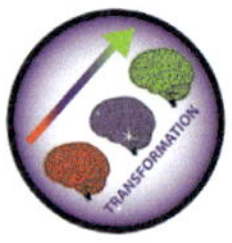 Change the Scene to Make It G.R.E.E.N.!: Help Julia Be On-Topic

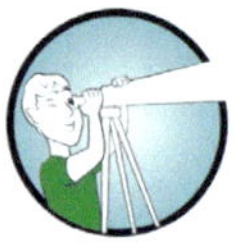

Survey this scene to see if Julia is talking about the same topic as everyone else.

Julia's uncle comes to speak to her class about being a veterinarian. While he is talking to the class, Julia asks him if he will drive her home after school.

1. What is the topic? ____________________

2. What is Julia talking about? ____________________

   ____

3. Circle whether Julia is **on-topic** or off-topic.

   on-topic off-topic

4. Circle what you think Julia's uncle and Julia's classmates think about Julia's action.

   A. It was **polite**.

   B. It was rude.

5. What would have been a **better** time for Julia to ask her question? ____________________

   ____

19.4 Being Respectful by Talking about Someone Else's Preferred Topic

It is often easier to talk about what we would like to talk about more than what someone else would prefer to talk about. However, it is an important skill to learn to talk about someone else's preferred topic because it shows we care about other people on our Team instead of only ourselves.

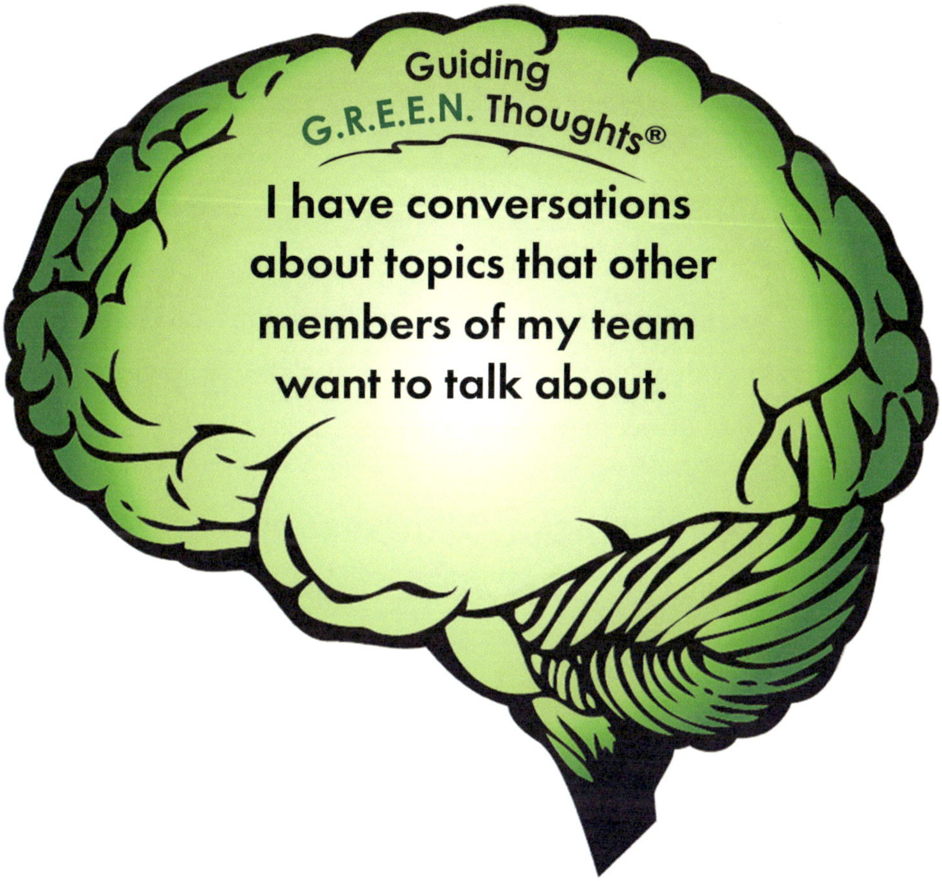

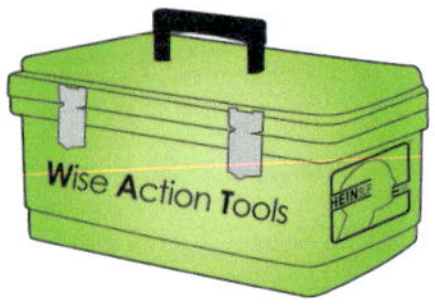

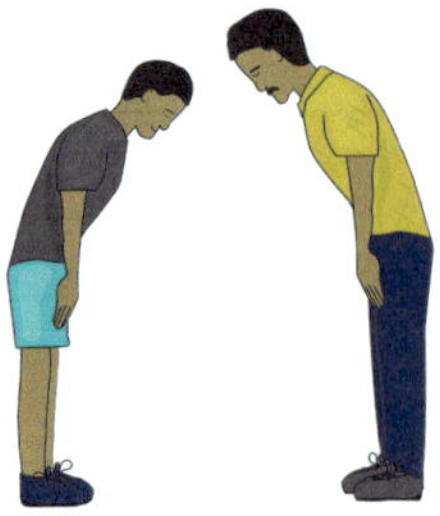

TAKE THE CONVERSATION POWER CHALLENGE!

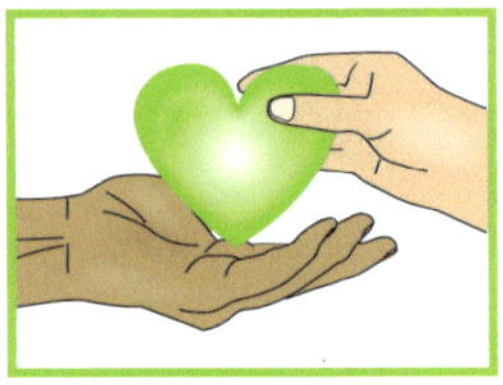

1. TALK ABOUT A TOPIC THAT YOUR CONVERSATION PARTNER LIKES TO TALK ABOUT—Challenge yourself to show that you **care** enough about someone else on one of your Teams by having a conversation with that person about a topic that is important to them. It may be a challenge for you because that topic may be one that has nothing to do with your own activities or interests.

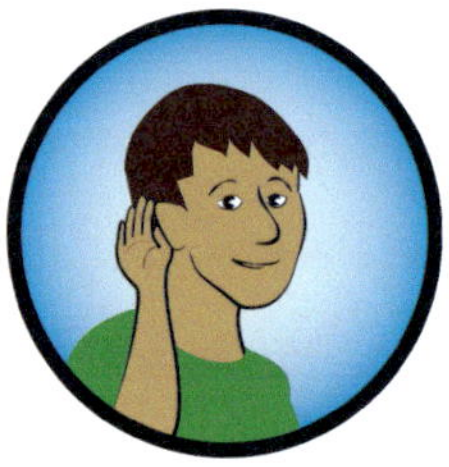

2. LISTEN—Carefully listen to what the other person is talking about so you can know what the topic is. "Capture" a detail or two that you can ask about when it is your turn. By doing your best to use your **power** to concentrate on the other person's topic, you are showing that you **care** about him or her.

3. MAKE COMMENTS AND ASK QUESTIONS—Show the other person you are **respectful** and **cooperative** by making comments and asking questions about something the other person said.

4. KEEP TRACK OF THE TOPICS THAT THE OTHER PERSON LIKES TO TALK ABOUT SO YOU CAN INITIATE CONVERSATIONS ABOUT THAT TOPIC!—You can use the **CARING CONVERSATION UPDATE SHEET** for each Team member with whom you will be having conversations. By continuing to add to this sheet you will have an updated log that will help you remember the different topics that your conversation partner thinks are important. By initiating asking about these topics, it will show your conversation partner that you care enough to remember what is interesting and important to them.

The more you practice having these conversations, the easier it will be to show your growing conversation **power**.

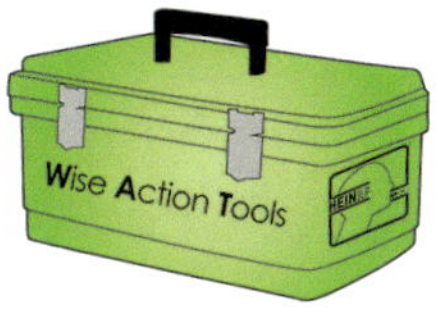

BUILDING MY CONVERSATION POWER BY PAYING ATTENTION, ASKING QUESTIONS & TAKING NOTES

1A. I AM TALKING TO ______________________________ Date ____________________

1B. I CHOOSE A TOPIC: This is a topic that I think this person would like to talk about today: ________

____

2. I ASK A QUESTION: I ask a question to learn something new about the topic:

   How is ____?

   or *Tell me what's new with* ____

3. I LISTEN AND TAKE NOTES: I use my **power** to listen carefully and write down an important detail about what was said: ____

   ____

4. I MAKE A COMMENT: (*Wow! That's interesting! That's great! Sounds good! Too bad.)* ______

   ____

5. I ASK A RELATED QUESTION: I ask another question about what the person just said:

   How do you feel about ____?

   Can you tell me more about ____?

   What ________________? *Where* __________________? *Why* __________________?

6. I LISTEN AND TAKE NOTES: I use my **power** to listen carefully and write down an important detail about what was said: ____

   ____

7. I MAKE A FINAL COMMENT THAT SHOWS I WAS LISTENING TO WHAT THE PERSON SAID:

   I politely end the conversation by saying one or more of the following:

   That's very interesting! Thanks for telling me about ______________________________

   I'm glad that ____

   or *I'm sorry that* ____

   and *I hope that* ____

(When we are done talking, I can draw a detailed picture to help me remember what my conversation partner said about this topic.)

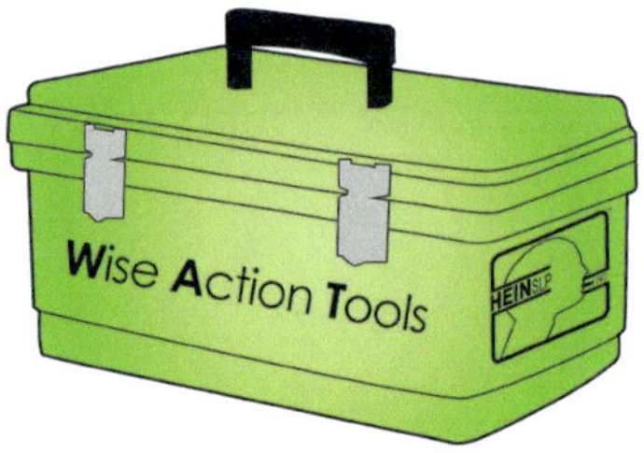

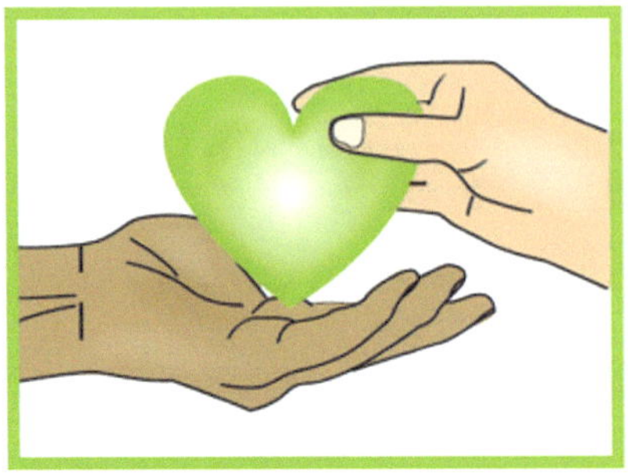

TOPICS FOR CARING CONVERSATIONS

I care about these people, so I keep track of the topics they care about. I can show I care by talking about these topics in my conversations with them.

Person I Care About	This Person Cares About These Topics

VOICE VOLUME CHART

WAY TOO LOUD!!!
MEDIUM LOUD
A LITTLE TOO LOUD
Just Right For The Room & The People
A little too soft
much too soft to be heard
I can't hear you!!

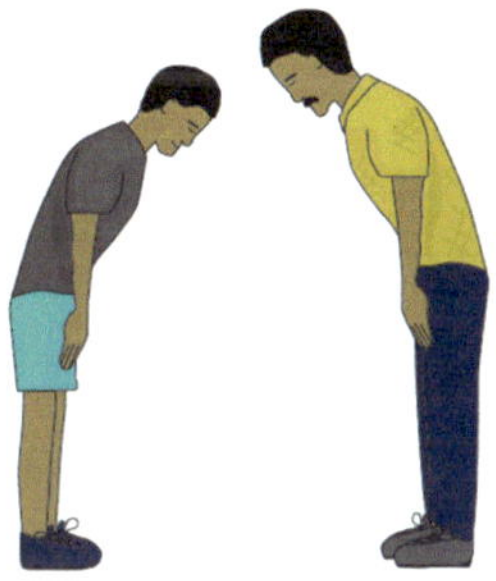

19.5 Why Choose the Best Voice Volume for Each Scene?

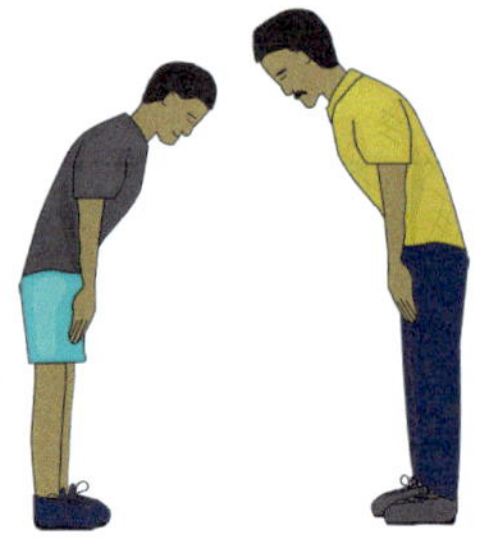

It is **respectful** to choose the best voice volume to match the scene.

If your voice is too loud, other people may think you are shouting at them. It is good to avoid shouting at other people.

On the other hand, if your voice is too soft, people will need to work hard to hear you. They might think you *don't* care whether they hear you.

It is not always easy to use a voice volume that is just right for the room and the people. Sometimes practice is needed to use a voice volume that is not too loud and not too soft.

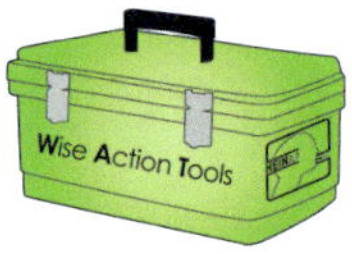

VOICE VOLUME CHART

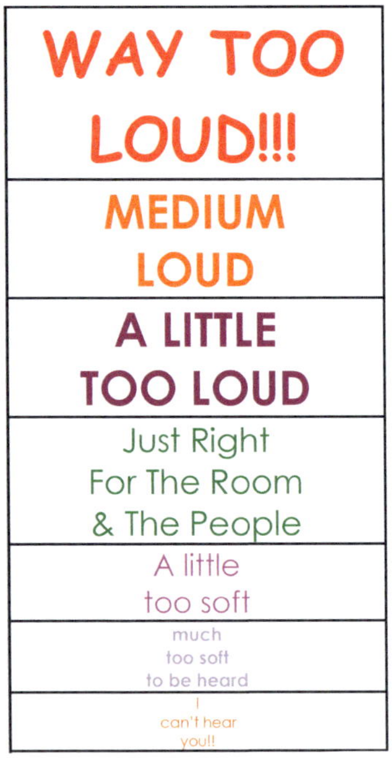

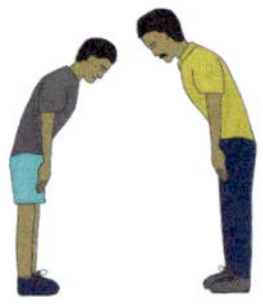

Growing G.R.E.E.N. InterActions HeinSLP, Inc. www.heinslpinc.com

19.6 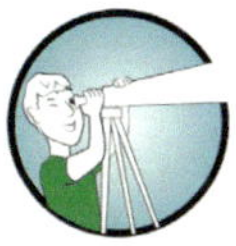 Survey the Scene: What Is the Best Voice Volume for This Situation? 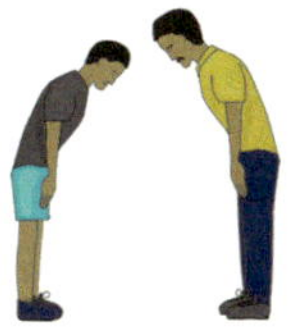

Survey the scene to see who else is with you and what they are doing. That helps you choose the volume you should use for your voice. You then can speak loudly or softly or somewhere in the middle so your voice volume matches the scene.

Circle how you should be controlling your voice when you are talking in these different situations.

1. In the classroom, asking a question while everyone is quietly working on their own assignments or projects.

   louder than usual　　　　softer than usual

2. In the classroom, when I have been asked to get in front of the class to share something I wrote.

   louder than usual　　　　softer than usual

3. At home, talking to my friend while another family member is sleeping in the next room.

   louder than usual　　　　softer than usual

4. At home, talking to my father who is on the other side of the yard.

   louder than usual　　　　softer than usual

5. In a quiet restaurant, talking to the person sitting next to me.

   louder than usual　　　　softer than usual

Practice using the best voice volume in situations such as those above. Check how you are doing by asking someone from your Team if your voice volume is just right or if you need to speak louder or softer.

19.7 Guiding G.R.E.E.N. Thoughts for a Respectful Tone of Voice

Having a **respectful** tone of voice is sometimes the hardest thing to work on, but it is one of the most important skills to learn. If you can learn to speak with a **respectful** tone of voice, you will discover many **positive** consequences. People will **respect** you more and will be glad to spend time being with you.

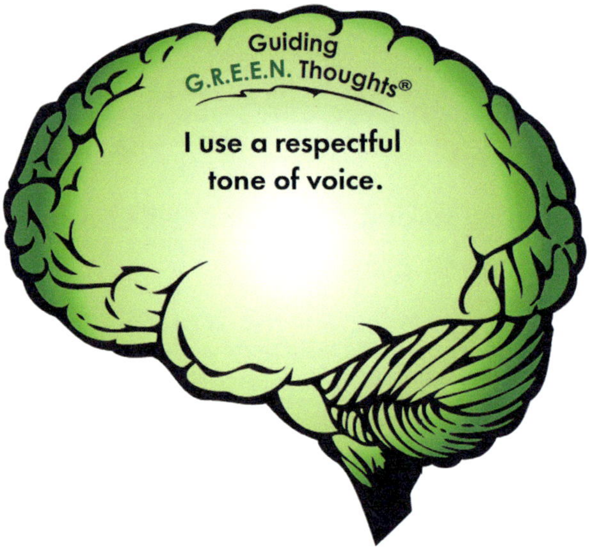

What is a **respectful** tone of voice?

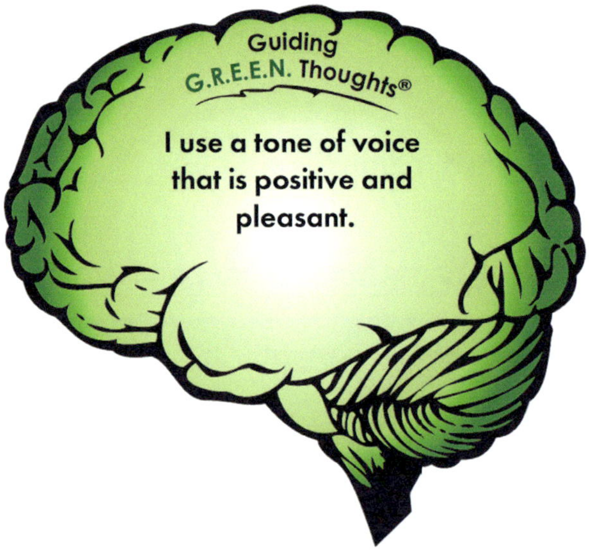

1. A **respectful** tone of voice is **positive** and **pleasant**.

   It is *not* negative, angry, annoyed, or irritated. Even if you feel like that on the "inside," it is best to have a neutral tone of voice on the "outside" so the other person can hear your words instead of just getting annoyed, irritated, or angry back at you!

Coach yourself to have as **positive** an attitude as you can about what the other person is saying to help you have a **respectful** tone of voice.

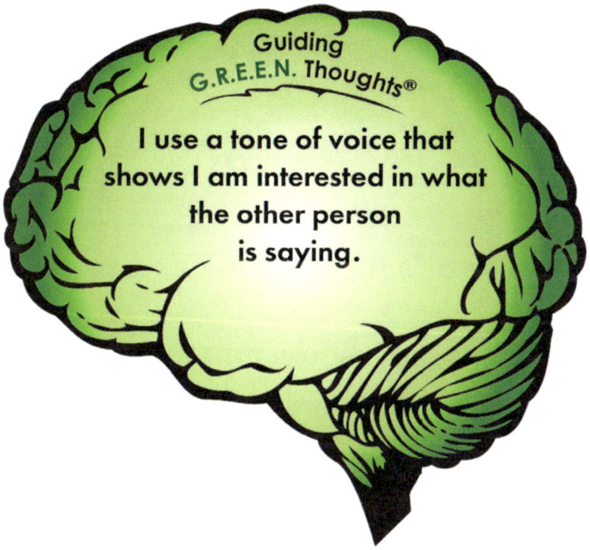

2. A **respectful** tone of voice shows you are **interested** in what the other person is saying. It is not showing you are bored.

   Coach yourself to **care** about what the other person is saying and it will help you have an **interested**, **respectful** tone of voice.

3. A **respectful** tone of voice is **sincere** and **truthful**.

   It is usually not joking or sarcastic, unless you know that the other person wants to act in a joking way, too.

   Coach yourself to be as **truthful** as you can about what you are saying. Show that your own words really matter by making them as **true** as possible.

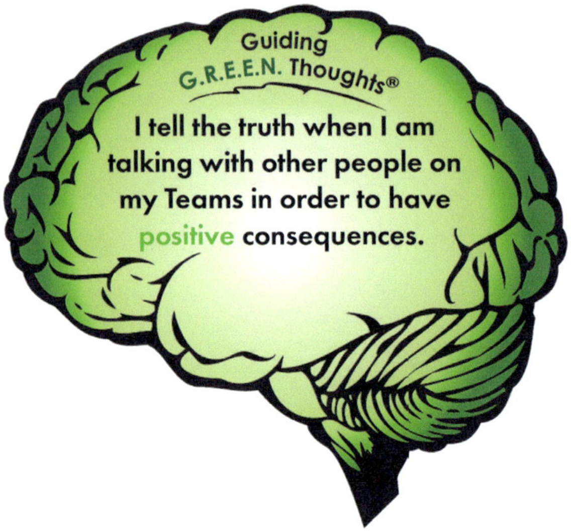

19.8 Telling the Truth Leads to Positive Consequences

We often are asked to talk about what we have been doing. When we are talking about our activities, it is important that we tell a **truthful** story.

Why should we tell a **truthful** story?

Telling the truth is one way to be **respectful** to our conversation partners. They expect us to **tell the truth** because it shows that we **care** about them. If they learn that we are *not* **telling the truth**, they will *not* **trust** and **respect** us. They will think that we are *not* ***showing good character*** in what we say and do. When people lose trust in us, they will *not* believe we will do what we say we are going to do. Our words will *not* mean much. It will be much harder to accomplish any of our **Common Team Goals** together.

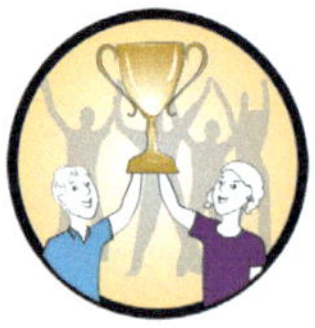

When we are part of a Team we should always **tell truthful stories** about what we have been doing. When we **tell the truth**, we can move together toward a **better** scene for the whole Team.

When we think about other people's characters, we describe what we think and feel about them. Do we feel safe with them? Do we think they can take responsibility for their actions? Do we trust them to be a good Team member? Do we trust that they **care** about us enough to **tell the truth**? Do we think they are working toward the Common Team Goal with us? Or are they only working on their own Personal Goals without caring how they might affect us?

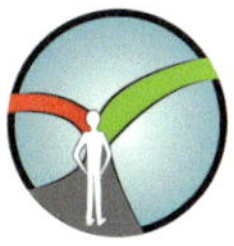

So the next time you are asked a question or telling someone a story, Think First! Consider whether you would like to be respected for having good character and telling the truth. Make the positive choice for yourself, your character, and your Team.

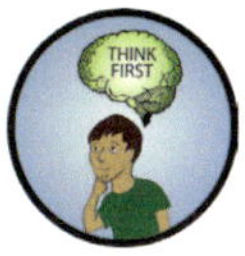

Reach for **Guiding G.R.E.E.N. Thoughts®** that remind you to make the best choice to **tell the truth** so you can have your **best life.**

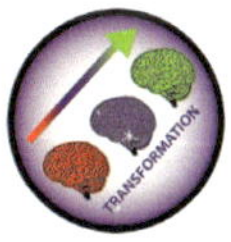

19.9 Change the Scene to Make It G.R.E.E.N.: Help Charlie Ask Politely Instead of Demand

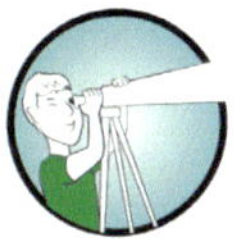

Survey this scene to see if Charlie is on the same topic as his mother. Also, see if he is **asking politely** for something or if he is demanding that his mother do something. See if he is forcing her to do something without asking if it is OK for her to do it.

Charlie's mother: *Charlie, please help your sister set the table for dinner.*

Charlie (answering in a demanding tone of voice): *I want to go get a new Nerf gun. Let's go right now!*

Charlie starts walking to the front door.

1. What is the topic that Charlie's mother is talking about? ____________________

   ____

2. What is Charlie talking about? ____

3. Circle whether Charlie is **on-topic** or off-topic.

   on-topic off-topic

4. Circle what you think Charlie's mother will think about words and action.

Charlie is acting **politely**

Charlie is acting rudely

5. What would have been a better time for Charlie to talk about getting a Nerf gun? ____

____

6. What do you think is a **better** way for Charlie to get a new Nerf gun?

A. Demand that his mother get him one.

B. Do what his mother is asking him to do now and then find another time to **ask politely** if he can get a new Nerf gun.

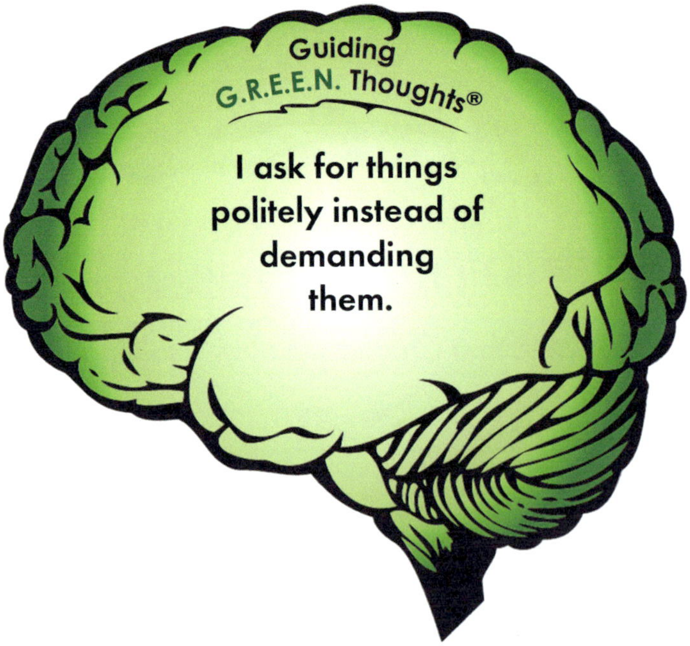

19.10 Survey the Scene: Can You Tell the Difference Between Politely Asking and Demanding?

Read the statements and questions below and circle whether you think the person who is speaking is politely asking for something or demanding it.

1. *I want that now!*

   politely asking   demanding

2. *Could we get it when you have the time?*

   politely asking   demanding

3. *Give it to me!*

   politely asking   demanding

4. *Could I have it please?*

   politely asking   demanding

5. *Come here right now!*

   politely asking   demanding

6. *Could you please come over here when you can? I need some help.*

   politely asking   demanding

19.11 Should I Be Serious or Funny in This Conversation?

When you are in a conversation, it is important to think about why you are talking to the other person. If you think about why you are talking to that other person, it helps your conversation stay on track. Are you trying to get something done and figure something out together, or are you trying to entertain each other?

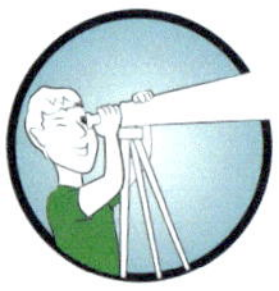

Survey the scene. Think about what you and the other person are trying to do right now.

Is It Time to Be Serious?

- Are you trying to be serious and get something done?
- Are you trying to learn something?
- Are you both trying to explain your ideas and points of view?

If you answered yes, then it is time to be serious. Stay on the serious topic and choose your best words and say them in a serious, **truthful** tone of voice without any joking.

Is It Time to Be Funny?

- Is it time to relax and be funny?
- Is it a break time and time to relax?
- Do you and the other person feel like joking together?

If you answered yes, then it is time to be funny. It is OK to tell jokes as long as the jokes *don't* hurt the other person's feelings.

It is important to remember that you need to pay attention to pick up clues to know if it is time to stop joking and **switch** to being more serious. This would be a time when you can use your **self-control**!

19.12 Read and Discuss: Sincere and Serious, or Sarcastic?

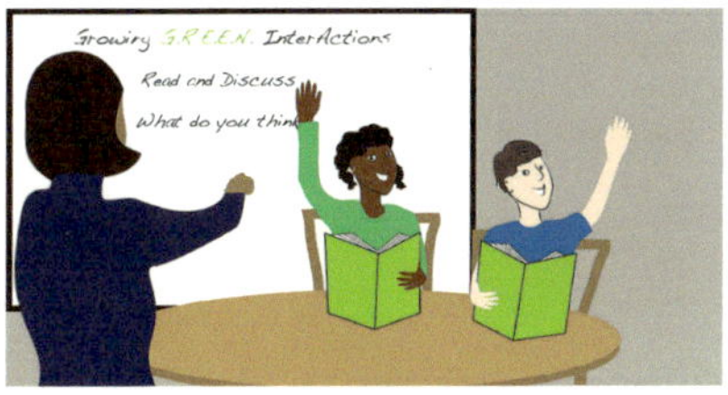

Are you using **truthful**, **helpful**, and **sincere** words, or are you saying words in a sarcastic tone of voice? When you are sarcastic, you say the opposite of what your words really mean. It is much easier to be **respectful** and **helpful** with others on your Teams if you *avoid* being sarcastic. If you are sarcastic, you are often not being **helpful** and are possibly making the other person feel confused or unsupported.

Being sarcastic confuses the other person because they don't know if you are **truthful** about what you are saying, or if you kidding, or if you are trying to being hurtful.

1. Do you prefer people being **sincere** and serious with you, or sarcastic? ____

   ____

   People get confused when other people are sarcastic with them because they are not sure what was really meant by the words that were said. Often when people are sarcastic, they then say, "only kidding." However, it is often too late because they may have already made the other person feel worse. You want to **support** the people on your Teams by letting them know you are on their side and are making choices to help them. If you are joking and being sarcastic, you might be hurting their feelings, so it is usually **better** to choose to act **sincerely** and **seriously**.

   If someone is sarcastic with you, you can hope that the other person is *not* trying to hurt your feelings on purpose. If a person is truly being mean, that is not funny. However, if the other person is just trying to be funny, you can learn to see how it is funny from that person's perspective and not get upset by what was said. It is a way to cope with the words that others say so that we can stay calm. You can learn to **navigate** successfully with a person who likes to be sarcastic with you.

2. Are you able to **navigate** the situation if someone says something sarcastic to you? What strategy do you use? ______________________________

   ____

19.13 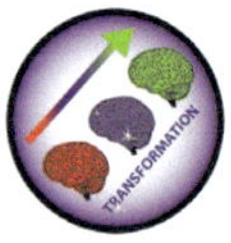 Change the Scene: What Can Be Said Instead of Sarcastic Words?

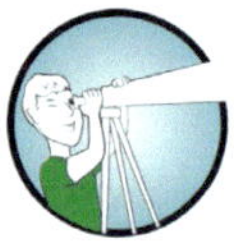

Survey the following scenes to find where Person A is using sarcastic words. Underline the sarcastic words in red. Decide if Person A is being **helpful** or hurtful to the other person, Person B. What can person A say to be even more **helpful** to Person B?

1. 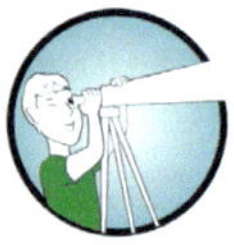 Tom was asked to help pass out the snacks in class even though his teacher knew he was occasionally clumsy. His teacher wanted him to have a turn passing out the peanut butter sandwiches because she knew how much he loved to help out.

   When he got to Peter's desk, Tom accidentally dropped the plate of sandwiches.

   Peter said, "Boy, you sure are talented!" Tom was embarrassed about dropping the snacks and was also confused about what Peter was really saying.

   A. Who is being sarcastic Person A? ______________________________

   B. Who is Person B? ______________________________

   C. 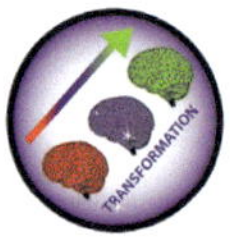 What can Person A say or do to be more **helpful** and **kind** to Person B? ______________________________

   ____

2. 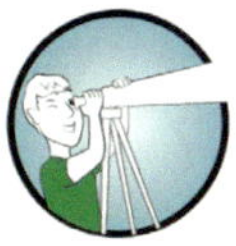

Bill was really thirsty. He asked his teacher to go to the water fountain. His teacher said he could go get a drink. Mark was already at the water fountain taking his own turn getting a drink. Bill, who was feeling as patient as a lit firecracker, said sarcastically to Mark, "I really love waiting for you. It is my favorite thing to do in the whole world." Mark was confused about what Bill was really saying and kept drinking.

A. Who is being sarcastic Person A? ______________________________

B. Who is Person B? ______________________________

C. 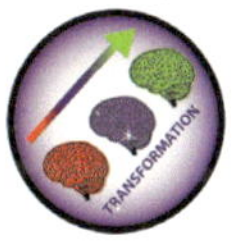

What can Person A say or do to be more **helpful** and **kind** to Person B? ______________________________

____

3. 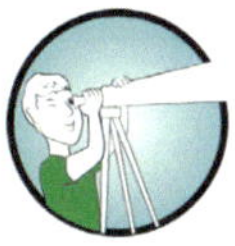

Ben Blake's older brother, Peter, was a great basketball player because he got to practice shooting hoops a lot with their father before Mr. Blake hurt his back two years ago in an accident. Unfortunately, Ben was not as lucky to have their dad practice with him after he got hurt. Ben wishes that Peter would teach him what he knows so he can learn to shoot hoops better. However, when Peter sees Ben trying to shoot baskets, he says, "Wow! You're so good at shooting for the moon!" Every time Peter says this, it makes Ben want to stop trying to shoot hoops.

A. Who is being sarcastic Person A? ______________________________

B. Who is Person B? ______________________________

C. 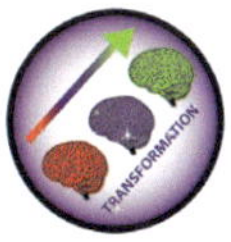

What can Person A say or do to be more **helpful** and **kind** to Person B? ______________________________

____

4. 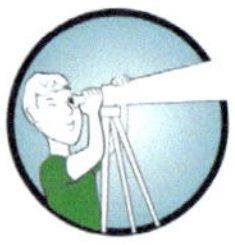 Bob was supposed to figure out how to answer the questions that the teacher had written on the board. He was really frustrated that he did not know how to answer the questions, but he blurted out loud to his teacher, Mrs. Garcia, "Why don't you ask harder questions?" The teacher ignored him because she thought the questions were hard enough and thought she should only answer his question when he was being **respectful** and raised his hand.

A. Who is being sarcastic Person A? ______________________________

B. Who is Person B? ______________________________

C. 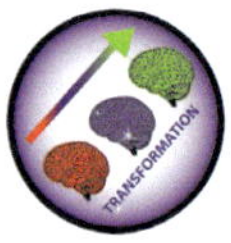

What can Person A say or do to be more **helpful** and **kind** to Person B while also requesting the help he needs? ____________

____

5. 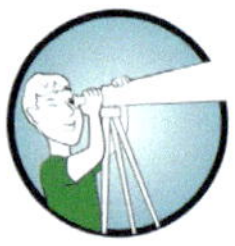 Scott and Kevin were playing chess. Kevin was a little nervous playing with Scott because Scott had a reputation for being a great chess player. Kevin had to really think about what moves to make so he would not have his chess pieces taken by Scott. During one of Kevin's turns, when he was really thinking about which move to make, Scott said, "Why don't you take all day? I have nothing better to do!"

A. Who is being sarcastic Person A? ______________________________

B. Who is Person B? ______________________________

C. 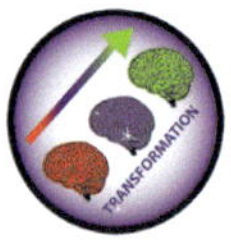

What can Person A say or do to be more **helpful** and **kind** to Person B? ______________________________

____

6. 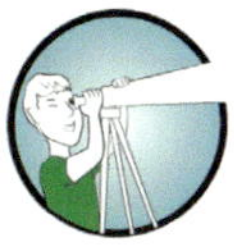 Tanika was at her cousin's birthday party. She was enjoying eating raspberry-frosted chocolate cake when her older sister, Monique, came to get her to bring her in the other room for a family photo. When Tanika heard she was going to be in a picture, she asked Monique, "How do I look?" Monique saw that Tanika had frosting in a couple of places on her face, but she said, "Your face is just perfect!" Tanika ran into the other room, ready to take her perfect picture, without cleaning her face.

   A. Who is being sarcastic Person A? ______________________

   B. Who is Person B?

   C. 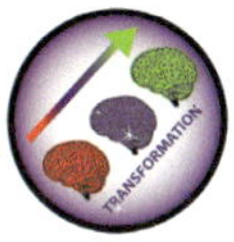

   What can Person A say or do to be more **helpful** and **kind** to Person B? ______________________

Possible answers to the questions in this section:

1. Ask, "Would you like some help picking those up?"

2. Just be patient and wait

3. Ask, "Would you like me to show you how to get better at shooting hoops?"

4. Raise his hand and ask for help in understanding the questions

5. Just be patient and wait quietly

6. Let her sister know she might want to clean her face with a napkin and get her one.

19.14 Quick G.R.E.E.N. Scenes: Practice Speaking Respectfully

Let's practice speaking **respectfully** by using a **G.R.E.E.N.** tone of voice when saying these **G.R.E.E.N.** action sentences.

Directions: Read the sentences below with a respectful tone of voice. People on your Team can let you know if you read each one with a G.R.E.E.N. tone of voice by giving you a thumbs up. See how many sentences you can read respectfully.

Use the clapboard when you are ready to start reading: Quiet on the set. Action!

1. I make the best choices for my Team when I am **thoughtful**.
2. I have the best conversations when I am **on-topic** with my conversation partners.
3. I support others when I am **kind**.
4. My Team can meet its **goals** when I am **helpful**.
5. I get along with others when I act **friendly**.
6. People appreciate being with me when I am **polite**.
7. I help my Team move forward when I am **positive**.
8. People feel better when my tone of voice is **caring**.
9. People can trust what I am saying when my tone of voice is **sincere**.

Total: How many sentences did you read with a **respectful** tone of voice? _______

Pick your two favorite sentences and practice saying them until you have them in your memory!!

19.15 Quick G.R.E.E.N. Scenes: Practice Answering Respectfully

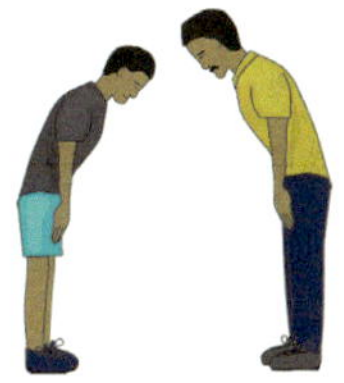

My name ________________________ Date ________________

In these Quick G.R.E.E.N. Scenes you get to practice using a respectful voice when you answer a question. You will get to tell the definitions of important G.R.E.E.N. words.

Directions: The **G.R.E.E.N.** Scene Director will ask what a word means. You read the answer and tell the definition of the word with a **respectful** tone of voice. The other people on the set can let you know if your tone of voice was **respectful** by giving you a **thumbs up** when they hear it. You will get a **positive** plus mark (+) if you were able to answer each question with **respectful** tone of voice. See if you can answer at least three questions with a **respectful** tone of voice. Follow the same procedure as in other Quick **G.R.E.E.N.** Scenes by having the Scene Director get the clapboard, and say when you are ready: "Quiet on the Set. Take One. Action!" You and the Scene Director should decide how many questions you expect to answer for each "take." You can have another chance to act in this Quick **G.R.E.E.N.** Scene if you want to get more plus marks by answering in a more **respectful** way or by answering more questions.

1. **What does it mean to act in a respectful way?**

   ___ *When you act in a **respectful** way, you are being **polite** and **considerate** of others.*

2. **What does it mean to be polite?**

   ___ *When you are **polite**, you are showing that you **respect** the other person by your words and actions. You are not being rude.*

3. **What does it mean to be kind?**

   ___ *When you are **kind**, you are acting in a **considerate** and **helpful** way.*

4. What does it mean to act in a positive way?

   ___ *When you act in a* ***positive*** *way, you are speaking and acting in a way to help things get* ***better****.*

5. What does it mean to act in a sincere way?

   ___ *When you act in a* ***sincere*** *way, you are being* ***honest*** *and* ***truthful*** *in what you say.*

Write the number of **positive** plus (+) marks you received during this "take."

____

19.16 Quick G.R.E.E.N. Scenes: Responding with G.R.E.E.N. Words and a G.R.E.E.N. Tone of Voice

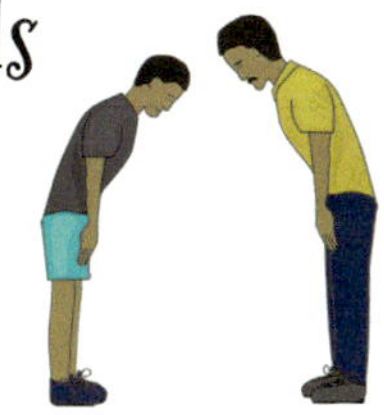

Directions: Listen to your conversation partner, then do your best to respond with respectful, G.R.E.E.N. words and a respectful, G.R.E.E.N. tone of voice. Your scene partner will let you know if your words were G.R.E.E.N. and if you sounded G.R.E.E.N. by circling the green positive plus (+) after each scene. You get two plus (+) marks for providing two responses in Quick G.R.E.E.N. Scene #3. See if you can get all five positive plus marks (+) for this set of Quick G.R.E.E.N. Scenes. (Follow the same script for using the clapboard that you find in section 19.14.)

1. Greeting people and having very simple conversations:

   A. 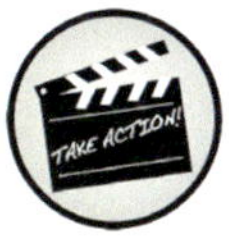

   Person A: *Hi! How are you?*

   B. Person B: *I'm ________________. How are you?* (+) G.R.E.E.N. tone

2. Asking for important information:

   A. 

   We are going to have an important game on Saturday, so make sure you get to the practice at the park on time today.

   B. *Excuse me. Could you please remind me what time practice is starting today?* (+) G.R.E.E.N. *tone*

3. Communicating that we care about the other person (in an empathetic, supportive tone of voice):

   A. 

   Person A: Last night, when my Dad was bringing in some heavy boxes from his car, Buster, our dog, got out the front gate and ran away. He didn't come back by the time I left for school this morning.

B. **Person B:** I'm sorry that ____
+ **G.R.E.E.N.** tone

I hope that ____
+ **G.R.E.E.N.** tone

4. Saying goodbye:

A. 

Person A: *It's good having you on the Team. Well, I must go. See you next time.*

B. *Person B:* ____
(Thank you! It's great being on this Team. See you next time!)

Date of this Quick G.R.E.E.N. Scene Exercise: ____________________

The role of Person A was played by: ____________________

The role of Person B was played by: ____________________

First take: The total number of (+) G.R.E.E.N. responses made by Person B with G.R.E.E.N. words AND a G.R.E.E.N. tone of voice

________/5

Second take: If there was a second take on this date, this was the second total number of (+) G.R.E.E.N. responses made by Person B with G.R.E.E.N. words AND a G.R.E.E.N. tone of voice.

________/5

If not all of my responses were G.R.E.E.N., I can always get better with practice. If I act out these Quick G.R.E.E.N. Scenes again, this will be my total score:

________/5

HEIN CONVERSATIONAL RATING SCALE

I have to think about:

- my choice of topic and if it is appropriate for my audience
- my choice of words and if they are appropriate for my audience
- my tone of voice
- my audience
- how much humor/teasing I can safely use with my audience and still be taken seriously when needed

G = General Audiences—What I say would be OK with Grandma or the school principal. I am on topic and am not saying anything odd, strange, mean, disgusting, or violent. No swear words are used at all. I get a lot of social points for being able to control my topic and my words. I am considered mature.

PG = Possible Guidance needed—What I want to say may be slightly funny or sarcastic. I need to know if my audience will appreciate my topic and words without my losing social points. With this style, I might be considered immature.

R = Restricted—The topic and word choice would offend most people. I can use this language only at special times with people who would appreciate my odd, strange, mean, disgusting, or violent topics. If I use this language in class or public, I will get in trouble and lose many social points. People will not trust that I can control myself and I will lose privileges and responsibilities. I should avoid saying things that are really off topic because people will consider them R-rated and will not want to have conversations with me in the future.

X = eXtremely Limited—These topics and words are so inappropriate, strange, odd, violent, disgusting, or mean that they really should not be said out loud. I should limit even thinking about these topics or words. Most people will be extremely offended, upset, or worried if they hear these words or topics, and I will get in serious trouble and lose all my social points.

19.17 Read and Discuss: Hein Conversational Rating Scale

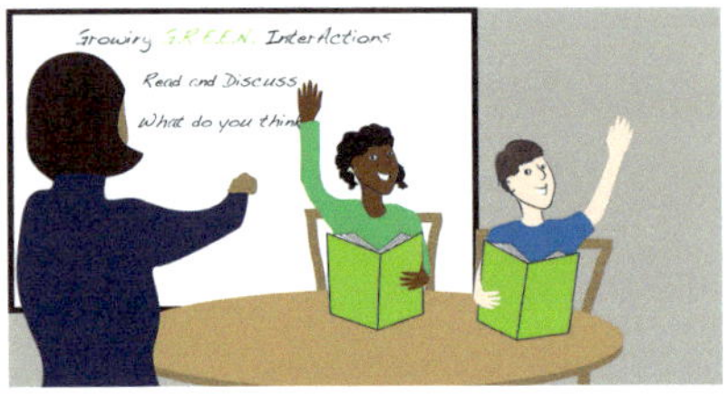

The Hein Conversation Rating Scale can be used to help Team members remind themselves and others about what to think about when choosing what to say. **Surveying the scene** is important so you can see who else is with you and know what topics to choose and what tone of voice or humor to use. In order to be certain that others will think you are acting **respectfully**, it is useful to practice having **G**-Rated conversations. You will not offend anyone or lose any social points if others can rate your conversation as "**G**."

It is useful to practice having "**G**"-Rated conversations with others. It means you are practicing having control over yourself. You are making sure to use words that help you **connect** with whoever is in the same scene at that moment. In order to get people to trust you and give you more responsibility in the jobs you are asked to do, it is necessary to learn to control your topics, words, and tone of voice. The more you practice this **self-control**, the easier it gets to do the next time and the next.

Some people use swear words without even thinking about whether they are offending people who do not like to hear those words. If you want to grow in your ability to build relationships with others, work to control your use of swear words or any other words that may offend others. You can make believe that these people are your customers and you would want them to feel comfortable in your store and come to your store again and again. If you can control yourself to have G-rated conversation, it is an important step toward being successful in any job or any relationship.

Answer the following questions:

1. If someone **politely** gives you feedback that your conversational rating has not been at the "**G**" level, and that person would like you to be speaking at a "**G**" level, could you accept the feedback and **switch** to a "**G**" level of conversation?

yes no

2. In your own life, in what situations do you think it is important to have "G"-Rated conversations? ____

   ____

3. Name three jobs you might like to have where it would be important to always have a "G" rating in your conversation.

   ____

   ____

4. Share an experience where you had **self-control** so that others considered you more mature, trustworthy, and responsible. ______________________

   ____

   ____

19.18 Change the Scene and Make It G.R.E.E.N.: Help Mark Be Respectful and Responsible

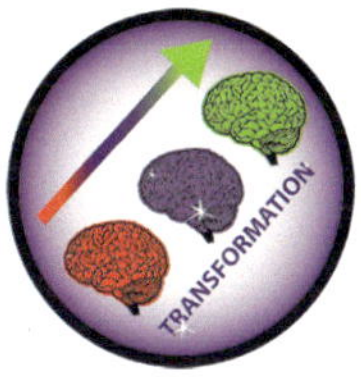

Mark's dad asked him to watch his younger brother, Scott, for a couple of hours while he went to a meeting. Mark's dad reminded Mark to make sure to avoid swearing in front of Scott so that Scott didn't get in trouble using the same words at school. He also asked if Mark could feed their dog, Ralph. Mark said he would be a good role model for his brother and would be responsible for feeding the dog.

Mark's dad left for his meeting. Mark sat in the living room and called his friend Lance. Scott was playing with his Legos on the floor in front of him. When he was on the phone, Scott talked about something that happened over the weekend and used swear words to tell how he felt about it. He also talked about an assignment that a teacher gave him and used swear words when describing the assignment. Mark talked on the phone the whole time that his dad was gone.

When Mark's dad came home, Mark ended his phone call. Mark's dad asked if Ralph had been fed. Mark realized he forgot what he was supposed to do, but answered, "No, what's the big deal, he's only a dog."

Scott came over to greet his father and told him something that he heard his older brother, Mark, say on the phone. Scott included some swear words that he heard his brother say.

Mark's disappointed dad said, "I thought I asked you not to use those kinds of words in front of your brother!"

Mark replied, "Well, he shouldn't have been listening to my conversation. Can't I have some privacy in this house?"

1. Is Mark saying it is OK to forget feeding the dog?

   yes no

2. In Mark's mind, is he making an excuse and rationalizing, telling himself it is OK to forget feeding a dog because it's only a pet?

   yes no

3. Is Mark saying it is OK to swear in front of his younger brother?

   yes no

4. Do you think Mark was paying attention to who else was in the scene when he was on the phone with his friend?

   yes no

5. Was Mark **respecting** his dad's words or was he ignoring them?

   respecting his dad's words   ignoring his dad's words

6. Would you want to have Mark work for you?

   yes   no

7. Can Mark be trusted to do what he says he will do?

   yes   no

8. Is Mark **taking responsibility for his actions** or is he thinking of excuses and rationalizing why his irresponsible actions did not matter?

   A. **taking responsibility** for his poor action choices

   B. rationalizing why his poor choices were OK

9. Can Mark learn from his mistakes if he does not take responsibility for his actions?

   yes   no

10. 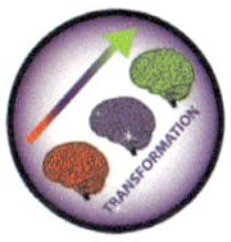

Change the end of the scene to make it more G.R.E.E.N. What could Mark have said to his Dad when he realized he had not done the things his father had asked him to do? He could have taken responsibility for his negative actions and said, "______________________________________

____"

11. What are some **Guiding G.R.E.E.N. Thoughts** that could have helped Mark avoid this **R.E.D.** situation in the first place? ______________________________

____

____

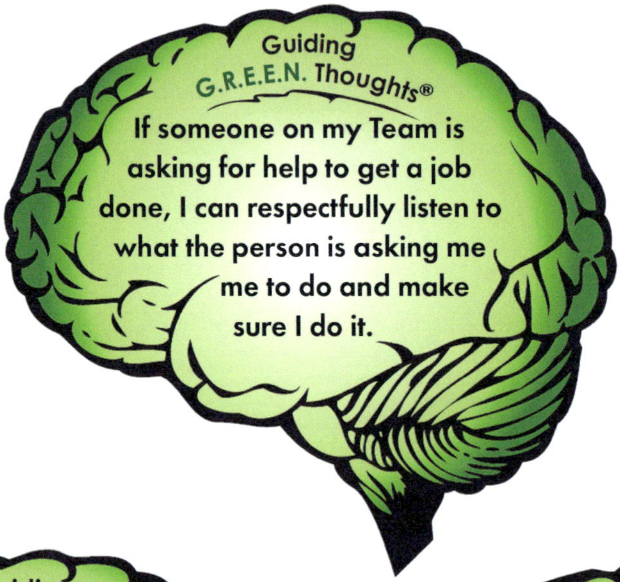

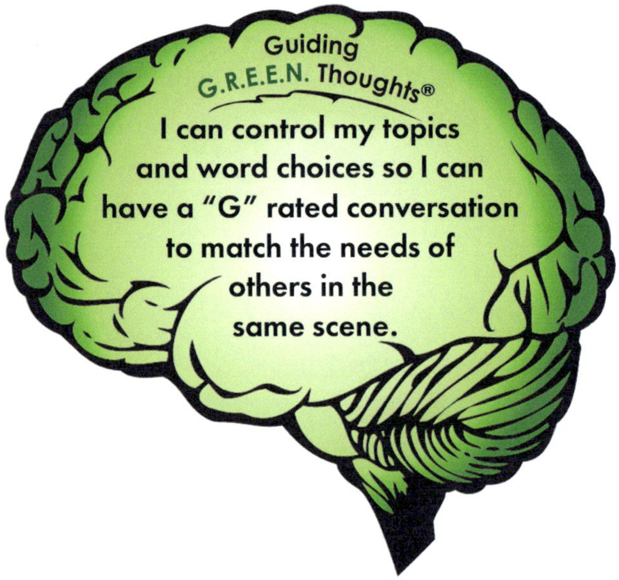

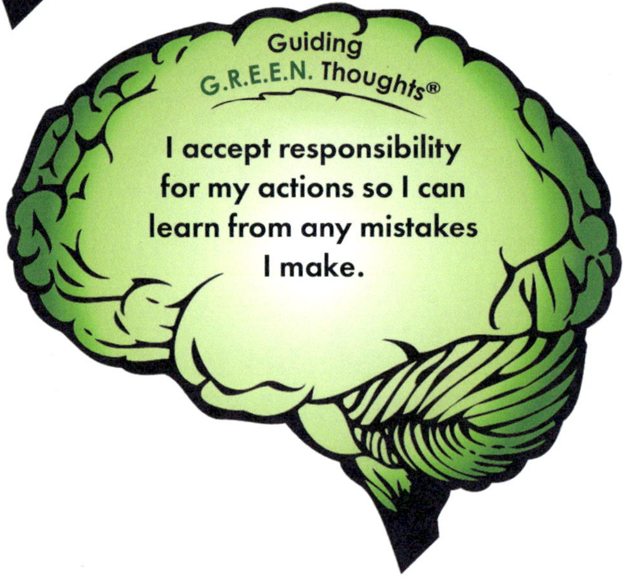

12. Are these Guiding **G.R.E.E.N.** Thoughts also useful for you so you can make the best choices in your own life scenes?

yes no

19.19 Survey the Scene: How Is Samantha Acting with Her School Team?

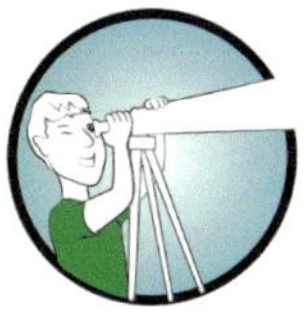

At Samantha's school, people got awards for being **respectful** and **helpful** to their peers. Every Friday, a couple of students from each class would get recognized at a school assembly for acting in a **G.R.E.E.N.** way. Even though Samantha said she wanted to have a job working with people when she grew up, she did not show people that she respected them. Whenever she could, she interrupted the teacher during lessons to tell her what other classmates were doing so she could get them in trouble. If she did not get an award for the week, she yelled at the teacher and threw things at the classmates that were going to get awards. When other people got awards at the assemblies, she booed them! As a consequence, she was no longer allowed to go to assemblies. She kicked and argued with the school staff when they told her that she could not go to the award assembly as long as she continued to act disrespectfully. She said, "This isn't fair," and then insulted the teachers by saying they did not know anything. She demanded that she should receive the next award and be recognized for her behavior because she knew how to act with other people.

Samantha's teacher repeatedly reminded her about how she could get an award as the other students did: "Samantha, students get awards when they are **respectful** and **helpful** in the classroom with everyone. When you learn to help the Class Team by acting this way, you will get an award, too."

1. We learn the point of view of Samantha's teacher by listening to what she just said. What is Samantha's teacher telling Samantha about her actions? ______________

   ____

2. Do you think Samantha was acting **respectful** and **G.R.E.E.N.** toward her teacher and classmates?

   yes no

3. Circle, underline, or highlight in red what Samantha said or did that you think was **R.E.D.** action.

4. What do you think is the **Common Team Goal** of the Class Team? ____________

   ____

5. Do you think Samantha was thinking of the **Common Team Goal** and the perspective of the other people on her Class Team?

yes no

19.20 Change the Scene: Help Samantha Be a More Respectful Team Member

1. If we give Samantha the chance to **rewind** the scene and make a **transformation** to act more **G.R.E.E.N.**, what **Guiding G.R.E.E.N. Thought** could she use to help her improve her actions?

Here are some Guiding G.R.E.E.N. Thoughts to choose from:

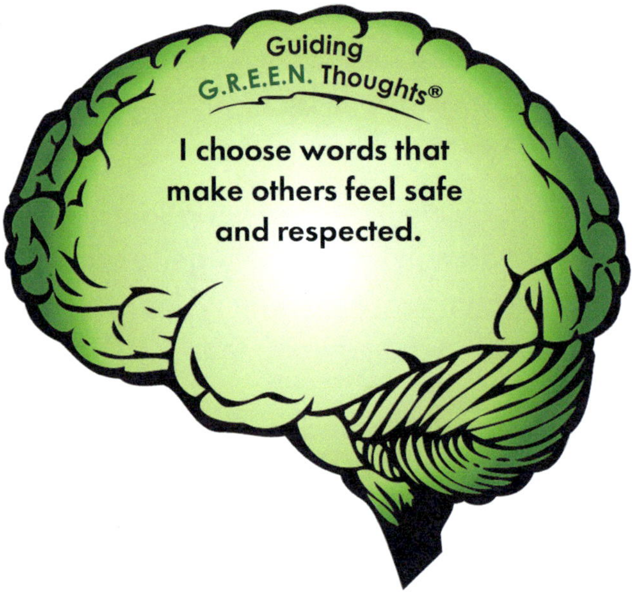

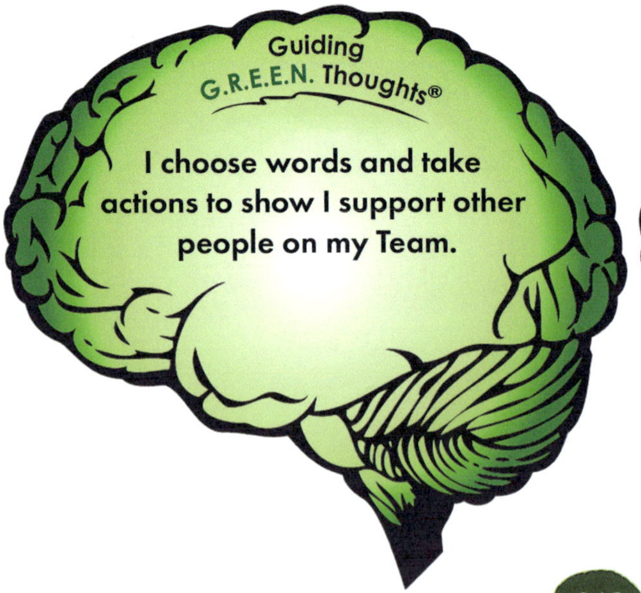

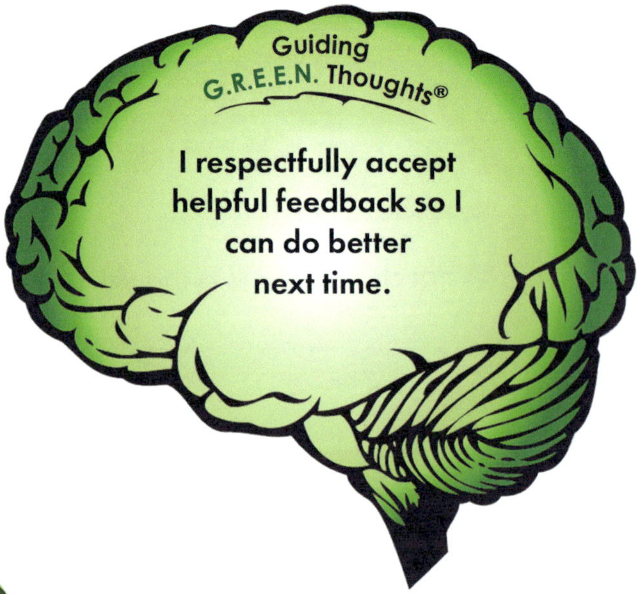

2. Look at Samantha's **R.E.D.** actions that you found. Write down four things she could do differently so her teacher and others on her Class Team would think she was acting in a more **respectful**, **G.R.E.E.N.** way.

   A. ______________________________

   B. ______________________________

   C. ______________________________

   D. ______________________________

19.21 Quick G.R.E.E.N. Scenes: Showing Samantha How to Be Respectful in Class

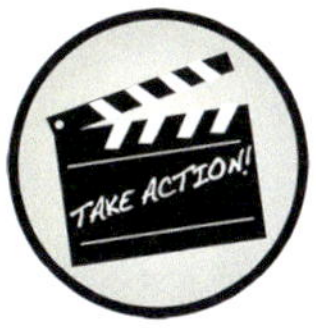

Act out the following **G.R.E.E.N.** Scenes to see how **respectful** you could be if you were Samantha and your teacher was saying each of the following things to you! You can be a role model to show Samantha how to act **G.R.E.E.N.** Use the clapboard for each scene.

1. **Teacher:** *Samantha, I would **appreciate** it if you stopped calling out and raised your hand instead during class lessons.*

   Samantha (Sam): *OK, I'll do my best. I'll put a note on my desk to help me remember.*

2. **Teacher:** *Class, I would like to announce that Tommy and Louisa will get awards this week for being **respectful** and **helpful.***

   Samantha (Sam), clapping hands: *"Congratulations! Good job!"*

3. **Teacher:** *Class, I would like you to not interrupt me when I am trying to teach you, unless you would like me to repeat something or explain something. If you need something repeated or explained, please raise your hand.*

   I would also really ***appreciate*** *it if you ignored any negative behavior of your classmates. If a student is misbehaving, let me handle it. You do your job of paying attention to me. You will really be helping the Class Team. Do you understand what I am saying?*

   Who can tell me one thing that I just said? Samantha (Sam), I see you have your hand raised. Please tell me something that I just said.

   Samantha (Sam): ____

   ____

   (Choose to say one of the things written below that the teacher said.)

   - I shouldn't interrupt you when you are teaching the class so you can stay on-topic.
   - I can raise my hand if I don't understand something or need something repeated.
   - I should ignore the negative behavior of my classmates and let you handle it.

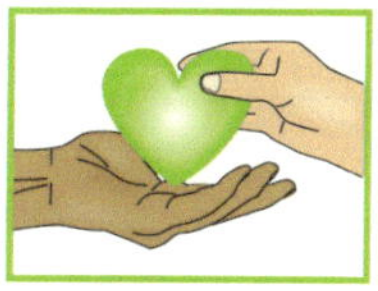

20 Learning How to Be More Empathetic

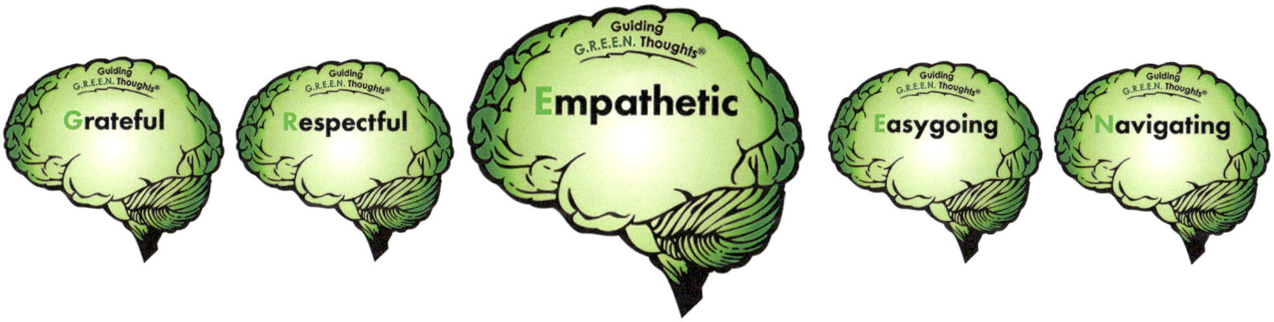

20.1 What Does It Mean to Be Empathetic?

When you show **empathy**, you are showing you are aware of how others around you feel. When you are **empathetic**, you say and do things that show you care about other people's feelings and want to help them.

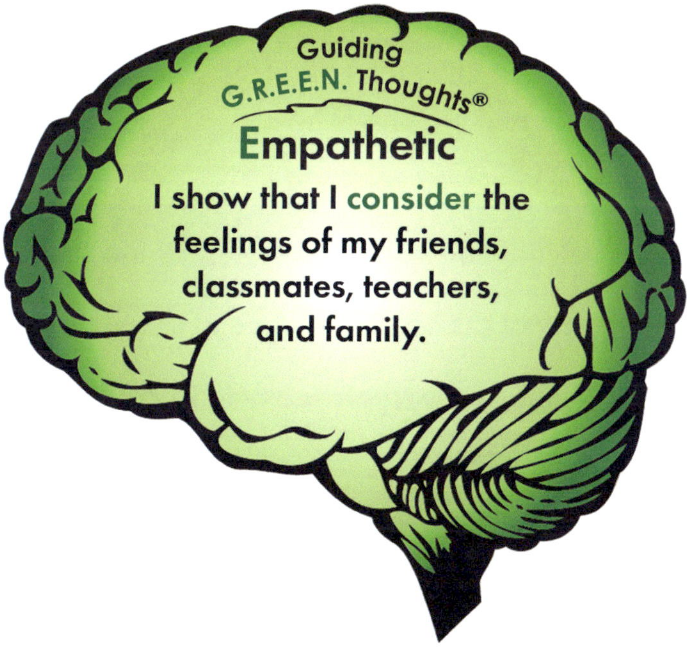

You are empathetic when you show that you are considerate of how others feel and help them as they try to achieve their own Personal Goals. Instead of only caring about your *own* feelings, you think about the feelings of your friends, classmates, and family. Make your best guess about how these people feel. Then think about their feelings as you choose your best actions.

20.2 How to Be Empathetic

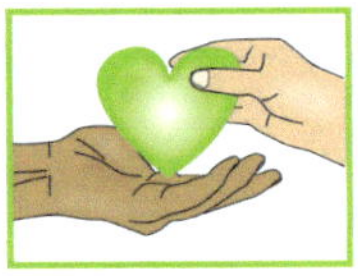

1. To be empathetic, you quietly Think First.

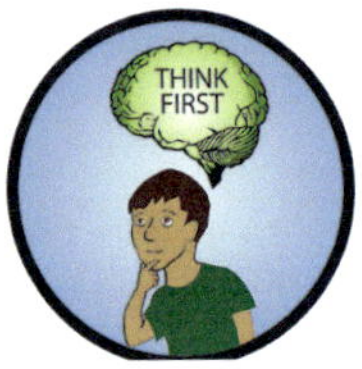

You use your self-control strategies to give yourself the time you need to Think First so you can figure out the best thing to say or do for everyone on your Team.

2. While you are taking the time to Think First, you survey the scene to notice who else is with you.

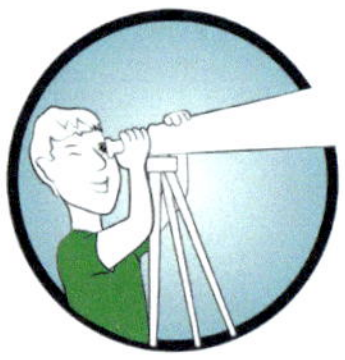

What is going on in this situation?

How is this person feeling?

Why might this person be feeling that way?

You make your best guess about what the people might be thinking or feeling.

3. The third step in being empathetic is making a good choice in what you say or do with the other person. This is how you can show you respect them and are supportive of their needs.

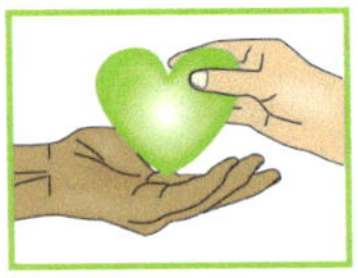

What can I do or say to make the scene better for this person?

What action could I take to show I am empathetic?

What empathetic comments could I make?

If you are not sure what you can say or do, you can ask directly how you could help the person in this scene:

How can I help you?

The other person may choose to accept your help or may not want your help at that time. It is good to show the person that you are there to help when and if they want you to help.

20.3 Why Act Empathetically?

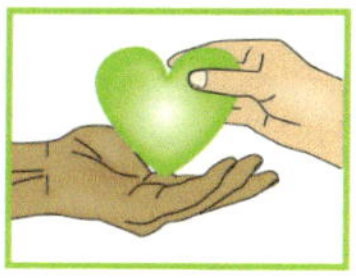

Why should you think about the other people in your life scenes and do things that show you **care** about them?

If you think about other people's feelings, you can act to help the scene be **good for everyone** in it. When you act **empathetically**, you show you are taking the time and effort to Think First and make **helpful** action choices that make things **better** for people on your Teams.

When you only think about yourself, there can be one or more of these negative consequences. The people on your Team:

- may think you *don't* care about them;
- might think you are ignoring their feelings;
- will *not* feel as if you are on their Team;
- may *not* want to care about you if you *don't* show you care about them;.
- may not want to spend time with you.

If you DO take the time and effort to think about other people and show that you care about their feelings, you are likely to experience **positive** consequences. The people on your Team:

- may want to spend more time with you;
- will think you care about them;
- will think that you can see how other people feel in different situations;
- will feel as if you are on their Team.

IT'S NOT ALL ABOUT ME

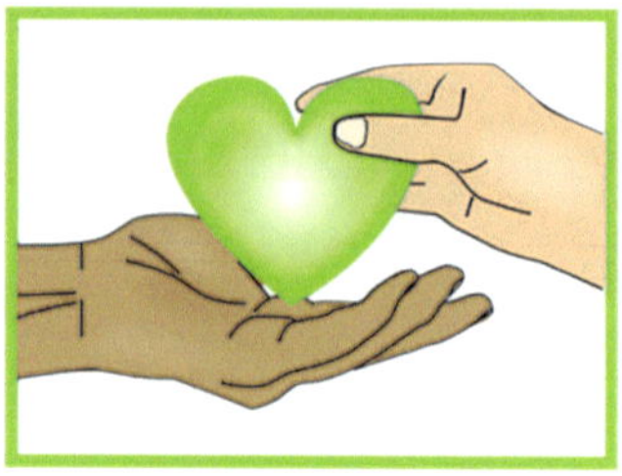

A Song for **Guiding G.R.E.E.N. Thoughts**®

By Herb Hein

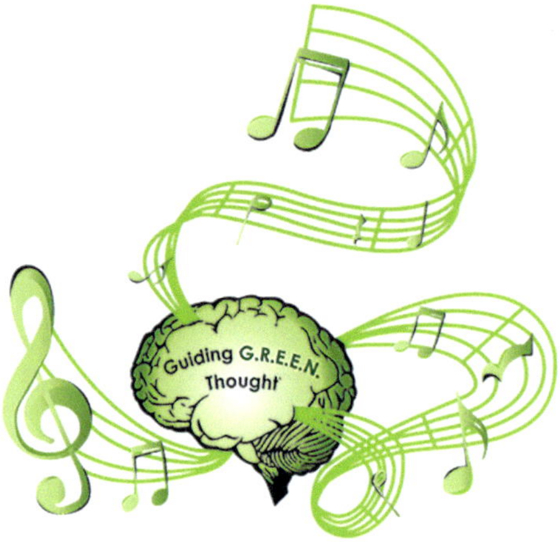

It's not all about me.

It's also about you.

It's not all about me.

I need to care about you.

I need to listen to you.

It's not all about me

because we're here together.

I try to know how you feel

to make things better for you.

It's good to care about you

to make things better for you.

20.4 Guiding G.R.E.E.N. Thoughts for Being Empathetic

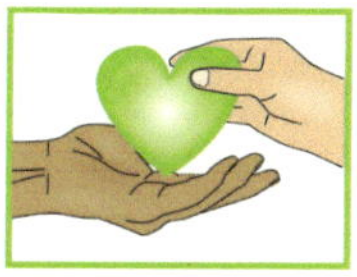

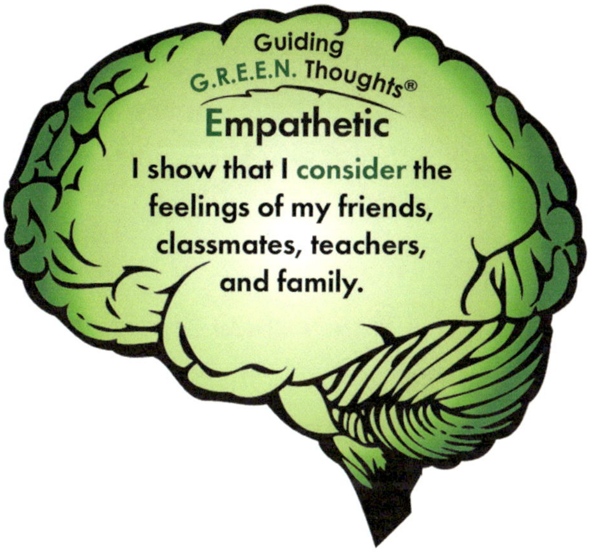

- I survey the scene to guess how people are feeling.
- In addition to focusing on my needs, I focus on what other people on my Team need.
- My words and my actions show others that I **care**.
- When my Team member seems upset, I stay calm and listen to their point of view.

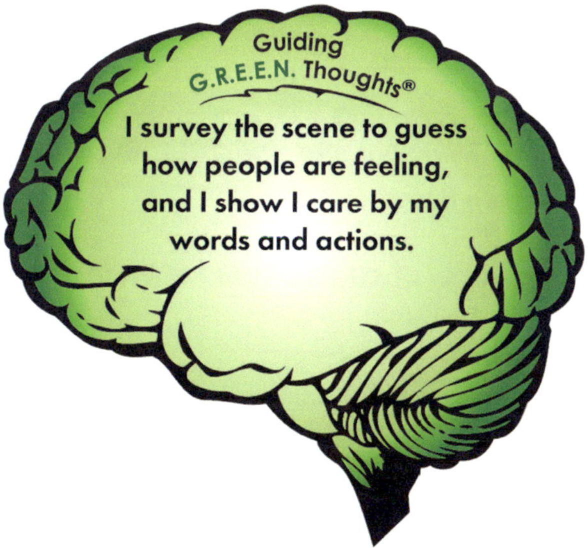

20.5 Underline Red or Green: Which Actions Show Empathy for Others?

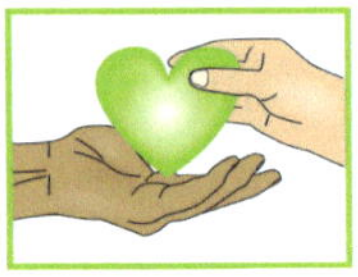

Directions: Which of the following actions show that you are putting your own feelings aside so that you can show empathy for someone else? Underline these empathetic behaviors green. They are green because they are helping you keep your relationship going, just as a green light tells drivers to keep going.

Underline the actions red if they show that you are *not* caring about how the person feels. They are red because they may stop the relationship from getting better and moving forward, just as a red light stops drivers from moving forward.

1. Your friend forgot her umbrella and it is raining. You offer to share yours with her.
2. You are racing to the finish line, and a boy is right next to you. You push him to the side and win.
3. You're watching TV and your mom says it's time for bed. You shut if off.
4. You are in class and the teacher is talking. You decide to talk to your friend.
5. Your classmate falls down and gets hurt. You laugh at him.
6. Your sister is doing her homework and she needs help. You have a lot of homework to do, but you help her anyway.
7. There is a new boy in school and he is lost. You help him find his class.
8. On your way to class you see that your teacher has dropped her books. You help her pick them up.
9. There are two pieces of candy. Your brother wants a piece. You take it all and don't share any of it with him.

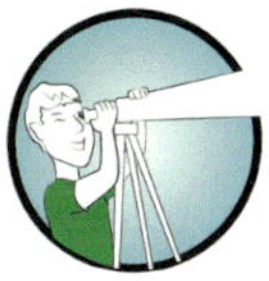
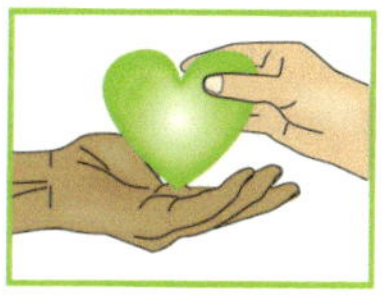

21 Survey the Scene: Infer How Others Feel

21.1 Making Inferences by Surveying the Scene

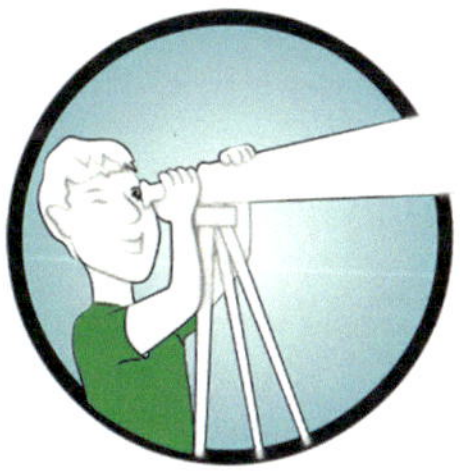

It is not always easy to see what is happening in the scenes around you. People often don't tell you exactly what they want or need. People usually don't say exactly how they feel.

So, how can you figure out what is going on? How can you know the best way to act with other people?

You can **survey the scene** to find clues that can help you notice what is happening. You can actively look for clues to understand how someone feels. When you use these clues to make your best guess about how the other person is feeling, you are making an inference about how they feel. You might not always be right when you make an inference, but you can still give it your best try.

When you are in a real situation with someone, you ask people about how they feel and why they feel that way. If you ask, you won't have guess:

How are you feeling?

Why do you feel that way?

The person may not know how they feel or may be unable to name the feeling, but at least the person can know that you **care**.

21.2 With Practice, You Can Notice How People Feel

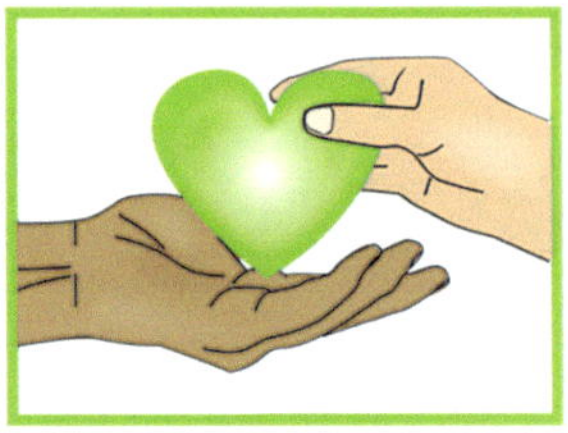

It is important to remember that people can have many different feelings. Sometimes people have different feelings on different days. Sometimes people change their feelings in the same day, depending on what is happening in their life scenes.

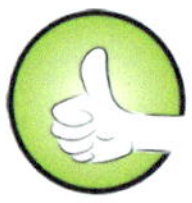

People might have happy, comfortable, **positive** feelings. They might be feeling as if they are moving **forward** toward their **goals**.

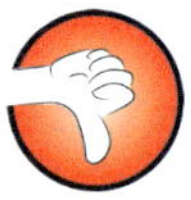

Or people might have sad, worried, uncomfortable, negative feelings. They might be feeling as if they are not meeting their **goals** in their life scene.

You can usually tell how someone is feeling from the words that person is saying. It is important to build the skill of making inferences about how other people feel so you can show you are an **empathetic** member of their Team. You can get better with practice.

21.3 How to Survey the Scene to Match Your Words with Their Feelings

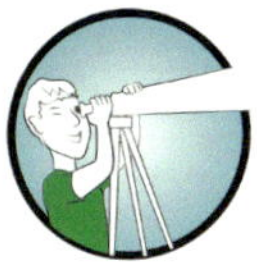

Survey the scene to learn how other people feel. Then choose things to say to match their feelings by following the steps below:

1. **Find clues for feelings.** Listen to what each person is saying to find clue words that help you guess how each person feels. Circle the clue words that help you tell what the person is feeling.

2. **What kinds of feelings are they?** Use the clue words to help you decide if the person is feeling good and happy, or if the person is feeling sad, worried, or bad.

3. **Choose empathetic words that match!** Think about what you can say that shows you were listening *and* that you **care** about how the other person is feeling. Choose words that match what the other person is saying so you can make a **relevant**, **empathetic** comment.

   If you hear words that make you think the person is feeling good and happy in some way, you can match those words and feelings by making a comment that starts with these words:

   Good for you! I am glad that ________________________________

   (add the words you heard that describe the good thing happening for this person)

   If you hear words that make you think that the person is feeling bad, worried, or sad in some way, you can match those words and feelings by making a comment that starts with these words:

   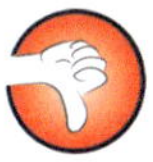

   I am sorry to hear that ________________________________

   (add the words you heard that describe the bad or sad thing happening for this person)

   I hope that ____

   (add what could get **better** for the person)

21.4 Survey the Scene and Choose Empathetic Words at Home

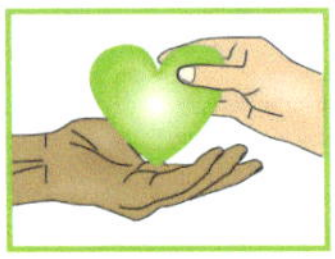

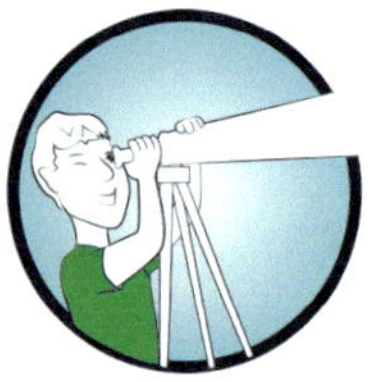

Directions: Practice surveying the scene by listening to or reading the sentences below and finding clue words to make an inference about how each person is feeling. Then write caring comments to show you were listening to what each person said.

1. *I can't find my keys.*

   A. How is this person feeling?

   happy   proud   bad   worried   sad

   B. What is something you can say to show you care?

   I'm sorry that ______________________________

   I hope that ______________________________

   or

   Good for you! I'm glad that ______________________________

---

2. *I think I am starting to feel sick.*

   A. How is this person feeling?

   happy   proud   bad   worried   sad

   B. What is something you can say to show you care?

   I'm sorry that ______________________________

   I hope that ______________________________

   or

   Good for you! I'm glad that ______________________________

3. *I am going to get an award tomorrow.*

   A. How is this person feeling?

   happy   proud   bad   worried   sad

   B. What is something you can say to show you **care**?

   I'm sorry that ______________________________

   I hope that ______________________________

   or

   Good for you! I'm glad that ______________________________

---

4. *I have so much work to do that I can't go to the movies with you tonight.*

   A. How is this person feeling?

   happy   proud   bad   worried   sad

   B. What is something you can say to show you **care**?

   I'm sorry that ______________________________

   I hope that ______________________________

   or

   Good for you! I'm glad that ______________________________

5. *The dentist said my teeth have no cavities!*

   A. How is this person feeling?

   happy   proud   bad   worried   sad

   B. What is something you can say to show you **care**?

   I'm sorry that ______________________________

   I hope that ______________________________

   or

   Good for you! I'm glad that ______________________________

---

6. *I don't have enough money to buy those new shoes right now.*

   A. How is this person feeling?

   happy   proud   bad   worried   sad

   B. What is something you can say to show you **care**?

   I'm sorry that ______________________________

   I hope that ______________________________

   or

   Good for you! I'm glad that ______________________________

7. *I gave Mom a present and she really liked it.*

   A. How is this person feeling?

   happy   proud   bad   worried   sad

   B. What is something you can say to show you **care**?

   I'm sorry that ______________________________

   I hope that ______________________________

   or

   Good for you! I'm glad that ______________________________

---

8. *I didn't do well at basketball practice today.*

   A. How is this person feeling?

   happy   proud   bad   worried   sad

   B. What is something you can say to show you **care**?

   I'm sorry that ______________________________

   I hope that ______________________________

   or

   Good for you! I'm glad that ______________________________

21.5 Survey the Scene and Choose Empathetic Words at School

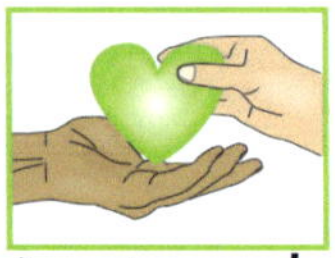

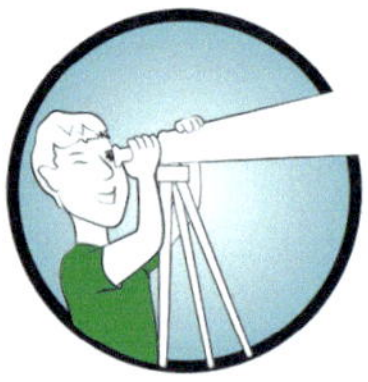

Directions: Pay attention to the words that each person is saying to make to make an inference about how that person is feeling. Think about why that person feels that way and then choose to say something that shows you care.

1. *I didn't do well on my test yesterday.*

   A. How is this person feeling?

   happy proud bad worried sad

   B. What is something you can say to show you care?

   I'm sorry that ______________________________

   I hope that ______________________________

   or

   Good for you! I'm glad that ______________________________

---

2. *I was chosen to be the captain of our basketball Team.*

   A. How is this person feeling?

   happy proud bad worried sad

   B. What is something you can say to show you care?

   I'm sorry that ______________________________

   I hope that ______________________________

   or

   Good for you! I'm glad that ______________________________

3. *My picture was chosen to be hung in the school office this month.*

   A. How is this person feeling?

   happy   proud   bad   worried   sad

   B. What is something you can say to show you **care**?

   I'm sorry that ______________________________

   I hope that ______________________________

   or

   Good for you! I'm glad that ______________________________

---

4. *Because of a meeting, I won't have time to eat lunch today.*

   A. How is this person feeling?

   happy   proud   bad   worried   sad

   B. What is something you can say to show you **care**?

   I'm sorry that ______________________________

   I hope that ______________________________

   or

   Good for you! I'm glad that ______________________________

5. *I didn't do well at basketball practice today.*

   A. How is this person feeling?

   happy proud bad worried sad

   B. What is something you can say to show you **care**?

   I'm sorry that ______________________________

   I hope that ______________________________

   or

   Good for you! I'm glad that ______________________________

---

6. *My school bus picked me up late today because there was so much traffic!*

   A. How is this person feeling?

   happy proud bad worried sad

   B. What is something you can say to show you **care**?

   I'm sorry that ______________________________

   I hope that ______________________________

   or

   Good for you! I'm glad that ______________________________

21.6 Survey the Scene and Choose Empathetic Words with Friends

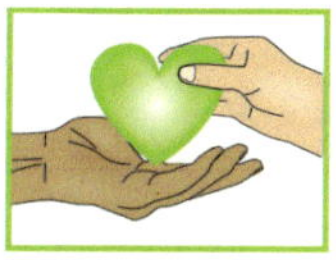

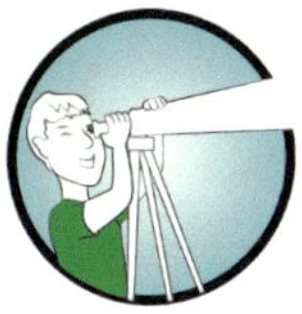

Directions: Pay attention to the words that each person is saying to make an inference about how that person is feeling. Think about why that person feels that way and then say something that shows you care.

1. *My mom gave me a reward for helping with chores.*

   A. How is this person feeling?

   happy   proud   bad   worried   sad

   B. What is something you can say to show you care?

   I'm sorry that ______________________________

   I hope that ______________________________

   or

   Good for you! I'm glad that ______________________________

---

2. *I can't go to the park with you because I must study for a test tomorrow. I didn't do so well on my last test.*

   A. How is this person feeling?

   happy   proud   bad   worried   sad

   B. What is something you can say to show you care?

   I'm sorry that ______________________________

   I hope that ______________________________

   or

   Good for you! I'm glad that ______________________________

3. *I didn't get to go to the beach on Saturday because our dog got sick and we had to take her to the vet.*

   A. How is this person feeling?

   happy   proud   bad   worried   sad

   B. What is something you can say to show you **care**?

   I'm sorry that ____

   I hope that ____

   or

   Good for you! I'm glad that ______________________________

---

4. *My dad said he was going to let me get a new video game this weekend because I did well on my report card.*

   A. How is this person feeling?

   happy   proud   bad   worried   sad

   B. What is something you can say to show you **care**?

   I'm sorry that ____

   I hope that ____

   or

   Good for you! I'm glad that ______________________________

5. *I won't get to play in the game tomorrow because I sprained my ankle.*

   A. How is this person feeling?

   happy   proud   bad   worried   sad

   B. What is something you can say to show you **care**?

   I'm sorry that ______________________________

   I hope that ______________________________

   or

   Good for you! I'm glad that ______________________________

21.7 Steps for Being Empathetic in Quick G.R.E.E.N. Scenes

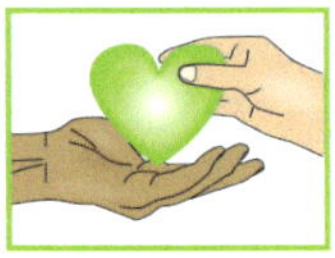

You have learned to make inferences about how other people feel. You also learned how to make comments that match their feelings. So now you can practice your skills as you act out these Quick **G.R.E.E.N.** Scenes. Person A will say something. If you are the person who is acting **empathetically** (Person B), you will be asked to make an **empathetic** comment. Person A will get to feel what it is like when people use words and a tone of voice to show they **care**. Person A and Person B can then **switch** roles so each person has a chance to act **empathetically**.

To be successful in each scene, Person B has to:

1. 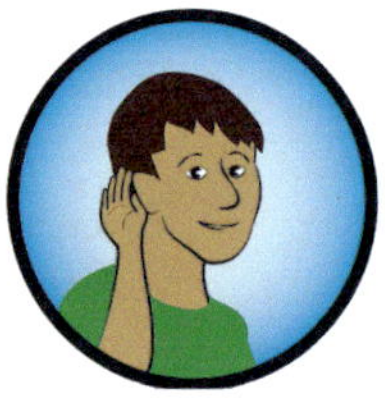 Listen to what the other person (Person A) says about their situation.

2. 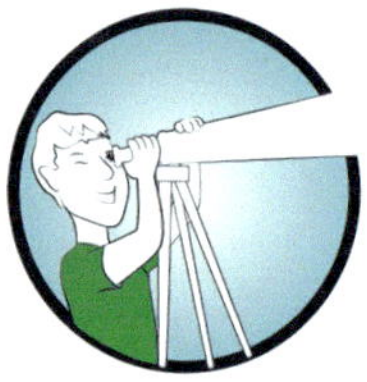 **Survey the scene** to guess how Person A is feeling.

3. 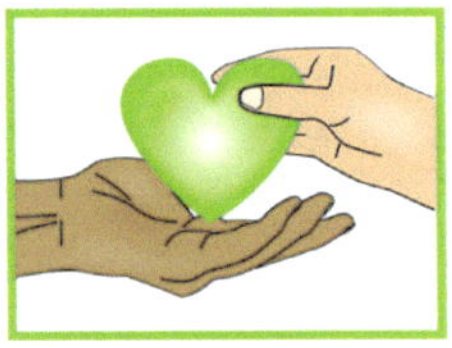 Make a **supportive** comment that matches how Person A is feeling.

21.8 Directions for Quick Empathetic G.R.E.E.N. Scenes

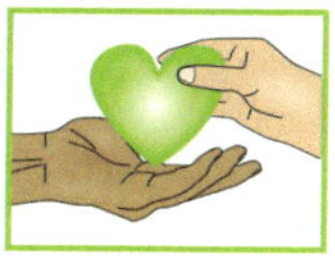

1. Get the G.R.E.E.N. Scene clapboard.

2. Two actors are chosen for these Quick G.R.E.E.N. Scenes.

3. For each scene the Director says "Quiet on the Set!" to signal to everyone else to be quiet and **pay attention to the scene**.

4. When everyone is quiet, the Director says "Action" and "claps" the clapboard.

5. Person A says the printed line and Person B makes a **supportive**, **empathetic** comment in a voice that shows they **care** about Person A.

6. After person B has had a chance to make a supportive comment with a **caring** voice, the Director claps the clapboard again and says, "Cut!"

7. Circle "yes" if Person B was successfully **empathetic**. Circle "no" if Person B was not. Person B can try again, with the Director saying "Take Two!" Write T 2 next to the clapboard for a scene that needed a second take. Circle "**yes**" if Person B was successfully **empathetic** on the second try.

8. Track how you do as **empathetic** person B using the tracking sheet (page 290).

21.9 Quick G.R.E.E.N. Scene Challenge: Making Supportive Comments with My Teams

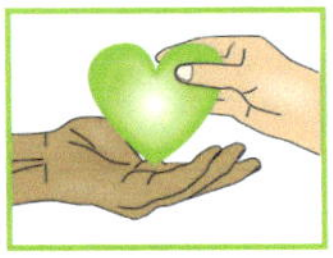

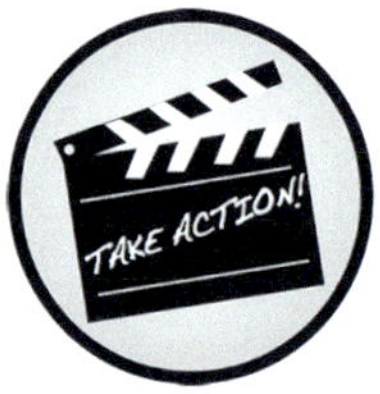

In real-life scenes, after making supportive comments, people usually ask supportive questions to know what is going on with other people. But for these scenes, when you are Person B, focus on taking that first empathetic step by making a supportive comment that shows you care. Use the steps in Section 21.3 for matching your words with how you think Person A is feeling. If you can't think of what to say, ask your Guide for help. Then see if you can remember to use the words they suggested in the scene.

21.10 Acting Empathetic at Home

Quick G.R.E.E.N. Scene #1

A. *I can't find my cell phone.*

B. Supportive comment made with caring voice:

yes no

Quick G.R.E.E.N. Scene #2

A. *I am starting to get a bad headache.*

B. Supportive comment made with caring voice:

yes no

Quick G.R.E.E.N. Scene #3

A. *I got my report card today and my grades were better than last time.*

B. **Supportive** comment made with **caring** voice:

yes no

Quick G.R.E.E.N. Scene #4

A. *I must finish a project that is due tomorrow so I can't play a game with you tonight.*

B. **Supportive** comment made with **caring** voice:

yes no

Quick G.R.E.E.N. Scene #5

A. *The doctor said my foot is good enough for me to run in the race on Friday.*

B. **Supportive** comment made with **caring** voice:

yes no

Quick G.R.E.E.N. Scene #6

A. *I don't have enough money to buy those new headphones now.*

B. **Supportive** comment made with **caring** voice:

yes no

Acting Empathetic at Home Total _____/6

21.11 Acting Empathetic at School

Quick G.R.E.E.N. Scene #1

A. *I didn't do well on my math quiz yesterday.*

B. **Supportive** comment made with **caring** voice:

yes no

Quick G.R.E.E.N. Scene #2

A. *I just found out I am student of the week in my class.*

B. **Supportive** comment made with **caring** voice:

yes no

Quick G.R.E.E.N. Scene #3

A. *I can't meet you for lunch because I must finish taking a test.*

B. **Supportive** comment made with **caring** voice:

yes no

Acting Empathetic at School Total ____/3

21.12 Acting Empathetic with Your Friend

Quick G.R.E.E.N. Scene #1

A. *My dad said I can start getting paid for doing some yard chores.*

B. **Supportive** comment made with **caring** voice:

yes no

Quick G.R.E.E.N. Scene #2

A. *I can't go to the park with you now because I must clean up my room.*

B. **Supportive** comment made with **caring** voice:

yes no

Quick G.R.E.E.N. Scene #3

A. *Our cat is really sick, so we are taking him to the vet this afternoon.*

B. **Supportive** comment made with **caring** voice:

yes no

Acting Empathetic with Your Friend Total ___/3

21.13 Quick G.R.E.E.N. Scene Tracking Sheet: How Well Did I Support My Teammates with Supportive Comments?

Date of this Quick G.R.E.E.N. Scene exercise ______________________________

The role of Person B was played by ______________________________________

Total number of **supportive** comments made by Person B with a **caring** voice:

At Home _______/6 At School ___/3 With Your Friend __/3 Total ____/12

Number of additional "takes" needed to have successful scenes for these Teams:

____

Circle any scenes that could not be performed successfully on this date.

I can always get even **better** with practice. If I act out these Quick G.R.E.E.N. Scenes again, this will be my total score: ______________________________

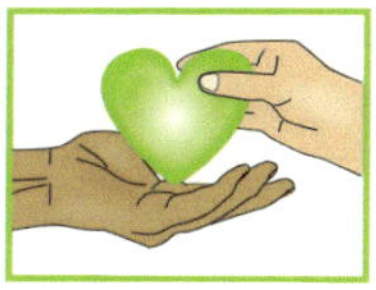

22 Expanding Empathy and Support with Peers

22.1 Expanding Your Vocabulary of Feelings

When you are with people on your Teams, you can listen to their words to guess how they feel. You can also look at their faces and watch their body movements to help you guess how they feel.

When you are reading a story, it is easy to tell how the characters feel when you can find specific words that describe their feelings. When there are no specific words to describe how they feel, you must make inferences about how the characters feel from other clues you can find. The clues from the story help you make your best guess about their feelings and what is making them feel that way.

As you try your best to describe how characters feel, challenge yourself to use new words. Instead of simple words such as "happy" or "sad," you can think of more descriptive words, such as "cheerful" or "disappointed." When you use different words to describe feelings in yourself and others you will be expanding your vocabulary of feelings. You will start to notice a wider range of feelings to help you understand people.

22.2 Survey the Scene and Choose Your Feeling Words: Situations 1–5

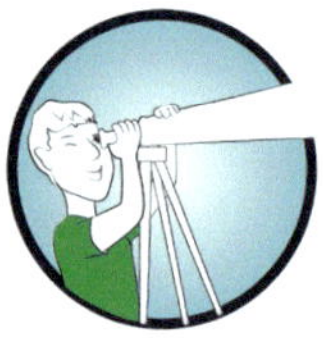

Directions: As you read each situation, underline the clue words that help you guess how each person is feeling. Then write down what you think each person is feeling and why they feel that way. Think of a supportive comment you might make to this person. Challenge yourself to choose words other than "happy" or "sad" when describing each person's feelings. You will be expanding your choice of feeling words. To describe the feelings of the characters in the following situations, you can choose from the vocabulary words on the bottom of this page.

1. Paul was riding his bike to his friend's house. He was smiling and whistling as he rode. He thought it was a perfect day.

2. Tom could not believe his eyes when he opened the front door of his house. All of his friends were there shouting, "Happy Birthday!"

3. Mark finished his slow climb up the ladder of the high diving board. He tried to keep his legs from shaking. He wanted to close his eyes, but knew he had to carefully watch his step as he moved toward the edge.

4. Sam knew he had worked really hard and deserved the perfect grade he got. His heart swelled as he watched his teacher put his A+ test paper on the bulletin board.

5. Jen had waited all week for this moment. She had worked so hard to make the team. She ran to read the list that had just been posted on the coach's door. She fought back tears when she saw that her name was not on the list.

Here are some word choices to help you describe the feelings of the characters in the scenes below:

content disappointed nervous excited proud surprised

Fill in the blanks to tell how you think each person in situations 1–5 was feeling and why they probably felt that way. Then write what you might say to the person if you were in the same scene.

1. Paul was probably feeling ______________________________

   because ______________________________

   This is what I could say to Paul if I knew him and wanted to show my **support** for how he was feeling as he rode by:

   It looks as if ______________________________

   I'm glad that ______________________________

2. Tom was probably feeling ______________________________

   because ______________________________

   This is what I could say to Tom if I was in the scene and wanted to show him I **cared** about how he was feeling:

   ____

3. Mark was probably feeling ______________________________

   because ______________________________

   This is what I could say to Mark if I was near him and wanted to show that I **cared** about him and wanted to **support** him:

   ____

4. Sam was probably feeling ______________________________

   because ______________________________

   This is what I could say to Sam if I was in the scene and wanted to show him that I **cared** about how he was feeling and wanted to **support** him:

   ____

5. Jen was probably feeling ______________________________

   because ______________________________

   This is what I could say to Jen if I was in the scene with her and wanted to show her that I **cared** about how she was feeling and wanted to **support** her:

   ____

Name ______________________ **Date** ______________

22.3 Survey the Scene and Choose Your Feeling Words: Situations 6–10

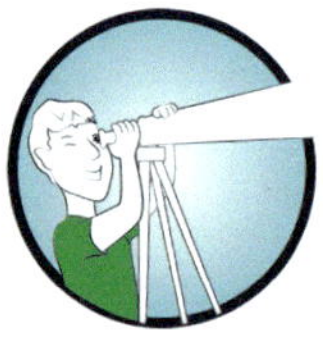

How are the people feeling in the following situations? Underline the words that help you make your best guess about their feelings. You will be making an inference about how they feel. To describe the feelings of the characters, you can choose from the vocabulary words provided on the bottom of the next page. Some characters might have two different feelings in the same situation.

6. Jim sat on the front step of his new house. He didn't know any other kids in the neighborhood and didn't see anybody who was his age. His mother and father and brother were at a meeting at his brother's new school. Jim sighed and thought about the friends he used to have in his old neighborhood.

7. All of Mike's good friends were with him in the car as his father drove to the movie theater. All the boys had waited six months since the last movie in their favorite superhero series came out. Tonight, the next movie in the series was playing for the first time and they would all see it together! Mike and his friends could hardly sit still.

8. Sandy had borrowed her mother's gold necklace to wear at the special school party. Unfortunately, after lunch recess, she noticed it was missing. The chain probably broke. Sandy did not know what to do. She started to cry, so her friend Tina asked her what was wrong. After Sandy told her, Tina tried to comfort her friend and told her that she would go and look for the necklace out in the field where they had been running around. Sandy could not believe it when Tina came back after about five minutes with the necklace in her hand. "You found it!" Sandy exclaimed, smiling broadly. "Thank you so, so much," she said. "You really saved the day," she added, giving her friend the biggest hug.

9. Melanie was watching her brother open his Christmas present. When he opened it up, she could not believe it was the cell phone that she wanted! She had asked her parents for one, but they said it was too expensive and she was not old enough to have one. Her brother always got what he wanted and she never did.

10. Billy's Dad had to go to the hospital in the middle of the night. His mother told him to watch his younger sister. He stayed up, unable to sleep, listening to every car pass by the house. He worried if his Dad would be OK, and could go to work tomorrow and then return home to coach his baseball team. To his surprise, the garage door opened at 5:00 in the morning and both his mother and his father got out of the car. His dad needed some medicine and needed to do special exercises, but he could soon continue to lead his regular life.

Here are vocabulary words to help you describe how the people might be feeling:

excited grateful jealous relieved lonely worried sad

Fill in the blanks to tell how each person feels and why you think they feel that way. Then write what you might say to the person if you were in the same scene.

6. Jim was probably feeling ______________________________

   because ______________________________

   This is what I could say to Jim when I was walking by if I lived on the same block and recognized that he was a new student at my school.

   ____

7. Mike was probably feeling ______________________________

   because ______________________________

   This is what I could say to Mike if I were one of his friends in the car with him:

   ____

8. At first, Sandy was probably feeling ______________________________

   because ______________________________

   At the end, Sandy was probably feeling ______________________________

   because ______________________________

   After Sandy told me what happened, this is what I could say to her to show that I **cared** about how she was feeling:

   ____

9. Melanie was probably feeling ______________________________

because ______________________________

If I was Melanie's brother in this situation, this is what I could say to her to show I was thinking about how she was feeling.

____

10. At first, Billy was probably feeling ______________________________

because ______________________________

At the end, Billy was probably feeling ______________________________

because ______________________________

This is what I could say to Billy to show I was thinking about how he was feeling if he told me what had happened.

____

Name ______________________________ **Date** ______________________________

22.4 Using Different Supportive Words to Match the Situation

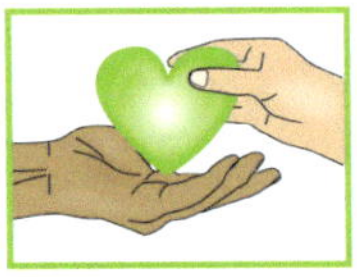

In order to make this a better world, one thing we can do is reach out to others around us and be supportive of them. When we are supportive, we are showing that we care about other people and their feelings. We support them in different ways depending on what has happened to them and how they feel. Sometimes, the person in need of support is not a close friend. They may be a peer (someone who is the same age or in the same group as you). They may not be your friend, but you can still show your support. If you show each other support, you *could* become friends.

Below are different situations and possible supportive phrases to say, as well as a blank line for you to add your own supportive words that would match the situation.

1. If they have just been successful, they are probably feeling *proud* of themselves. We can congratulate them right now by saying:

   It's great that you ______________________________

   I'm glad that you ______________________________

   or ______________________________

2. If they made a little bit of progress, we can help them feel encouraged by supporting the progress they have made. We could say: ____________________

   ____

   You are getting better! You are getting closer to the target.

   I bet you will do even better next time.

   or ______________________________

3. If they are really struggling to do something, or if something bad has happened, they might be feeling *discouraged* or *worried*. We can support them by saying:

   I'm sorry that ______________________________

   Would you like some help? How can I help you?

   or ______________________________

22.5 Survey the Scene and Choose the Best Words for Each Situation

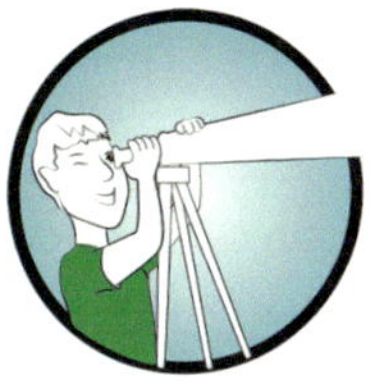

Think about how each person is feeling. Then think about what you could say to show your support. Remember to match your words with how the other person is feeling. You can get an idea of what to say by referring to Section 22.4.

1. **Carlos:** *I am having such trouble shooting the ball into the basket. I think our team is losing because of me.*

   Carlos is probably feeling ________________________________

   so I would show support by saying: ________________________

   ____

2. **Robert:** *I have been getting Cs and Ds in my science class, so I decided to not watch TV or play games on my computer all weekend and studied for my science test instead. I ended up getting a B+.*

   Robert is probably feeling ________________________________

   so I would show support by saying: ________________________

   ____

3. **Erica:** *My brother and I used to fight all the time so our parents had to get us some counseling help. With the counselor's help, we learned to be calm and listen to each other. Now we get along much better.*

   Erica is probably feeling ________________________________

   so I would show support by saying: ________________________

   ____

22.6 Directions for Quick G.R.E.E.N. Scenes for Supporting Peers

Now that you have learned more about how to show **support** for your peers, let's act out these Quick **G.R.E.E.N.** Scenes:

1. Get the **G.R.E.E.N.** Scene clapboard. Two actors are chosen for these Quick **G.R.E.E.N.** Scenes.

2. For each scene the Director says "Quiet on the Set!" to signal to everyone else to be quiet and **pay attention to the scene**.

3. When everyone is quiet, the Director "claps" the clapboard and says "Action."

4. Person A says the printed line and Person B makes a supportive, **empathetic** comment in a voice that shows they **care** about Person A. Person B can remember what was written in Section 22.5 to help know what **empathetic** words to use.

5. After Person B has had a chance to make a **supportive** comment with a **caring** voice, the Director claps the clapboard again and says, "Cut!"

6. Circle "yes" if Person B was successfully **empathetic**. Circle "no" if Person B was not able to make a **supportive** comment. Person B could try again, with the Director saying "Take Two!" Write T 2 next to the clapboard for a scene that needed a second take. Circle "yes" if Person B was successfully **empathetic** on the second try.

7. Keep track of how **empathetic** you are as person B on your "How **Supportive** Was I?" tracking sheet (Section 22.8).

8. To be successful in each scene, Person B has to

   A. Listen to what the other person (Person A) says.

   B. **Survey the scene** to guess how Person A is feeling.

   C. Make a **supportive** comment to *match* how Person A is feeling. Use what was written for responses in Section 22.5.

22.7 Quick G.R.E.E.N. Scenes: Showing Support for Peers!

Quick G.R.E.E.N. Scene #1

A. **Carlos:** *I am having such trouble shooting the ball into the basket. I think our team is losing because of me.*

B. Comments from empathetic, supportive peer: ______________________

____

yes no

Quick G.R.E.E.N. Scene #2

A. **Robert:** *I have been getting Cs and Ds in my science class so I decided to not watch TV or play games on my computer all weekend and studied for my science test instead. I ended up getting a B+.*

B. Comments from empathetic, supportive peer: ______________________

____

yes no

Quick G.R.E.E.N. Scene #3

A. **Erica:** *My brother and I used to fight all the time so our parents had to go get us some counseling help. With the counselor's help, we learned to be calm and listen to each other. Now we get along much better.*

B. Comments from empathetic, supportive peer: ______________________

____

yes no

22.8 Keeping Track: How Supportive Was I with My Peers?

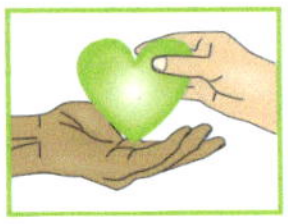

Date of Quick G.R.E.E.N. Scene Exercise: ______________________

The role of Person B was played by ______________________

Total number of **relevant**, **supportive**, **empathetic** comments made by Person B with a **caring** voice:

Showing Support for a Peer _____/3

Number of additional "takes" needed to have successful, supportive G.R.E.E.N. scenes: _________

Circle any scenes that could not be performed successfully on this date.

If Person B was not able to be successful in all the scenes on this date, they should have the chance to fill out the following about how they will perform next time after some practice.

I can always get even **better** with practice. If I act out these Quick G.R.E.E.N. Scenes again, this will be my total score: ______________________

22.9 Choosing a Supportive Scene for Eddie

Eddie had been going to a school where he did not get to have recess or P.E. He did not have much experience catching, kicking, and throwing balls, so he was not good at doing these things. However, when he got to a new school, he was looking forward to having recess and P.E. so he could practice getting better. When his classmates saw him catching or throwing balls, they saw that he was not as good as they were. Each of his classmates had two choices when Eddie asked if he could join in their ball game.

Eddie: *Hey, can I join your game?*

Eddie's classmates have two choices. You decide what choice you would make:

	Choice #1 *You Are Not Good Enough!*	Choice #2 *I'll Help You Get Better*
Which choice do you make?	Tell Eddie he is not good enough to play with you: *"No! You can't play with me because you are not good enough!"*	You tell Eddie he can play with you and that you will help him learn how to get better at the game: *"Yes! You can join the game. First, let me show you how to throw and catch better. You can practice with me."*
Predict what happened next. What will be the negative or positive consequence of each choice?		

Choice Checker for Responding to Eddie's Question:

	Choice #1 *You Are Not Good Enough!*	Choice #2 *I'll Help You Get Better*
	"No! You can't play with me because you are not good enough!"	*"Yes! You can join the game. First, let me show you how to throw and catch better. You can practice with me."*
Does this choice show self-control? Are you Thinking First before you speak?	yes no	yes no
If you make this choice, are you being empathetic? Are you caring about Eddie's feelings?	yes no	yes no
If you make this choice, are your words and actions helping the Class Team?	yes no	yes no

Circle the choice that has the most "yes" answers:

Choice #1: Telling Eddie, "You are not good enough!"

Choice #2: Telling Eddie, "I'll help you get better."

22.10 G.R.E.E.N. Scene #10: Write a Supportive Scene for Eddie

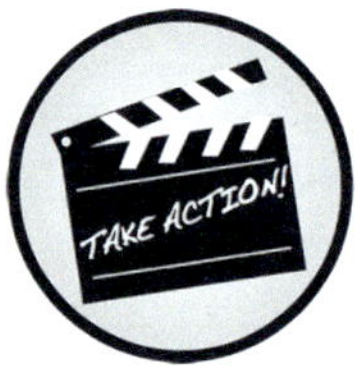

On the previous pages, you made the choice to show that you could Think First, be **empathetic**, and **support** both your peer and your Class Team with what you chose to say and do.

Now you can write out and act out this best choice scene:

Eddie: Hey, can I join your game?

You: ____

Eddie: ____

You: ____

Eddie: ____

To make the best **G.R.E.E.N.** Scene, follow the steps and use the Wise Action Tools noted in Sections 12.2 through 12.5.

22.11 Read and Discuss: Really Winning by Showing Good Sportsmanship

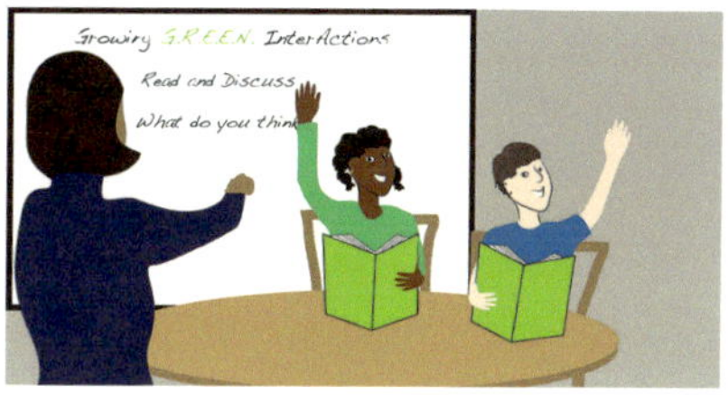

Let's talk about what it means to have good sportsmanship. When you are playing a game, you work hard to win. The truth is that each game always has a winner and loser. The winners of the game may feel happy and excited. The person or team that has lost may be feeling upset about losing. It is considered rude and bad sportsmanship if the winner says something to make the loser feel worse about the loss. Instead, the winner can say something **supportive**—for instance, that it was a good game and that they enjoyed playing.

Good *Game!*

I enjoyed playing with you!

Also, the winner can say that they look forward to playing another game with the other person in the future.

I look forward to playing with you again.

If you lose a game, it is **good sportsmanship** to just accept that you lost and to thank the other team for playing with you. If you have a bad attitude, people won't want to play with you again. If you have a **good attitude**, people will want to choose to play with you next time. Then you will have another chance to play, and maybe you will win the next time.

There is an expression that says, "It doesn't matter if you win or lose, it's how you play the game." This encourages you to focus on doing your best and having fun playing, instead of focusing only on whether you win or lose. It also encourages you to always show **good sportsmanship**.

- These are some words that describe actions of someone who shows **good sportsmanship**.

fair polite respectful courteous mature magnanimous

gracious generous honest resilient cheerful

- These are words that describe actions of someone who shows bad sportsmanship.

bragging arrogant boastful disrespectful

impolite egotistic immature gloating

- Here are some words used to describe **positive** feelings that come from **good sportsmanship**:

happy proud safe comfortable respected relaxed balanced

- Here are some words that can be used to describe negative feelings that come from bad sportsmanship:

sad mad resentful discouraged bitter envious humiliated

Practice showing that you can have good sportsmanship:

You just won the game. What can you say to the person you played against?

____

____

You just lost the game. What can you say to the person you played against?

____

____

22.12 Survey the Scene: What to Say after the Game

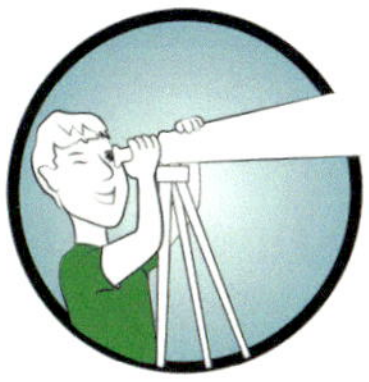

Find clues to make your best guess about how Peter feels in these two different scenes and why he might feel that way.

Directions:

1. Circle any words that tell you how Peter felt.
2. Underline with a **green** pencil if John said something to make Peter feel **better.**
3. Underline with a red pencil if John said something to make Peter feel worse.
4. Fill in the spaces below with your best guesses.

R.E.D. Scene: Peter and John both worked really hard to win when they were playing chess. Peter did not win the game. John won the game. John said, "I won and you lost. I'm the winner and you are such a loser!" Peter didn't want to play with John again.

In this scene, Peter was probably feeling ______________________________

because ____

G.R.E.E.N. Scene: Peter and John both worked really hard to win when they were playing chess. Peter did not win the game. John won the game. John said to Peter, "Good game!" and "It was nice playing with you." "I look forward to playing with you again!" Peter wanted to keep playing with John.

In this scene, Peter was probably feeling ______________________________

because ____

You really win by showing **good sportsmanship**!

22.13 Showing Empathy by Making Comments and Asking Questions

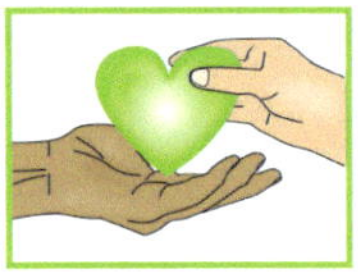

When you see that a person is sad, upset, worried, or frustrated, you can make comments to **support** them. You also can ask a question to show that you care about what happened.

Comments That Might Be Made

These are some **supportive**, **empathetic** comments that might be made when the other person is telling about something sad or challenging that happened to them:

Too bad!

I feel sorry for you!

That sounds terrible!

What a challenge!

Wow! You must have felt ________________________________

Questions You Might Ask to Show You Care about the Other Person:

How did it happen?

When did it happen?

What happened next?

How can I help you?

22.14 Building a Bridge to a Related Topic in an Empathetic Conversation

Sometimes you have had an experience that you think is similar to the other person's experience. You may want to share what happened to you if it helps show that you had the same kinds of feelings as the person you are talking to.

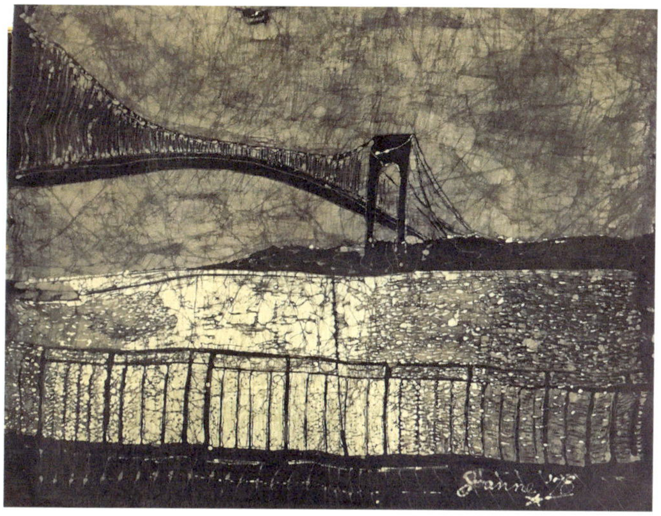

You may want to share what you did to **navigate** the situation and cope with it or solve it. You might share a useful strategy for the other person to try. If your experience is related to the person's problem, and if the other person wants to hear about it, it might be **helpful** to share your similar experiences.

You can ask the person if they want to hear about your similar experience. You can say something such as this:

Something similar happened to me. Would you like me to tell you what happened?

or

I had that kind of experience before. Can I tell you what happened?

If the person says "yes," then you can go ahead and *briefly* tell how your experience related to the other person's experience. After sharing your experience, you then return to talking about what happened to the other person. You make a bridge from their experience to your experience and then return on the bridge, back to their experience.

If the person says "no," then you *don't* share your experience. The person may not be ready to think about anything except their own story. So you just continue talking about what happened to the other person and do not share your own story.

At the end of the conversation, it shows you were really listening and really care if you are able to say something that shows you remember the main problem that the other person is having. You can say, "**I'm sorry that** . . . (the person is going through the challenging situation)." Then you can say that, "**I hope** (the situation gets better soon)."

22.15 Take These Steps for an Empathetic Conversation:

1. Listen carefully to the other person to learn what happened.
2. Make a **supportive** comment:

   I'm sorry that is happening to you.

   I'm sorry to hear that ______________________________

3. Then ask a relevant question and listen to the answer:

   Why did that happen? What will happen now?

4. If the person wants to hear it, you can share a similar experience that you had: ______________________________

   Something similar happened to me. Would you like me to tell you about it?

5. Return to talking about the other person's situation.
6. End the conversation by referring back to their problem and making a **supportive** comment:

   I'm sorry that ______________________________
   (Tell what the main problem was.)

   I hope that ______________________________
   (Tell how the situation might get **better**.)

22.16 Fill in the Blanks: Steps to Take in an Empathetic Conversation

Fill in the blanks with words that can be said in an empathetic conversation. (The answers can be found in Section 22.15.)

1. I carefully ________________ to the other person to learn what happened.

2. Make a ____ comment:

   I'm sorry that is happening to you.

   I'm sorry that happened to you.

3. Then ask a relevant ______________________ and listen to the answer:

   Why did that happen? What will happen now?

4. If the person wants to hear it, share a _________________ experience that you had:

   Something similar happened to me. Would you like me to tell you about it, and tell you what I did?

5. ___________ to talking about the other person's situation.

6. End the conversation by referring back to their ________________________ and making a ____ comment.

   I'm sorry that ____
   (Tell what the main problem was.)

   I hope that ____
   (Tell how the situation might get ________________.)

22.17 G.R.E.E.N. Scene #11: Write It and Act It Out: No One to Play With

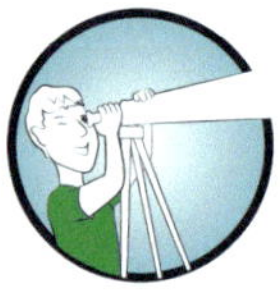

1. **Survey the scene** to make an inference about how the person feels and why the person feels that way. Find and underline the clue words that can help you make your best guess about how this person is feeling.

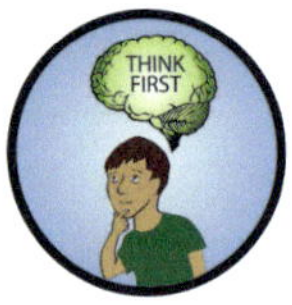

2. Think about what you could say or do to help this person feel **better**.

3. Fill in the script lines and then act them out.
4. To make the best **G.R.E.E.N.** Scene, follow the steps and use the Wise Action Tools found in Sections 12.2 through 12.5.

Person A—New neighbor: *I just moved here and I don't have anyone to play with. I used to have people to shoot baskets or ride bikes with. I'm getting really bored. I miss my old friends and my old neighborhood.*

Person B—Helpful, empathetic neighbor: ________________________________

Person A—New neighbor: ________________________________

Person B—Helpful, empathetic neighbor: ________________________________

Person A—New neighbor: ________________________________

22.18 G.R.E.E.N. Scene #12: Write It and Act It Out: Help! I Lost the Key!

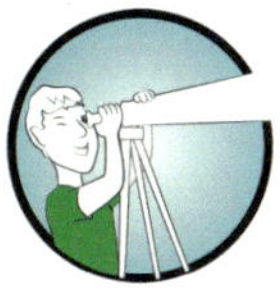

1. **Survey the scene** to make an inference about how the person feels and why the person feels that way. Find and underline the clue words that can help you make your best guess about how this person is feeling.

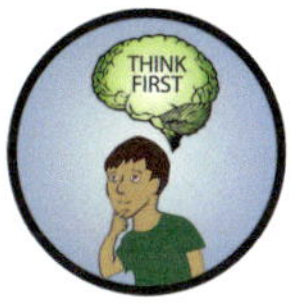

2. Think about what you could say or do to help this person feel **better**.

3. Fill in the script lines and then act them out.
4. Follow the steps and use the Wise Action Tools found in Sections 12.2 through 12.5 to make the best G.R.E.E.N. Scene.

Person A—Schoolmate on playground: *I don't know what to do! My father let me borrow this antique key that he got when he was a kid. I had it in my pocket before I went on the swings and on the climbing bars. It's almost time for me to leave the park, but I can't find the key anywhere! I'm gonna get in so much trouble if I lost it.*

Person B—Helpful, empathetic schoolmate: ________________________________

____

Person A—Schoolmate on playground: ________________________________

Person B—Helpful, empathetic schoolmate: ________________________________

____

22.19 G.R.E.E.N. Scene #13: Write It and Act It Out: Help Me Carry the Load!

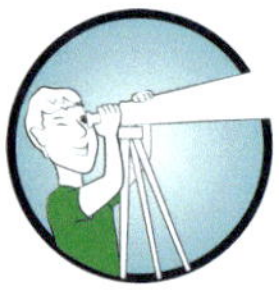

1. **Survey the scene** to make an inference about how the person feels and why the person feels that way. Find and underline the clue words that can help you make your best guess about how this person is feeling.

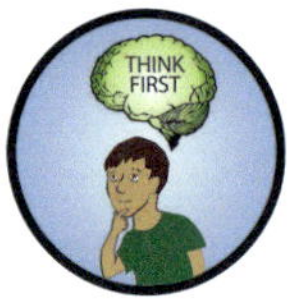

2. Think about what you could say or do to help this person feel **better**.

3. Fill in the script lines and then act them out.

4. Follow the steps and use the Wise Action Tools found in Sections 12.2 through 12.5 to make the best G.R.E.E.N. Scene.

Person A—Pat: *My classmate was supposed to help me carry these ten books to the classroom, but he decided to go play on the playground instead. He's going to get in trouble, but I think I will end up getting in trouble, too! My teacher was counting on us bringing these books to class so she could start teaching the next lesson with them. I know she's gonna need these books in 5 minutes. I think I can carry only 4 books at a time and I'm gonna be late if I must make more than one trip.*

Person B—Helpful, empathetic schoolmate: ______________________________

____

Person A—Pat: ____

Person B—Helpful, empathetic schoolmate: ______________________________

22.20 G.R.E.E.N. Scene #14: Write It and Act It Out: Please Help Me Remember

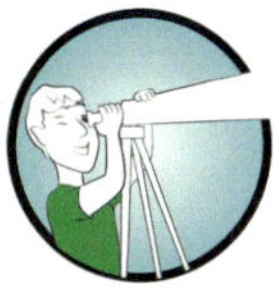

1. **Survey the scene** to make an inference about how the person feels and why the person feels that way. Find and underline the clue words that can help you make your best guess about how this person feels.

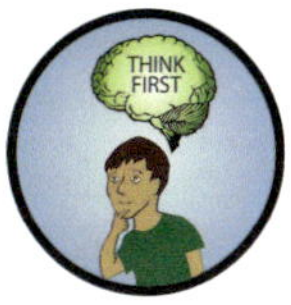

2. Think about what you could say or do to help this person feel **better**.

3. Can you think of a memory strategy that might help Sam? Fill in the script lines and then act them out.

4. Follow the steps and use the Wise Action Tools found in Sections 12.2 through 12.5 to make the best G.R.E.E.N. Scene.

Person A—Sam: *We got a new dog two weeks ago. It is so cute. I love to take it for walks around the block. I get to have it sleep in my room at night. However, my mother said that I am not doing my part to take care of it. My dad says I need to learn responsibility. They say that I must make sure it has water to drink, but I never remember to check its water bowl! My mother says that if I can't remember to give the dog water, then we may be unable to keep it. It's hopeless! I have a terrible memory. I won't be able to keep my dog!*

Person B—Helpful, empathetic friend: ______________________________

____

Person A—Sam: ______________________________________

Person B—Helpful, empathetic schoolmate: ______________________

Person A—Sam: ______________________________________

22.21 G.R.E.E.N. Scene #15: Write It and Act It Out: Please Help Me Play Better

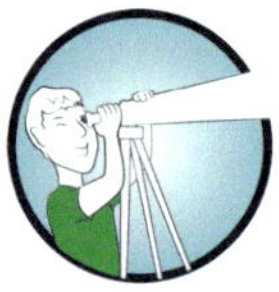

1. **Survey the scene** to make an inference about how the person feels and why the person feels that way. Find and underline the clue words that can help you make your best guess about how this person feels.

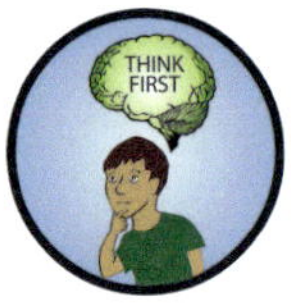

2. Think about what you could say or do to help this person feel **better**.

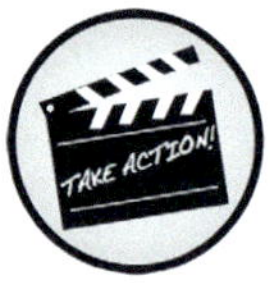

3. Fill in the script lines and then act them out.
4. Follow the steps and use the Wise Action Tools found in Sections 12.2 through 12.5 to make the best **G.R.E.E.N.** Scene.

Person A—Scott: *My brother keeps laughing at me when I try to throw a softball to him. It makes it even harder to concentrate on doing a good job. I want to practice throwing and catching so I can get on a softball team at my school, but I can't practice with my brother because I know all he wants to do is laugh at me. I'm never going to learn to throw and catch well.*

Person B—Helpful, empathetic friend: ______________________________

____

Person A—Scott: ______________________________

Person B—Helpful, empathetic schoolmate: ______________________________

Person A—Scott: ______________________________

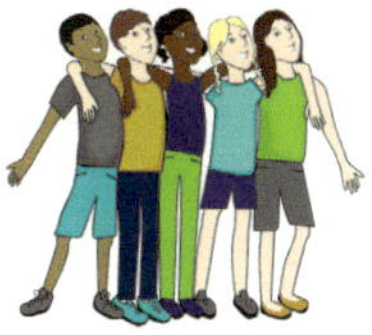

23 Being Easygoing

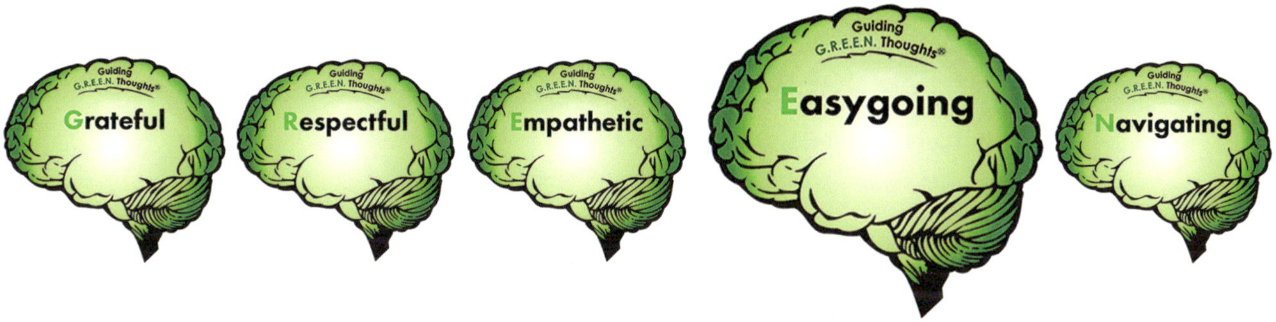

23.1 What Is Easygoing?

When you are **easygoing**, you work easily and peacefully with people on your Team so you can meet your **goals**. You all **cooperate** together. You **take turns** and **share** with others. When you are **easygoing**, you **compromise** with others so that you meet your **Personal Goals** while others meet their **Personal Goals**. When you are **easygoing**, you remember the **Common Team Goals** and **cooperate** to meet your Team **goals**, too. Your actions are good for you and your Team.

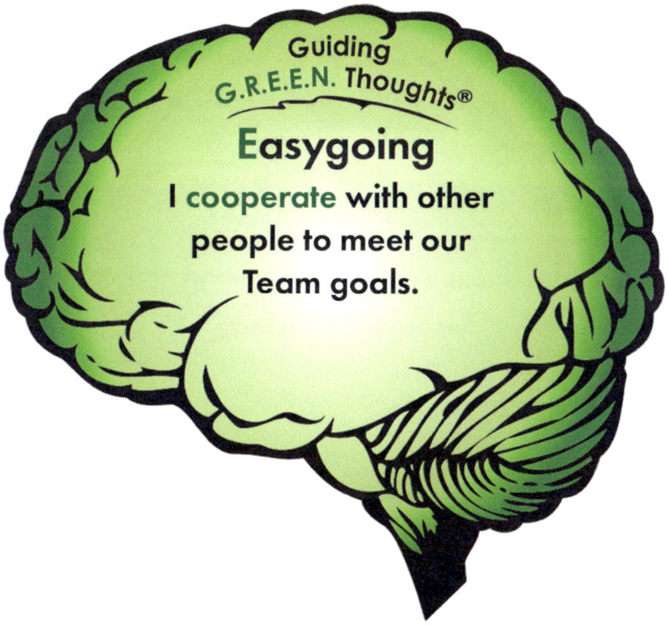

23.2 Guiding G.R.E.E.N. Thoughts: Ways to Be Easygoing

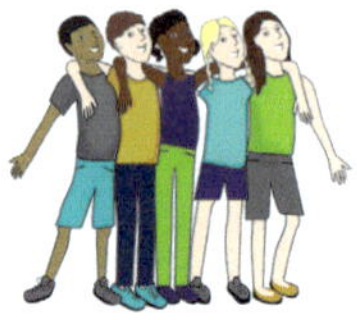

- I **cooperate** with other people on my Team to meet **Common Team Goals**
- I listen to directions and follow them.
- I choose to act in a way that is **safe**, **logical**, and **good for all**.
- I have a **positive** attitude.
- I am **patient** and **open-minded** to learn what other people want or need.
- I **wait** patiently for others to share their ideas.
- I **take turns** listening to and talking with others on my Teams in order to have **cooperative conversations**.
- I **compromise**.

COOPERATION'S IN THE AIR

A Song for **Guiding G.R.E.E.N. Thoughts**®

by Herb Hein

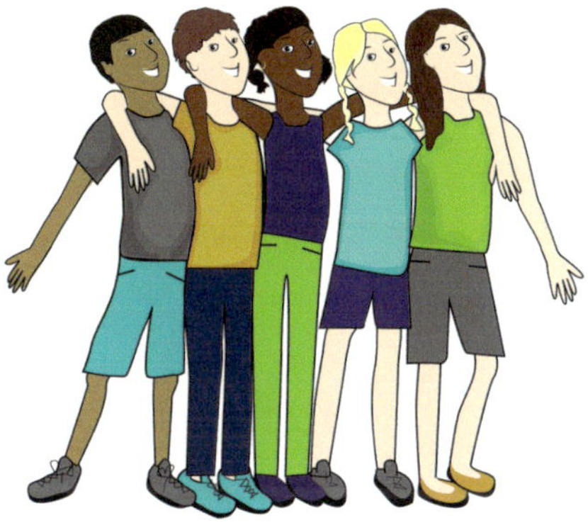

It can be so easy to get along with you.

It can be so easy to get along with you

because we learn to care,

because we learn to share,

because we learn it feels so good

when cooperation's in the air!

It can be so easy to get along with you.

It can be so easy to get along with you.

23.3 Change the Scene to Make It G.R.E.E.N.: Please Help Steve Cooperate!

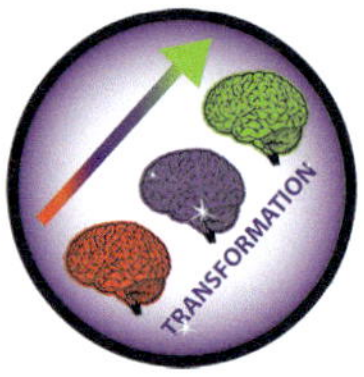

Remember when you learned about being **R.E.D.**? It means being **R**ude, **E**gocentric & **D**isruptive. **R.E.D.** action does *not* help the Team move **forward**. Let's **survey the scene** to notice the **R.E.D.** action. Then let's think about how to **change the scene** to make it **G.R.E.E.N.**

1. Read the paragraph below. Underline in red where Steve's action is *not* being **helpful** to the Team because it shows someone *not* being **easygoing** and **cooperative**.

   Steve does not like to listen to his teacher. When she asks him to stop making loud noises, he tells her, "No!" When the teacher asks why Steve is making the noises, Steve says, "I am making loud noises because I feel like it, and it's fun!"

2. Circle which Team Steve should be thinking about in this scene.

   Home Team   Classroom Team   Friendship Team   Sports Team

3. Is Steve **helping** or hurting the Team?   **helping**   hurting

4. Circle the **Common Team Goals** below that you think Steve should be thinking about in this scene.

   A. We all **cooperate** so that our classroom is a place where we can all work and learn.

   B. We easily **accept feedback** from other Team members.

   C. We distract each other, so we don't finish our work.

   D. We all **respect** one another and **cooperate** so everyone can focus and do their best work.

5. Complete this **Guiding G.R.E.E.N. Thought** to help Steve **cooperate better** in his classroom. You can help him make the best choice from the following:

   A. **change** my actions

   B. continue the bothersome action

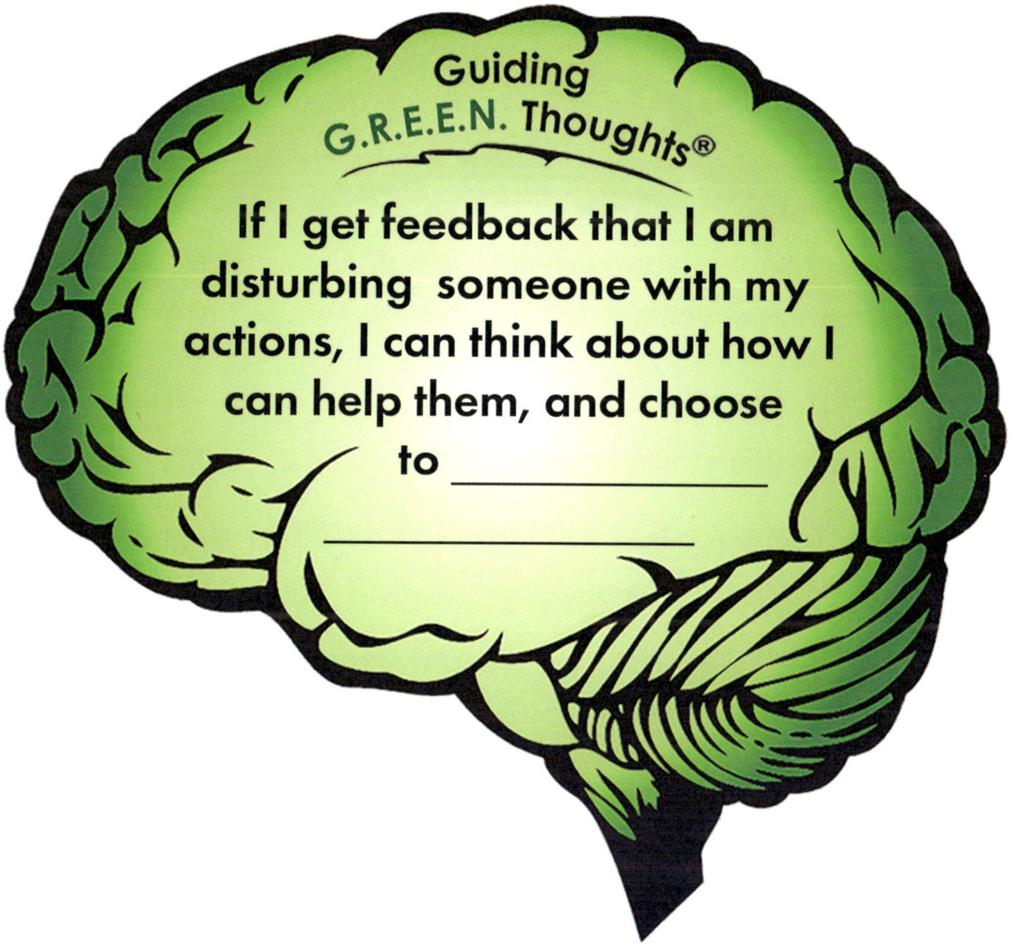

What about you? If you get feedback that you are disturbing someone with your actions, are you able to **cooperate** with a **positive attitude** and **change** your actions?

yes no

23.4 G.R.E.E.N. Scene #16: I Cooperate with a Positive Attitude

Let's **rewind** the scene so Steve can act **helpful.** Underline in **green** where Steve's action is **helpful.** Then act out the **G.R.E.E.N.** Scene. Follow the steps and use the Wise Action Tools found in Sections 12.2 through 12.5 to make the best **G.R.E.E.N.** Scene.

Narrator: Steve enjoys humming, and he sometimes forgets that he should not hum in his classroom.

One day, his teacher hears him humming during independent work time, so she asks him to stop.

Teacher: *Steve, please stop humming. It is disturbing your classmates, who are concentrating on their work.*

Narrator: Steve remembers that he wants to **cooperate** with his teacher and his classmates, so he stops what he was doing.

Steve: "Sorry, I didn't realize I was being so loud. I'll do my best to remember to be quiet so I don't disturb the others."

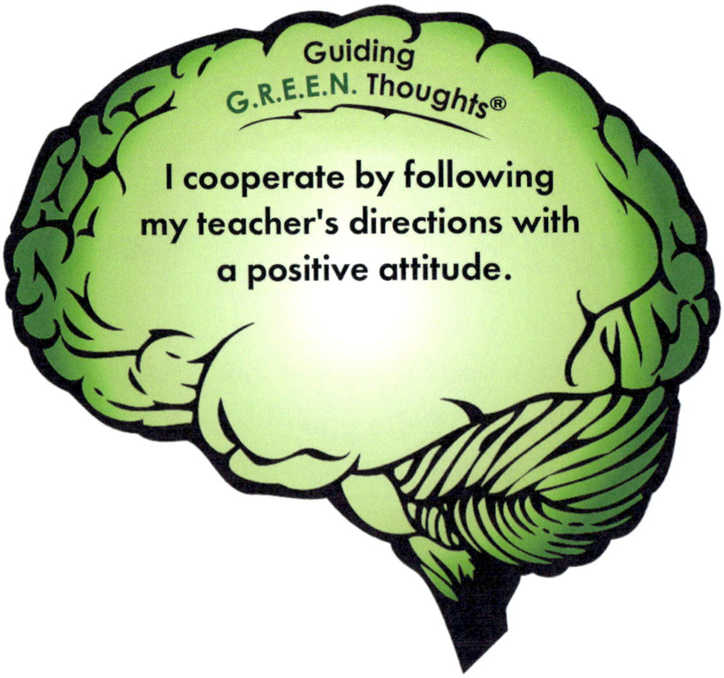

23.5 Change the Scene to Make It G.R.E.E.N.: Please Help Marco Share!

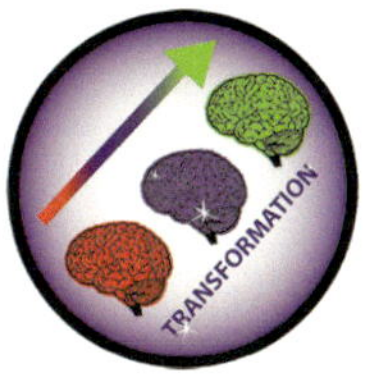

R.E.D. action stops the Team from moving **forward**. Let's **survey this scene** to notice the **R.E.D.** action. Then let's think about how to **change the scene** to make it **G.R.E.E.N.**

1. Read the paragraph below. Underline in red any action you think is *not* being **helpful** to the Team because it shows that someone is *not* **cooperating**.

   Marco does not like to share. When his classroom heads out to recess, he grabs the only classroom ball and holds on to it. When he is outside, his classmates ask him to pass the ball to them, but he just bounces it to himself and moves away from them. When his teacher asks him to share, he says, "I got it first! It's mine!"

2. Circle which Team Marco should be thinking about in this scene.

   Home Team   Classroom Team   Friendship Team   Sports Team

3. Is Marco **helping** or hurting the Team?

   helping   hurting

4. Circle the **Common Team Goals** 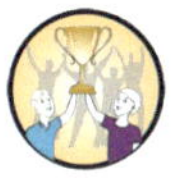 that Marco should be thinking about in this scene.

   A. We **share** and **take turns**.

   B. We get to school on time.

   C. We stay quiet when it is time to get our work done.

   D. We take action to **cooperate** well with one another.

5. Circle the classroom rules Marco should be following so his Classroom Team can be **easygoing**:

   A. **Take turns** doing important or fun things if we all can't do them at the same time.

   B. Ask for help when you need it.

   C. We **share** the things we have in the classroom in a fair way.

6. Complete this **Guiding G.R.E.E.N. Thought** to help Marco **cooperate better** with his classmates. You can make the best choice from the following words:

   A. **share**

   B. not share

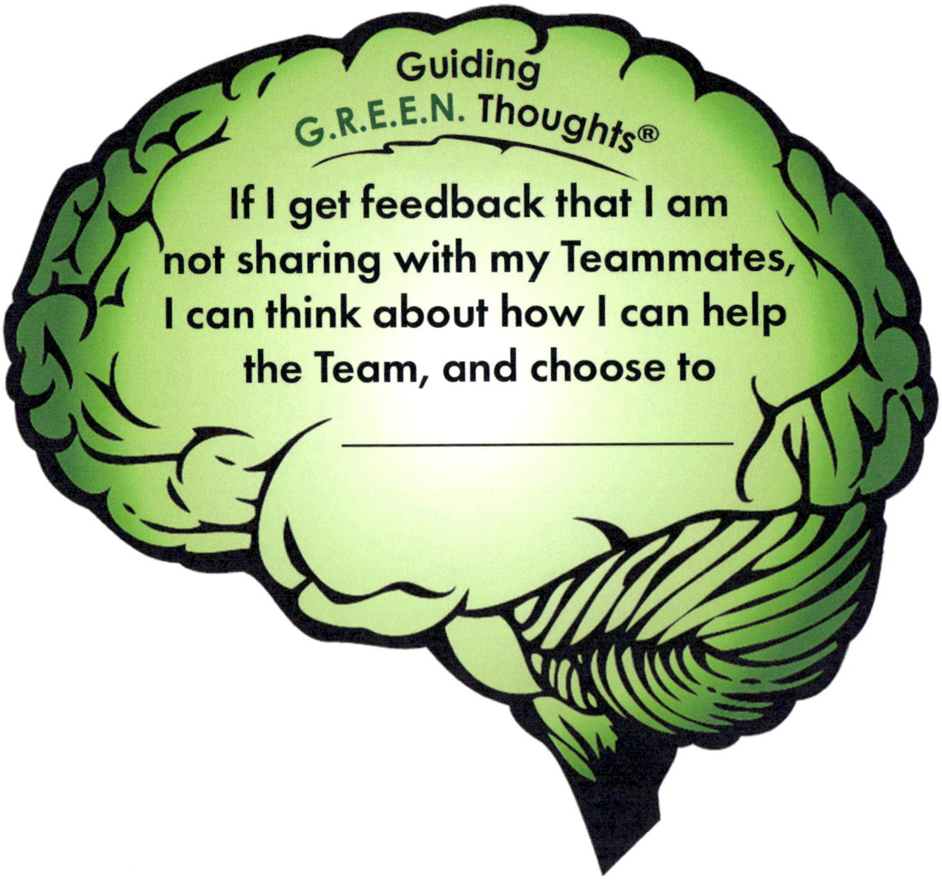

23.6 Scene #17: I Share the Ball with My Team

Let's **rewind** the scene so Marco can act **cooperatively**. Underline in **green** where it shows that Marco's actions are **cooperative**. Then act out the **G.R.E.E.N.** Scene. Follow the steps and use the Wise Action Tools found in Sections 12.2 through 12.5 to make the best **G.R.E.E.N.** Scene.

Narrator: It is time for recess. Everyone starts to line up at the door. Marco gets the ball. The class walks outside.

Marco's classmate Rick: *Marco, can we take turns passing the ball to each other?*

Marco: *Sure. Let's see who else wants to play Pass the Ball with us.*

Rick: *Who else wants to play with the ball?*

Narrator: Two other classmates say they want to.

Marco: *Great! Let's get in a circle and I'll pass it to Rick and then he'll pass it to next person. Let's see how many times we can pass it around without missing.*

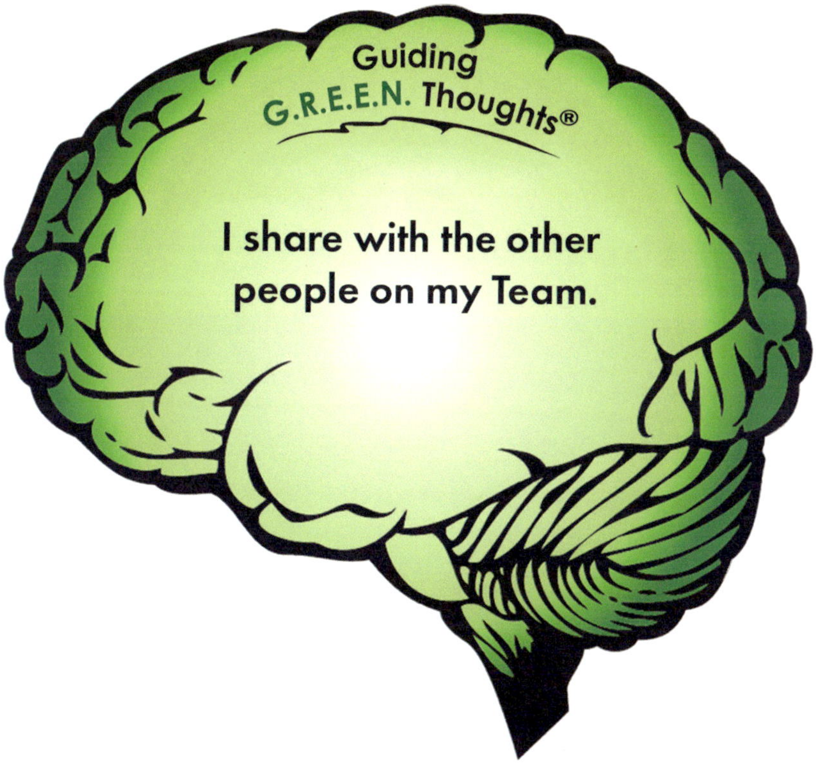

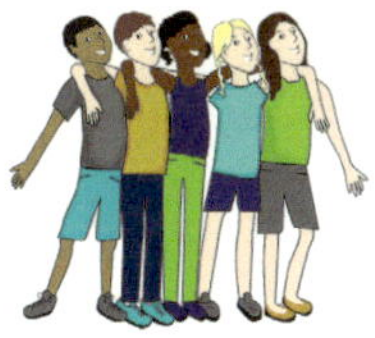

24 Take Steps to Make Connections with Teams

Take a step forward to connect →

I took steps to *disconnect* from other people.	-4	-3	-2	-1	0	+1	+2	+3	+4	I took steps to make positive civilized connections with other people.

← Take a step backward to disconnect

24.1 Thinking of Being on Friendship Teams

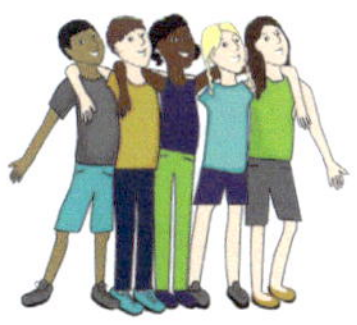

Humans mostly are social creatures. This means we usually like to be with other people. Most humans like to build friendships. But it is not always easy to make friends or keep friends. It is easier to know how to make and keep friends if you think that you are on a Team with them. It makes life enjoyable when we know that we have friends and are on the same Friendship Team with them.

24.2 Read and Discuss: Why Do Humans Have Friends?

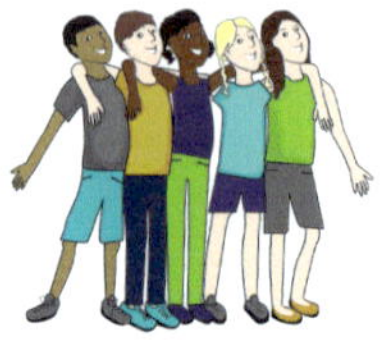

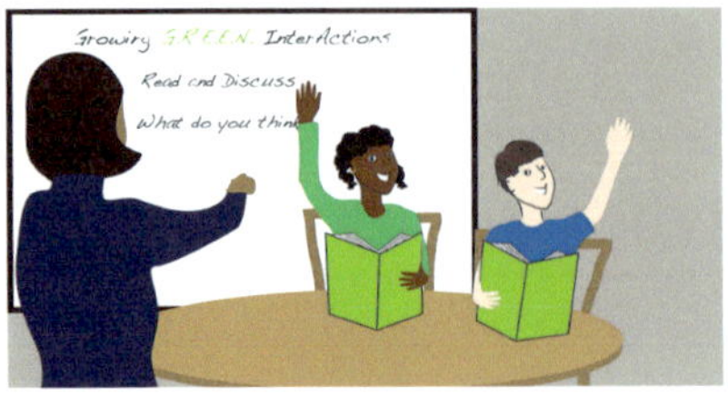

Many humans like to have friends around them so they won't feel lonely. Many humans like to share experiences with other people. Friends enjoy doing many things together and enjoy talking about all kinds of things together.

Let's list more reasons why it is good to make friends and keep friends?

What are the **positive** consequences of having friends? Friends can

- support you
- encourage you
- agree with you
- challenge you to be your best
- help you when you're feeling sad or worried
- laugh with you
- play with you
- converse with you
- share things with you
- introduce you to new people, places, ideas, etc.

Add your own ideas! ____

____

When you realize that friendships are important to you, you learn to take action to make friends and keep them. You can learn to **connect** to your Friendship Team in a **positive** way.

Hopefully, you can expect your friends to act **positive** and **helpful** with you. You also want your friends to trust you to act **positive** and **helpful** with them. When friends act **positive** and **helpful** with each other, it usually feels great. Friends make the effort to **care** about each other and **help** each other out.

24.3 What Common Team Goals Can You Share with Your Friends?

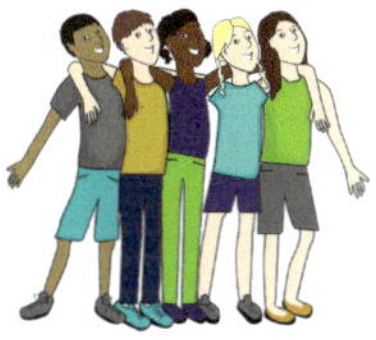

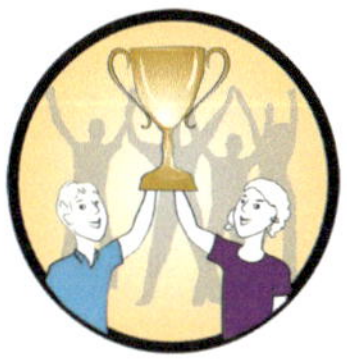

Can you think of some **Common Friendship Team Goals**? What kinds of **goals** can be achieved when friends are working together on the same Team?

1. We act **supportive** and **respectful** with one another.

2. We show that we **care** by making sure we *don't* hurt one another's feelings.

3. We enjoy spending time being together and doing things that we both like to do.

4. We **take turns** talking to one another and **sharing** ideas.

5. ____

6. ____

When you think about your friendships and **Common Friendship Team Goals**, you can build **powerful** friendships! You can build strong connections with your friends by carefully choosing your words and actions to **support** your Friendship Team!

"Go Friendship Team!"

YOU ARE A FRIEND OF MINE

A Song for **Guiding G.R.E.E.N. Thoughts**®

By Herb Hein

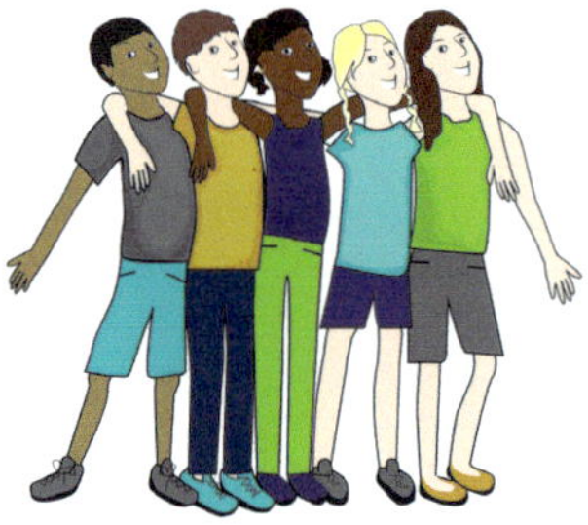

You are a friend of mine.
You help make my life worth living.
You are a friend of mine.
We walk down the same path.
We walk down the same path for a while.
We walk down the same path for a while,
or maybe longer.
You are a friend of mine.
We sit down and talk together.
You are a friend of mine.
You listen to my stories.
I listen to what you have to say.
We help when times are bad
and then we're there to share
when we're soaring.
I feel alive when I'm with you;
You bring out the best in me.
I feel alive when I'm with;
I bring out the best in you.
You are a friend of mine.
You help make my life worth living.
You are a friend of mine.
We walk down the same path.
We walk down the same path for a while.
We walk down the same path for a while,
or maybe longer.

24.4 Survey the Scene: Are They Connecting to Friendship Teams or Disconnecting from Them?

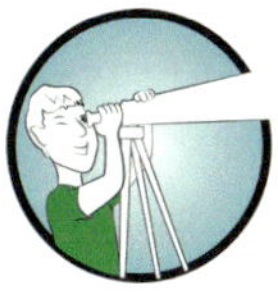

Survey the scene to see what kinds of choices some people are making.

- Are they choosing to **build** and **connect** with **respectful**, **empathetic**, and **supportive** words and actions to make their Friendship Teams **stronger**?
- Are they choosing to disconnect and break from their Friendship Teams, making them weaker with their rude, egocentric, and unsupportive words and actions?
- Are they making their friendships **stronger** or weaker?

Directions: Circle the words that tell if the person's behavior is a friendship connector or a friendship disconnector. Think about what might happen next in each situation. Will the consequences of each action choice be positive or negative?

1. Alex demands that his friend only plays the games that Alex wants to play.

   friendship connector friendship disconnector

2. Alex takes turns with his friend to decide what they will do together.

   friendship connector friendship disconnector

3. Stephanie says that she already knows everything about all her subjects and does not need her friend to tell her anything.

   friendship connector friendship disconnector

4. Stephanie says that even though she already knows a lot about her subjects, she would still like to hear what her friend knows about them.

   friendship connector friendship disconnector

5. When his friend asks him to be quiet while he is finishing his homework, Robbie listens, respects that his friend needs quiet time to work, and waits quietly.

   friendship connector friendship disconnector

6. When his friend asks him to be quiet while he is finishing his homework, Robbie laughs at his friend and makes fun of him.

   friendship connector friendship disconnector

7. Peter makes sure that he and his brother take turns when playing games. He thinks this is fair.

   friendship connector friendship disconnector

8. Peter likes to take extra turns when playing games and makes his brother beg to have a turn. He does not care whether his brother thinks this is fair.

   friendship connector friendship disconnector

What do you think makes an action a **friendship connector** action? ___________

____

24.5 Using the Connection Direction Tracker: Am I Moving Forward or Backward with My Team?

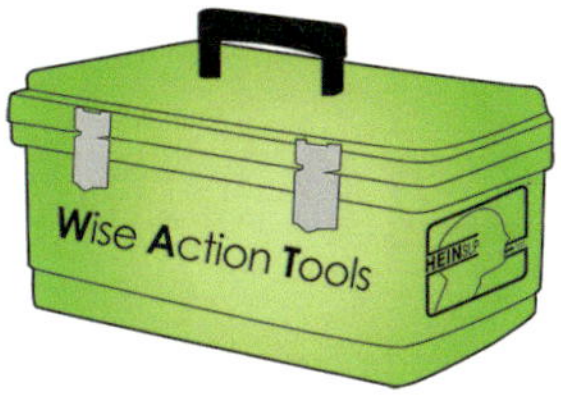

On the next exercise, you can use the Connection Direction Tracker to track each action you make and show whether it moves in a direction to **connect** with the Team or moves in a direction to disconnect or break from the Team.

Start on the Connection Direction Tracker by putting a token in the middle on zero (0).

If you make a **helpful, respectful**, or **empathetic** comment, the other person will know that you **care**. To show this, you will take a step **forward** and move your token one space to the right. Your words or actions **connected** you to the Team!

However, if you make an impulsive or hurtful comment, the other person will feel sad or unsafe. To show this, you will take a step backward and move your token one space to the left, to show that your words or actions disconnected you from the Team.

CONNECTION DIRECTION TRACKER

AM I MOVING FORWARD, OR BACKWARD, WITH MY TEAM?

Take a step forward to connect →

I took steps to *disconnect* from other people.	-4	-3	-2	-1	0	+1	+2	+3	+4	I took steps to make positive civilized connections with other people.

← Take a step backward to disconnect

If you were given the chance to act four times with your Team, where would your token end up? Do you think the location of the token would show that you moved **forward** with your Team, backward with your Team, or would you end up back in the middle on zero? The Connection Direction Tracker lets you see if you are consistently acting as if you want the Team to move **forward** or if you only sometimes act in this **Team-connecting** way.

Each time you start to do an exercise in this section, start at the zero location until you start taking actions to show your Teammates if you are **connecting** or disconnecting from them. Before you take action, the other person does not yet know whether you can be trusted to be a good Team member. But if you make a **helpful, respectful**, **empathetic** comment to show that you **care**, you can take a step **forward** to **connect**. Your words or actions helped make a stronger Team connection.

However, if you make an impulsive, hurtful comment that makes the other person feel sad or unsafe, take one step backward. Your words or action disconnected you from the rest of the Team.

Help make a strong Team by consistently moving **forward** on the Connection Direction Tracker with your words or actions. You will have a chance to see how well you can **connect** by acting in Quick **G.R.E.E.N.** Scenes for different Teams. Start in the zero (0) space and then do your best to keep moving toward the goal of (+4) by consistently taking action to move the Team **forward**. You can have as many turns to act in these Quick **G.R.E.E.N.** Scenes until you are able to move each Team **forward** four times with your **connecting** words.

Follow the directions for Quick **G.R.E.E.N.** Scenes (1–6 in Section 21.8).

Take a step forward to connect →

I took steps to *disconnect* from other people.	-4	-3	-2	-1	0	+1	+2	+3	+4	I took steps to make positive civilized connections with other people.

← Take a step backward to disconnect

24.6 Quick G.R.E.E.N. Scenes: Connecting on a Home Team

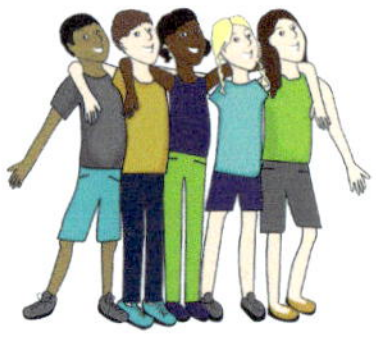

Directions:

1. Act out these Quick **G.R.E.E.N.** Scenes. In each scene a person will say something to you. Think of something to say that will make you be a Home Team connector. (If you want help knowing what to say, you can find some **helpful G.R.E.E.N.** comments below each line.)

2. Use your Connection Direction Tracker with the Quick **G.R.E.E.N.** Scenes to see how well you can build connections on a Home Team.

3. Start with your token on zero. Then, after you act out each scene, move your token one step **forward** or one step backward depending on what you said. Ask for feedback from the others you are with during this exercise. Do they think you moved in a **forward-connecting** or a backward–disconnecting direction? Take the challenge to **connect** as much as possible in each scene. Where is your token at the end?

Home Scene #1

Father: *Can* you help *me bring down the trash?*

You: ____

Possible Home Team-Connector comments: *Yes. Let me put on some shoes.* Then I'll meet you outside.

Home Scene #2

Mother: *Could* you help *me find my keys?*

You: ____

Possible Home Team-Connector comments: *Sure. Where did* you *have them last?*

Home Scene #3

Brother: *Could I please have a turn?*

You: ____

Possible Home Team-Connector comments: *OK, I'll be finished with my turn in one minute.*

Home Scene #4

Sister: *Could* you *turn that down? I'm trying to sleep.*

You: ____

Possible Home Team-Connector comments: *Sure. Sorry for bothering you.*

Take a step forward to connect →

I took steps to *disconnect* from other people.	-4	-3	-2	-1	0	+1	+2	+3	+4	I took steps to make positive civilized connections with other people.

← Take a step backward to disconnect

Where is your token at the end of the four Home interactions?

Mark it with an X.

Name ______________________________ Date ____________________

24.7 Quick G.R.E.E.N. Scenes: Connecting on a Classroom Team

Directions:

1. Act out these Quick G.R.E.E.N. Scenes. In each scene a person will say something to you. Think of something to say that will make you be a Classroom Team connector. (If you want help knowing what to say, you can find some **helpful, G.R.E.E.N.** comments below each line.)

2. Use your Connection Direction Tracker with the Quick **G.R.E.E.N.** Scenes to see how well you can build connections on a Classroom Team.

3. Start with your token on zero. Then, after you act out each scene, move your token one step **forward** or one step backward depending on what you said. Ask for feedback from the others you are with during this exercise. Do they think you moved in a **forward-connecting** or a backward-disconnecting direction? Take the challenge to **connect** as much as possible in each scene. Where is your token at the end?

School Scene #1

Teacher: *Please rewrite the sentence you wrote so that we can read it.*

You: ____

Possible **Classroom Team-Connector comments:** *OK, Sorry. I wrote it really fast.*

School Scene #2

Classmate: Could you please stop shaking the desk?

You: ____

Possible **Classroom Team-Connector comments:** *OK, Sorry. I didn't realize I was shaking it.*

School Scene #3

Classmate: *Can we take turns shooting baskets?*

You: ____

Possible **Classroom Team-Connector comments:** *Sure. Let me finish taking this shot.*

School Scene #4

Teacher: *Could you please share your book with Jeremy?*

You: ____

Possible **Classroom Team-Connector comments:** *Yes, of course.*

Take a step forward to connect →

I took steps to *disconnect* from other people.	-4	-3	-2	-1	0	+1	+2	+3	+4	I took steps to make positive civilized connections with other people.

← Take a step backward to disconnect

Where is your token at the end of the four Classroom interactions?

Mark it with an X.

Name ______________________________ Date ____________________

24.8 Quick G.R.E.E.N. Scenes: Connecting on Friendship Teams

Directions:

1. Act out these Quick **G.R.E.E.N.** Scenes. In each scene a person will say something to you. Think of something to say that will make you be a Friendship Team connector. (If you want help knowing what to say, you can find **helpful G.R.E.E.N.** comments below each line.)

2. Use your Connection Direction Tracker with the Quick **G.R.E.E.N.** Scenes to see how well you can build connections on a Friendship Team.

3. Start with your token on zero. Then, after you act out each scene, move your token one step **forward** or one step backward depending on what you said.

Ask for feedback from the others you are with during this exercise. Do they think you moved in a **forward-connecting** or a backward-disconnecting direction? Take the challenge to **connect** as much as possible in each scene. Where is your token at the end?

Friendship Scene #1

Friend in line at lunchtime: *I can't wait to eat. I'm really hungry.*

You: ____

Possible Friendship-Connector **comments:** *Me, too. I wonder what our choices are today.*

Friendship Scene #2

Friend in the backyard: *I am really afraid of spiders.*

You: ____

Possible Friendship-Connector **comments:** *I'm afraid of some things, too.*

Friendship Scene #3

Friend: *I'm worried about the spelling test I have tomorrow.*

You: ____

Possible Friendship-Connector **comments:** *I'm sorry to hear that. Can I help you study your words?*

Friendship Scene #4

Friend: *I just got this new sweatshirt for my birthday yesterday.*

You: ____

Possible Friendship-Connector comments: *That looks really comfortable. Happy Birthday!*

Take a step forward to connect →

I took steps to *disconnect* from other people.	-4	-3	-2	-1	0	+1	+2	+3	+4	I took steps to make positive civilized connections with other people.

← Take a step backward to disconnect

Where is your token at the end of the four Friendship interactions?

Mark it with an X.

Name ______________________________ Date ____________________

24.9 Survey the Scene at Dinnertime—Scene #1: Who Is Connecting on the Home Team?

Take a step forward to connect →

I took steps to *disconnect* from other people.	-4	-3	-2	-1	0	+1	+2	+3	+4	I took steps to make positive civilized connections with other people.

← Take a step backward to disconnect

Directions: Circle in green when you notice that someone said something or did something to connect with the Team and help the Team reach its goal. Circle in red if someone said something or did something that disconnected from the Team and blocked the Team so it couldn't move forward to reach its goal. Move a token on the Connection Direction Tracker to show the steps Rob took in Scene #1 to connect or disconnect from his Home Team.

Scene #1

Rob *and* Mark were kicking the ball back *and* forth with each other in the backyard. They enjoyed taking turns. Their mother came to the door *and* told them she was almost done cooking dinner. It was time to come in *and* wash up. She asked them to please set the table. The boys stopped playing. They came in the house, washed their hands, *and* set the table. Then they sat down to eat dinner with their mother. They enjoyed talking to each other while they were eating dinner. When the boys were done, they thanked their mother for dinner *and* put their dishes in the sink. Then they asked if they could go back outside to play. Their mother said "yes." She was proud of how her sons were acting.

Questions about Scene #1

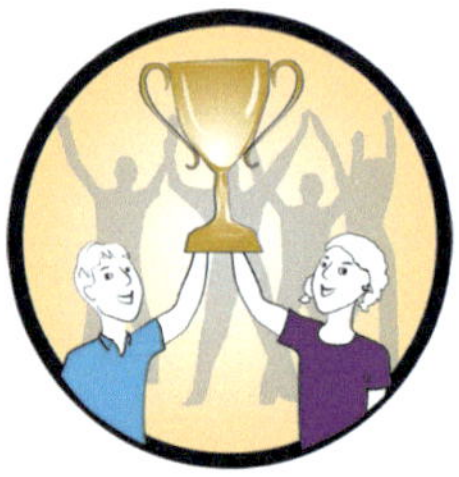

1. What do you think the Common Team Goal might be for this Home Team? ______________________________

____

____

2. Are both boys helping the family meet the Common Team Goal?

yes   no

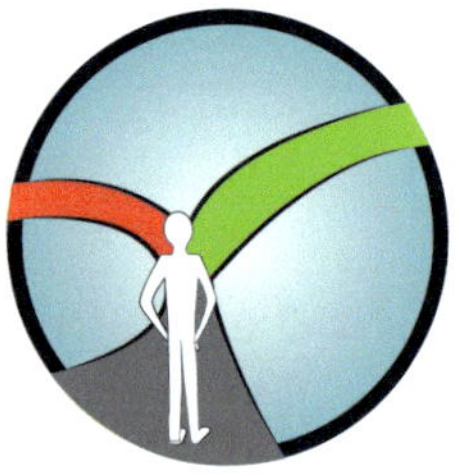

3. What are the boys choosing to do to help the Team?

____

____

4. What is the mother doing to help the Team? ______________________________

____

5. What did the boys do to show their mother that they appreciated her cooking dinner for them? ______________________________

____

24.10 Survey the Scene at Dinnertime—Scene #2: Who Is Disconnecting from the Home Team?

Take a step forward to connect →

I took steps to *disconnect* from other people.	-4	-3	-2	-1	0	+1	+2	+3	+4	I took steps to make positive civilized connections with other people.

← Take a step backward to disconnect

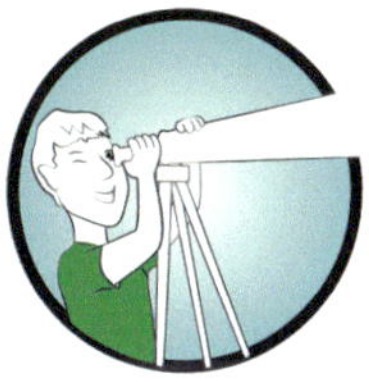

Directions: Circle in green when you notice that someone said something or did something to connect with the Team and help the Team reach its goal. Circle in red if someone said something or did something that disconnected from the Team and blocked the Team so it couldn't move forward to reach its goal. Move a token on the Connection Direction Tracker to show the steps Rob took in Scene #2 to connnect or disconnect from his Home Team.

Scene #2

Mark wanted to share the ball with his brother, Rob. Rob did not want to share the ball. He was holding on to it and making noises that he thought were funny. Their mother came to the door and told them she was almost done cooking dinner. It was time to come in and wash up. She asked them to please set the table. Mark came in, washed his hands, and started to set the table. Rob ran around the house making funny noises. He did not wash his hands. He did not help set the table. He did not sit down at the table. His mother asked him to please do what she had asked him to do so they could all sit down to dinner and talk about their day. When Rob still did not sit down, the mother sat down with Mark to eat dinner before it got cold.

Questions about Scene #2

1. What do you think the **Common Team Goal** might be for this Home Team?

____

____

2. Is Rob **helping** the family meet the **Common Team Goal**?

yes no

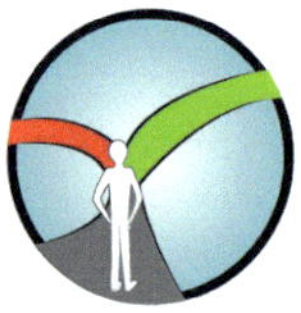

3. Is Mark making choices to **help** the Home Team?

yes no

4. What is the mother doing to **help** everyone meet the **Common Team Goal**?

____

____

5. Let's **rewind** the scene to make it more **G.R.E.E.N.** and **better** for the Team. What **changes** could any of the characters make in their actions so everyone could be **helping** the Home Team? ________________________________

____

____

6. What is the best scene for showing everyone **connecting** on this Home Team?

Scene #1

Scene #2

Name ________________________________ Date ________________

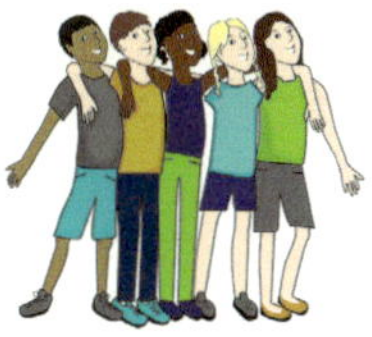

25 Being Easygoing When You Have Mixed Feelings

25.1 Read and Discuss: Having Mixed Feelings

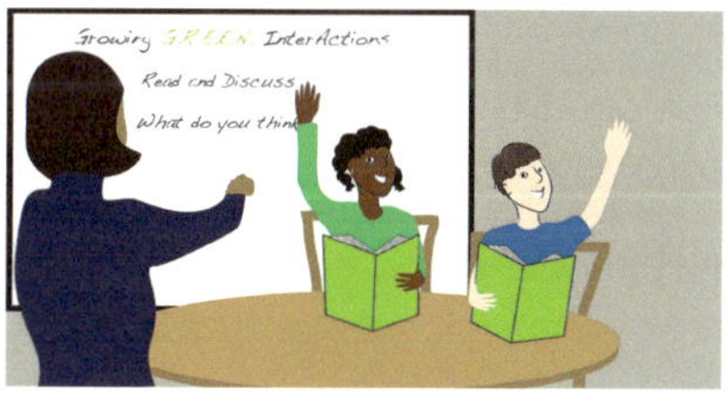

When you are in a real-life situation, you may have several different feelings. Sometimes it is hard to figure out those feelings.

On top of that, some feelings "inside" you may be different from the best ones shown to people on the "outside." Your "negative inside" feelings might lead you to think or act **R.E.D.** At the same time, you may be working hard to act **positive** and **G.R.E.E.N.** on the "outside" with the people around you. This gets confusing! It is important to be aware of these mixed feelings and understand them so you can have the **self-control** needed to choose to act on your **positive** feelings so they can lead to **positive** consequences for you and your Teams.

It is often hard to figure out what these mixed feelings are, but you can do your best to name these feelings and figure out why you have them. When you can Think First to do your best to figure out how you feel, it can help you make the best choices in what you say and do when you are with others. Thinking First to help you figure out your mixed feelings helps you avoid disconnecting from your Teams and having negative consequences. Even though you might have some negative feelings on the "inside," you can help yourself find some **positive** feelings that will help you make **better** action choices on the "outside" with others. You can then work to make these **positive** feelings stronger so you can keep **connecting** with your Team with **G.R.E.E.N.** action. You can feel proud of yourself for your **self-control**.

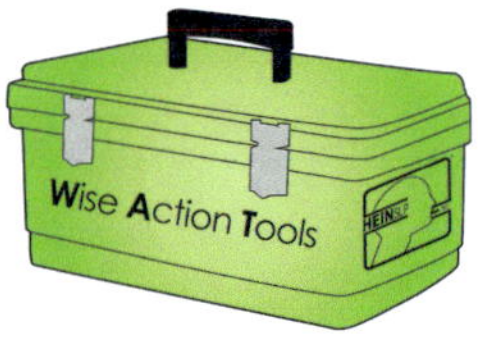

NAME MIXED FEELINGS AND THINK OF ACTION CONSEQUENCES

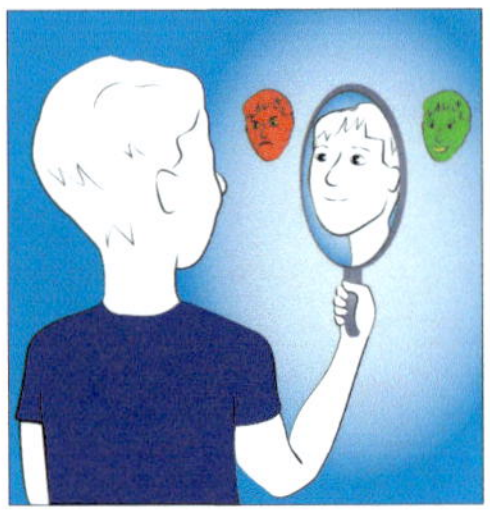

1. I put on my brakes to get self-control!
2. I Think First!
3. I name my mixed feelings.
4. I think of the positive & negative consequences of acting upon outside and inside feelings.
5. I think about how I help myself and my Team when I act upon my positive outside feelings instead of my negative inside feelings.

1. Name my inside negative feelings: What name can I give to these negative feelings? ____________________ 2. Why could I be feeling these feelings? ____________________ ____________________	1. Name my possible outside positive feelings: What name can I give to these positive feelings? ____________________ 2. Why could I be feeling these feelings? ____________________ ____________________
3. Negative consequences of showing my negative feelings: What would the negative consequences be if I acted upon these negative feelings by acting **R.E.D.**? ____________________ ____________________ ____________________	3. Positive consequences of showing my positive feelings: What would the positive consequences be if I acted upon these positive feelings by acting **G.R.E.E.N.**? ____________________ ____________________ ____________________
4. I take action to find ways to weaken these negative feelings to *avoid* acting **R.E.D.**	4. I work to strengthen these positive feelings so it is easier to take **G.R.E.E.N.** action with my Team?

25.2 Using Wise Action Tools to Take Positive Outside Action

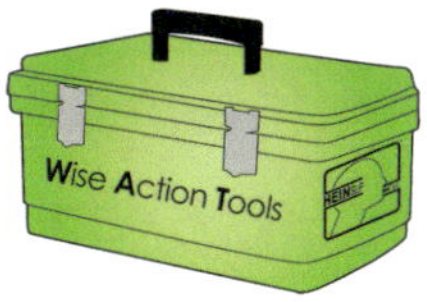

Here is a review of some Wise Action Tools that can help you act on **positive** feelings to take **G.R.E.E.N.** action with your Team!

1. Calm yourself. Brake to take a 5 break. 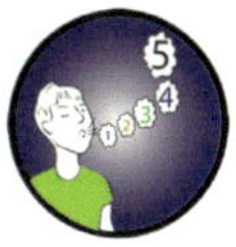

2. Think First. 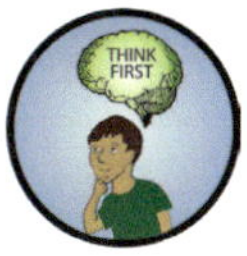

3. Think about choices you can make with your actions and the consequences of positive versus negative action. 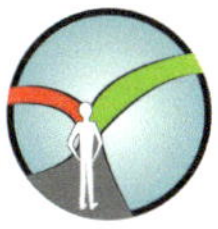

4. Think about **Guiding G.R.E.E.N. Thoughts** to guide your actions. Find words to help you think thoughts that can guide you to make the best choice for yourself and your Team. 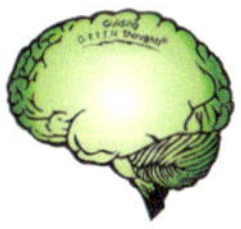

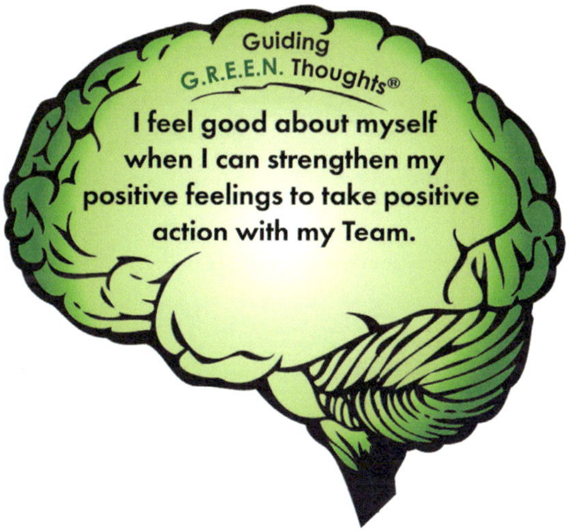

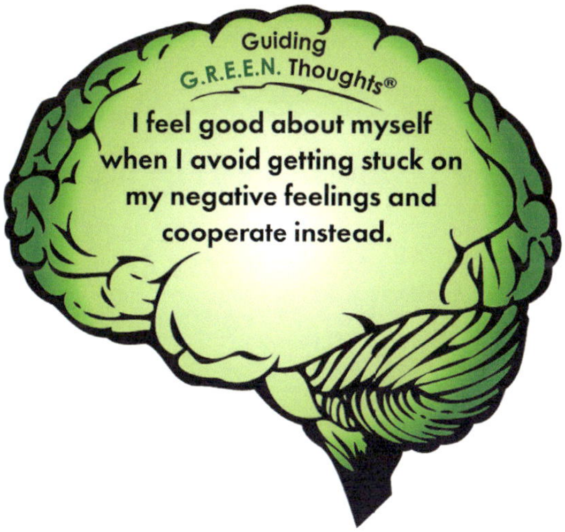

5. Use the "**Name Mixed Feelings and Think of Action Consequences**" sheet to name and write about your inside versus **outside** feelings and the consequences of acting on each. Then use your **power** to only show your **positive** feelings, actions, and words on the **outside** while keeping negative feelings on the inside.

6. Draw and write about your inside and **outside** feelings and actions by using the Wise Action Tool called "**Show Positive Outside Action Control**" found in the next section.

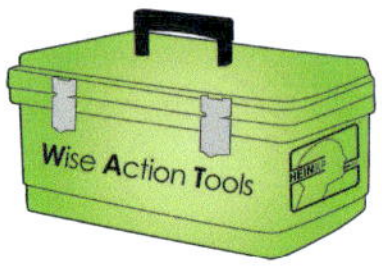

25.3 Drawing Your Choices to Help Show Positive Outside Action Control!

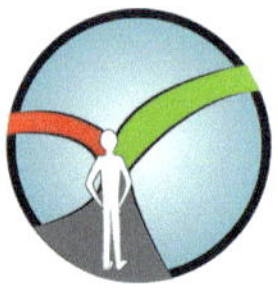

If you have positive and negative feelings at the same time, you can picture yourself having these different feelings in two different scenes. This will help you have the **self-control power** needed to only show the **positive** action that is best for you and your Team. You can take these steps when using the Wise Action Tool to "**Show Positive Outside Action Control**!"

1. Think First of what the negative consequences would be if you showed your negative actions on the outside. Within the negative inside box, write and draw the negative feelings and actions that are best kept "inside." Show how these actions negatively affect others on your Teams. What are the others with you in this scene thinking about you or saying to you? Add thought and word bubbles to show what you and the other people in this scene are thinking or saying.

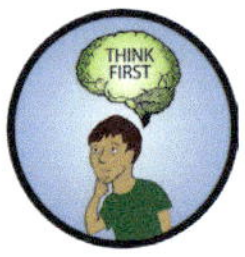

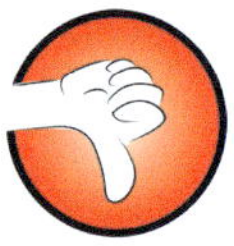

2. After you fill in the negative inside box, write and draw the **positive** feelings and actions that are best shown on the "**outside**."

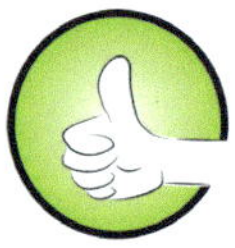

Show the **positive** consequences of choosing to show your **positive outside** action control with your Teams. What are others thinking about you or saying to you in this **positive outside** scene? What are you thinking about yourself? Add thought and word bubbles to show what you and the other people in this scene are thinking and/or saying.

3. Use your **self-control power** by remembering what you have put in the two sections of this Wise Action Tool. Then cover up the negative inside box with your hand so you cannot see it. This will help you choose to avoid acting this way in the scenes of your life.

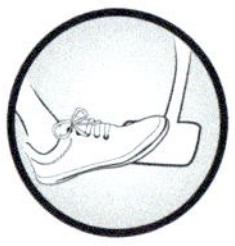

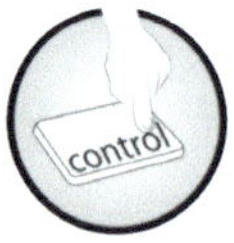

Now use your **self-control power** to focus on what happens in the **positive outside** action scene where you find yourself saying **positive** words and taking **positive** actions on the outside with your Team.

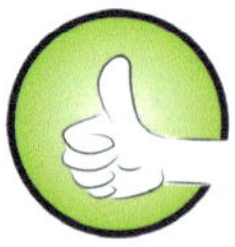

SHOW POSITIVE OUTSIDE ACTION CONTROL!

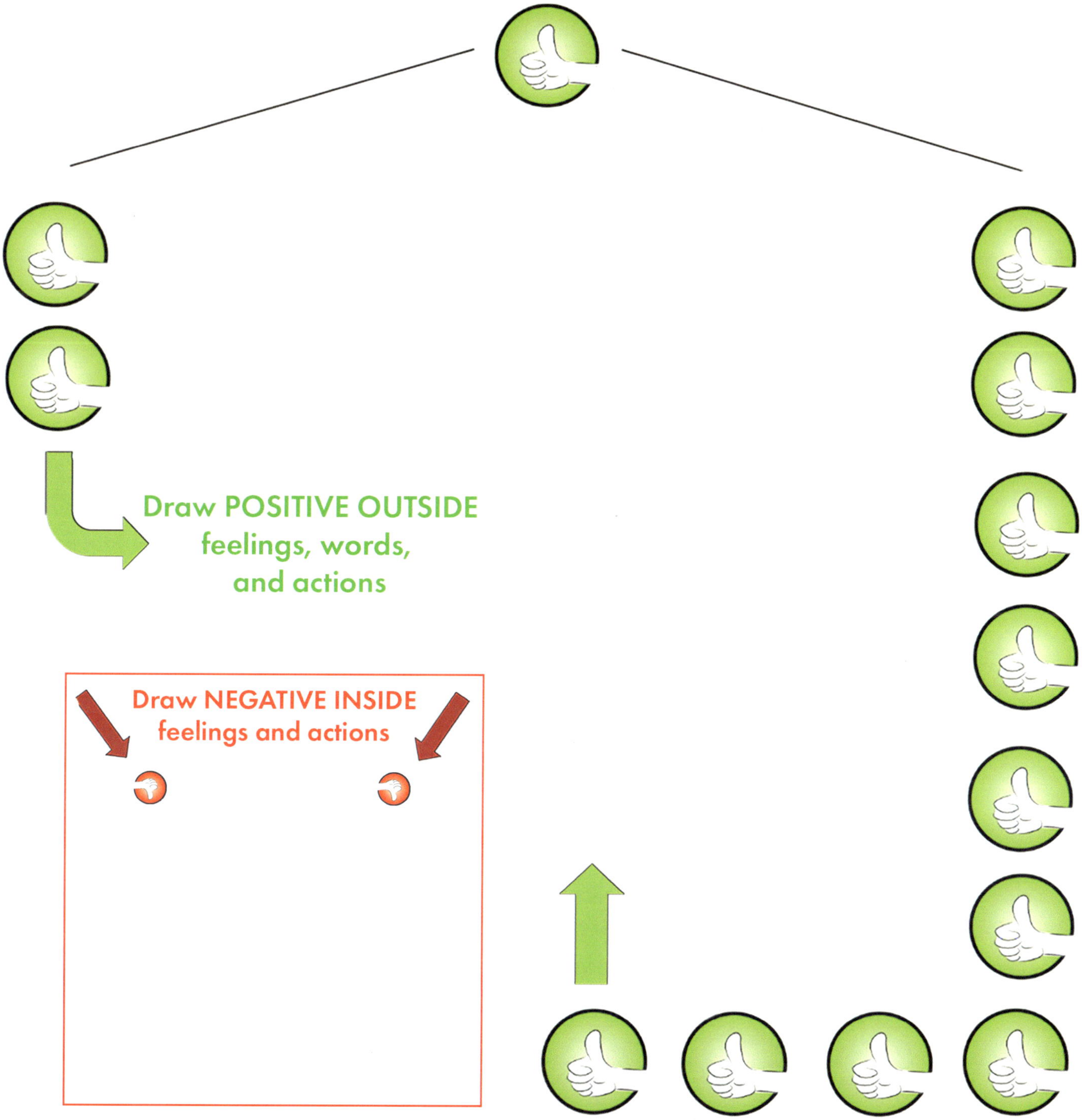

25.4 Show Positive Outside Action Control to Act Generous, Not Jealous

Imagine yourself in the following situation. What would your feelings be? Which feelings would be **better** to keep on the "inside" and which **positive** feelings would be **better** to show on the "outside" with your Teams? You might continue having both kinds of feelings, but you can use your **self-control** to show only **positive outside** feelings with your **G.R.E.E.N.** actions.

The situation: You feel happy to be playing with your friend John. You are passing a ball back and forth. He is listening to your stories and making you laugh when he tells you his stories. You enjoy his company so much that you feel surprised and annoyed when Steven comes over to join your game. You don't really want to play with anyone else and really don't want Steven playing with John and taking away his attention from you. You are starting to think that you want to tell Steven to go away and leave you both alone. Let's Think First about how you might be feeling on the "inside."

1. How would you be acting If you showed you *didn't* want to share toys or games?

   selfish and greedy or **generous**

2. How would you be acting If you showed you *didn't* want to share the time you spent playing with John with one of his other friends?

   selfish and greedy or **generous**

3. What do you think about selfish, greedy people? ______________________

   ____

4. If you were in this situation, you might be having jealous feelings whenever John gave his attention to Steven by talking to him. When you feel jealous, you want to have what the other person has. When you feel jealous, you may not be feeling **grateful** for what you already have. You may *not* be acting **grateful** for the attention you are already getting from John while he is also giving Steven some attention. Instead of acting jealous, you might develop your **transformation** skills by showing yourself and others you can act and feel **generous**! When you are feeling **generous**, you are feeling comfortable when freely giving to others. You would be acting **generous** with Steven by being willing to

share the fun of being friends with John. If you acted in this **generous** way, it is more likely that Steven would enjoy your company and want to be your friend too! By showing your **positive outside** action **control** to show your **outside generous** feelings instead of any inside jealous feelings, both John and Steven would enjoy being with you more.

What does it mean to be jealous? ______________________________

____

What do you think John would think about you if you started to act in a jealous way when he was talking to Steven? ______________________________

____

What does it mean to be generous? ______________________________

____

What do you think John would think about you if you started to act in a **generous** way to **share** John's friendship with Steven? ______________________________

____

Would it be OK to have some inside jealous feelings about Steven, but to only show **generous outside** action with both Steven and John? yes no

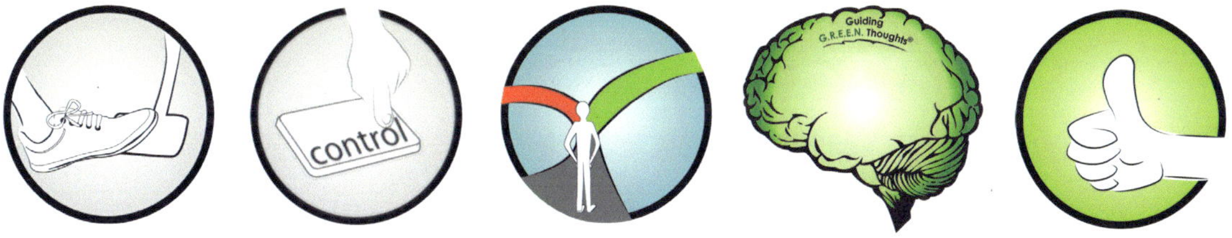

You can put on the brakes, show **self-control**, and quietly think of some **Guiding G.R.E.E.N. Thoughts** that might help you feel and act more **positive** about what is going on in this scene or any scene. You can then focus on your **positive** feelings and **positive** actions to act **G.R.E.E.N.** and **generous** on the "outside" with your friend and his other friend. You would be showing your **Positive Outside** Action **Control**!

25.5 Guiding G.R.E.E.N. Thoughts about Sharing While Controlling Selfish, Jealous Feelings

In thinking about this friendship situation, you successfully **put on the brakes** and showed **self-control** when you noticed yourself feeling selfish and jealous. If you were in the scene, what are some **Guiding G.R.E.E.N. Thoughts** that could help you act more **G.R.E.E.N.** and share time playing with both John and Steven?

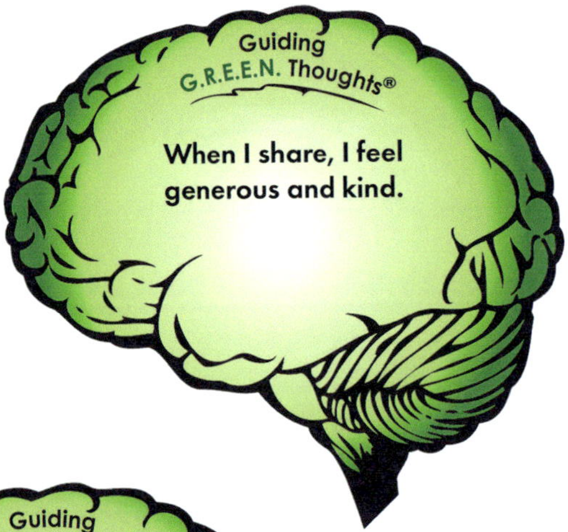

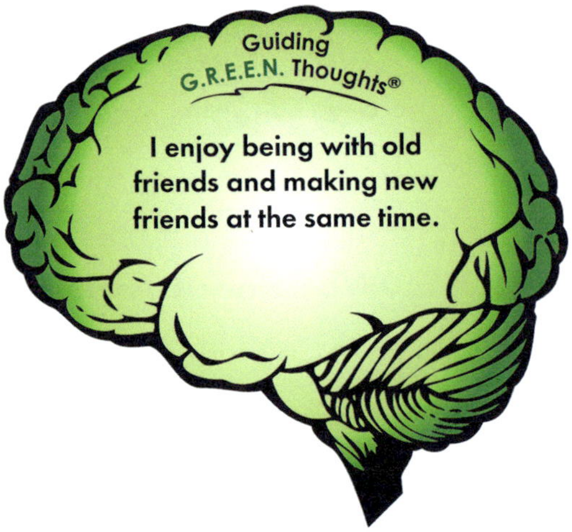

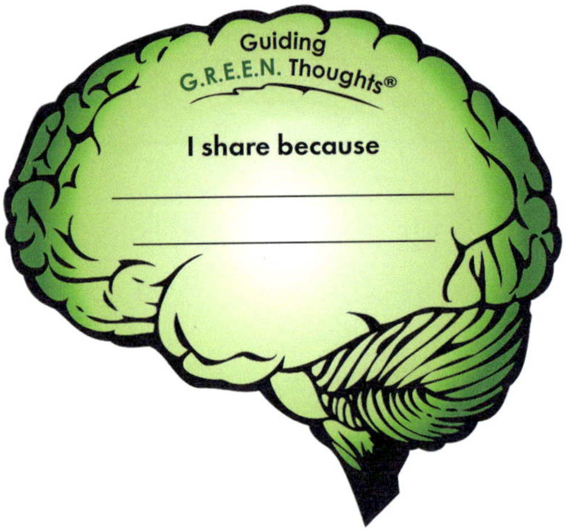

My own Guiding G.R.E.E.N. Thought for this scene:

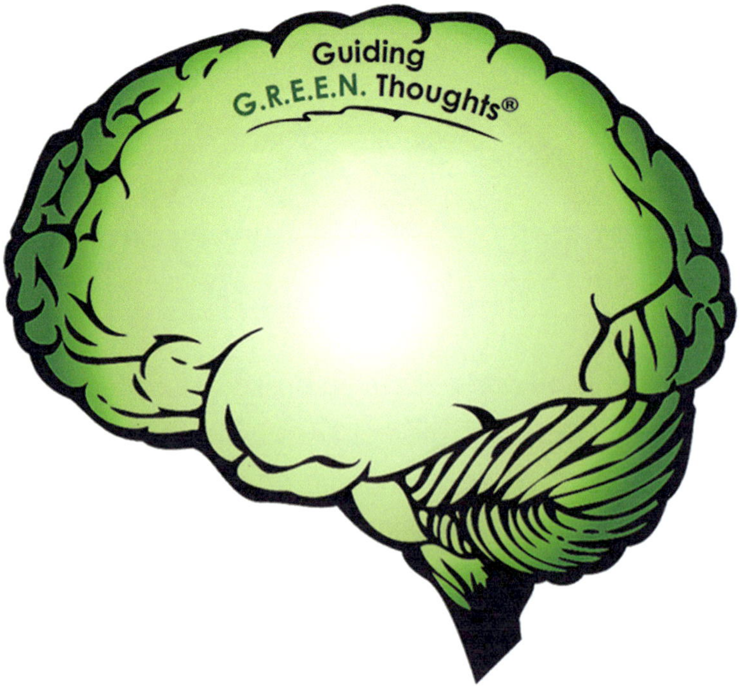

25.6 G.R.E.E.N. Scene #17: I Act Friendly with My Friend's Other Friend

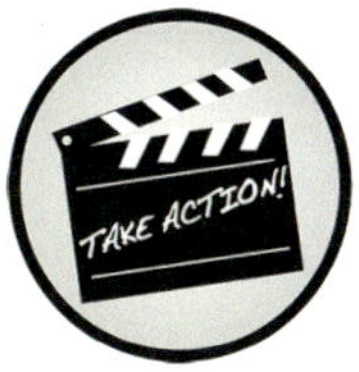

Why Act Out This Scene?

This scene can help you practice acting **positive** and **G.R.E.E.N.** on the "outside," even though you may have negative feelings on the "inside." You will find the **power** to move **forward** with your Friendship Team by focusing on the most **positive** feelings inside you. You can use a **Guiding G.R.E.E.N. Thought** from the previous page to help you succeed at acting **positive** on the "outside" to move **forward** with your friend.

Follow the steps and use the Wise Action Tools found in Sections 12.2 through 12.5 to make the best G.R.E.E.N. Scene. Get a bouncy ball to use in this scene.

Narrator: You and your friend Luis are bouncing a ball back and forth to practice your passing skills. You would like to just continue playing with Luis. One of his friends, Francisco, who you never met before, comes over and wants to play with both of you. If you forget to Think First you might tell Luis that you don't want Francisco to join you. But then you think a **Guiding G.R.E.E.N. Thought** that reminds you that it's better for your Friendship Team to act **open-minded** and **generous** by **sharing** Luis's friendship with Francisco.

Luis's other friend, Francisco: *Hey, Luis, good to see you. Can I play with you guys?*

Luis: *Yes. I think so (turning to talk to you). Is that cool with you?*

You: *Um—yeah, sure it is.*

Francisco: *Great. My name is Francisco. What is your name?*

You: *My name is* ______________________________. *Nice to meet you, Francisco.*
(say your name)

Francisco: *It's nice to meet you, too.*

You: *We were passing the ball to each other. Now we can make a bigger circle.*

Francisco: *Sounds good.*

Luis: *I'm glad we all get a chance to play together.*

Can you act only G.R.E.E.N. and generous, successfully sharing your friendship on the "outside," even though you might still have some greedy and jealous feelings on the "inside"?

yes no

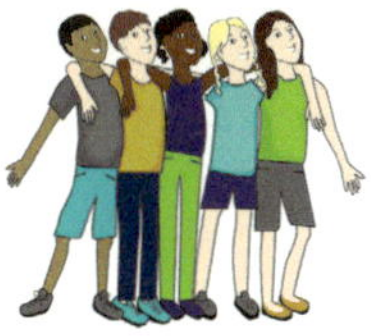

26 Sharing Points of View

26.1 Read and Discuss: Different People Have Different Points of View

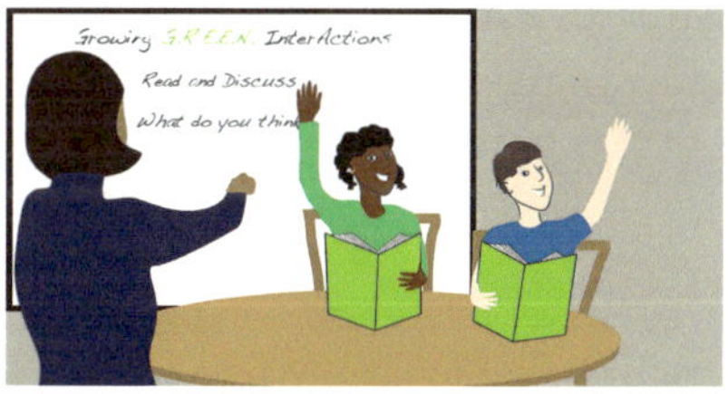

A point of view is how someone looks at something or how someone thinks about it. Different people often see and think about things differently. These different points of view come from the different experiences we each have in our lives. People have different points of view about foods, games, movies, school, people, and situations. A mother, father, brother, and sister may have different points of view about something happening in their family. A teacher and a student may have different points of view about a situation in the classroom or playground.

We each think about the world from our own points of view. However, it is important also to think about the points of view of the other people on our Teams:

- What is the other person on my Team thinking?
- What is the other person thinking about my words and actions?

The more you understand about the other person's point of view, the more **respectful** and **easygoing** you can be with that person.

Questions to Discuss:

1. What are some situations where you might have a different point of view than someone else on your Team?
2. How do you share your point of view with others?

26.2 Survey the Scene: Different Points of View about Waiting in Line

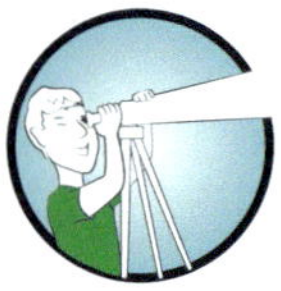

Survey the scene in this situation so you can think about different points of view.

Here is the situation: A line of four people are waiting to warm up food in the microwave. Bill is really hungry and only has five minutes to eat his lunch. Bill cuts ahead of Tom so he can be next to heat up his food.

1. What do you think Bill was thinking? What is his point of view? ____________

   ____

2. What do you think Tom thinks about Bill's actions? What is Tom's point of view in this situation? ________________________________

   ____

3. What are other people in the line thinking? ____________________

   ____

4. Do you think Bill is showing people that he is **respecting** them by thinking about their needs and feelings?

   yes no

5. Let's **rewind** the scene and help Bill think about what he could do differently so he could share *his* point of view and also consider *their* point of view?

   A. Could he have explained something to the other people in line before he cut in front of them?

      yes no

      What could he explain to them?

      ____

   B. Could he ask them for their **help** after he tells them his situation?

      yes no

      What could he ask them? ______________________________

      ____

   C. After Bill uses your help in explaining his situation, what could the other people do to **help** Bill? ______________________________

      ____

26.3 Survey the Scene: Different Points of View about Setting the Table

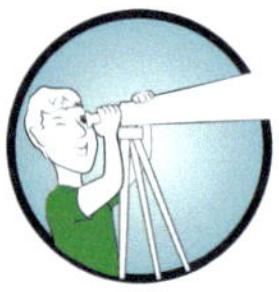

Survey the scene in this situation so you can think about different points of view.

Here is the situation: It is 7:00 p.m. Carlos's mom is cooking dinner. Carlos is playing a video game. Carlos's mom asks him to set the table because it is almost time to eat and setting the table is his chore. Carlos wants to keep playing his game. He does not want to stop because he has two minutes to finish the level he is on. He does not say anything and does not get up to help his mom.

1. What do you think Carlos is thinking? What is his point of view? ____________

   ____

2. What do you think Carlos's mom is thinking about Carlos's action or non-action? What is her point of view in this situation? ______________________

   ____

3. Do you think how Carlos is acting toward his mother shows **respect** for her needs and feelings?

   yes no

4. Is he showing his Home Team that he is **cooperative**, **respectful**, and **easy-going**?

   yes no

5. Let's **rewind** the scene and help Carlos think about what he could do differently. How can he share his point of view and also show he is thinking about his mother's point of view?

   What is the best way to tell his mother that he will help her and also let her know what he needs?

   A. *Not right now.*

   B. *I'll be right there, mom. I will be finished here in two minutes.*

   C. *I must finish this.*

6. What will Carlos's mother know after Carlos says the words you chose for him? ____

   ____

7. How do you think Carlos's mother would feel after Carlos says the words you chose for him? ____

   ____

8. If Carlos says those words and gets up in two minutes to help his mother set the table, will he be acting in a **cooperative** and **easygoing** way?

   yes no

26.4 The Necessary Ingredients for a Cooperative Conversation

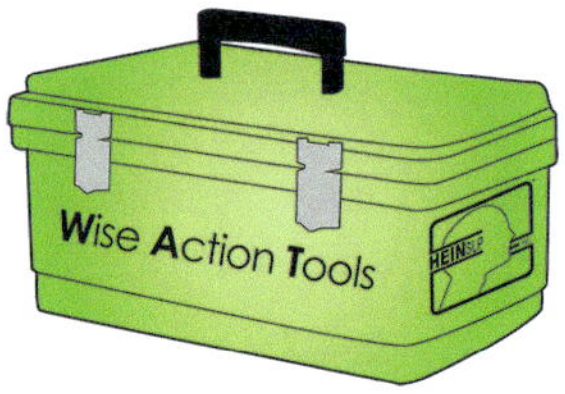

It is important to communicate well with the people on your Teams. But it is not always easy to know what other people want or how to get along easily with them.

The only way to understand others is by having conversations. When you have a conversation, you listen to their point of view to find out what they want or need. Then the other person can listen to you so you can tell them what you want or need. Listening to each other's point of view will lead to a **cooperative conversation**.

When you **cooperate** with each other, you can determine how you both can get some or all of your needs met. Practice having **cooperative conversations**. When you have **cooperative conversations** with your Teammates, you are **supporting** one another to meet **Common Team Goals** and **Personal Goals**. When you learn to have **cooperative conversations**, you will find that you can have better relationships with the people in your life. When you have **cooperative conversations**, you **transform** the situation so everyone on the Team can win!

For a **cooperative conversation**, the necessary ingredients are that all people in the conversation:

1. are allowed to have the time to take a turn to tell what they need;
2. show they **care** about the other person by **patiently listening** to the other person's point of view;
3. work together to find a way to meet each other's needs;
4. will use **respectful** words to **navigate** around challenges that come up during the conversation;
5. will stay **flexible** to new ideas and solutions they might not have thought of on their own.

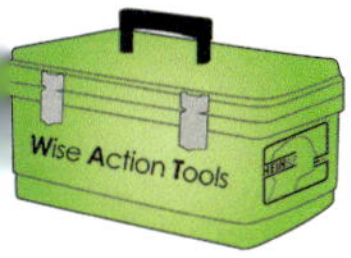

COOPERATIVE CONVERSATION INGREDIENTS CHECKLIST

Name ______________________________ Date ______________________

Think about the ingredients needed in a Cooperative Conversation. Mark this checklist to show whether Persons #1 and #2 have included those ingredients.

Situation Topic: ____

____

Common Team Goal ____

____

Ingredients for a Cooperative Conversation	Name of Person #1: ____________	Name of Person #2: ____________	Did both people work cooperatively?
1. Calmly and respectfully *tell* what each person needs.	Did this person calmly and respecttfully use words to say what was needed? yes no	Did this person calmly and respecttfully use words to say what was needed? yes no	Did both people have a chance to *tell* what they wanted or needed? yes no
2. Respectfully and patiently listen to what each person needs.	Did this person respectfully and patiently listen to what the other person needed? yes no	Did this person respectfully and patiently listen to what the other person needed? yes no	Did both people listen to find out what the other person wanted or needed? yes no
3. Respectfully and patiently use words to *share ideas, making a plan* to meet *both* people's needs. Both people win!	Did this person say some-thing to help the other person feel that their needs will be met? yes no	Did this person say some-thing to help the other person feel that their needs will be met? yes no	Did both pople work together to flexibly find a way to meet each other's needs? yes no

Are all ingredients included? yes no

If not, circle the ingredients to add to make the next conversation more cooperative.

26.5 Survey the Scene: Is This a Cooperative Conversation?

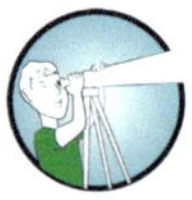

Conversation #1—Sharing the Computer

Using a Cooperative Conversation Ingredients Checklist (from the Wise Action Tools), see whether Conversation #1 about sharing the computer is a **cooperative conversation**.

Narrator: Jesse is playing a video game on his computer. His younger brother, Mark, does not have his own computer. Mark wants to play a video game on Jesse's computer.

Mark: *Jesse, let me play a game on your computer now!*

Jesse: *No. Go away. I'm playing a game.*

Mark: *I'm going to tell Mom that you're not* sharing.

Jesse: *This is my computer. I don't need to share with you.*

Mark: *I never get to play video games at home.*

Jesse: *That's not my problem. Leave me alone.*

Mark: *I'm telling Mom.*

1. What does Mark want or need? ______________________________________

   ____

2. Is Mark asking Jesse in a **calm** and **respectful** way?

   yes no

3. Is Mark getting his needs met?

   yes no

Conversation #2—*Sharing the Computer*

Using a **Cooperative Conversation** Ingredients Checklist (from the Wise Action Tools), see whether Conversation #1 about sharing the computer is a **cooperative conversation**.

Narrator: Jesse is playing a video game on his computer. His younger brother, Mark, does not have his own computer. Mark wants to play a video game on Jesse's computer.

Mark: *Jesse, since I don't have my own computer, could I please take a turn playing a game when you are done playing your game.*

Jesse: *Why don't you have your own computer?*

Mark: *Mom and Dad said I'm too young to have my own, so can you share yours with me a little?*

Jesse: *Will you be careful and not bang on the keyboard like you did the last time I let you borrow it?*

Mark: *Yes, I promise to be* **careful** *with your stuff.*

Jesse: *OK, Let me finish this game. I've been waiting to play this all day. Come back in 15 minutes. Then you can play for half an hour. After that I will need my computer back to look something up for my homework, OK?*

Mark: *OK, I'll come back in 15 minutes. I promise I will be* **careful** *with your computer. I really* **appreciate** *you sharing with me. Thank you.*

Jesse: *You're welcome. I'll let you have your turn in 15 minutes.*

4. What did Mark want or need? ______________________________

____

5. Circle words Mark said in conversation #2 to help make it a **cooperative conversation**.

6. What did Jesse want or need? ______________________________

____

7. Circle words Jesse said to help make it a **cooperative conversation**.

8. How did they both get their needs met? ______________________________

____

26.6 Survey the Scene: Can Everyone Get Their Needs Met When Justin Gets Home?

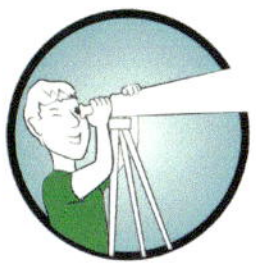

Directions: Survey the scene to see what is happening in the following situation. Underline clues that will help you think about the different points of view of the different characters.

Justin just spent his day at school. He had really worked hard to control himself so he would not lose any points for "bad behavior."

He was looking forward to going on a field trip at the end of the week and knew that he couldn't go if he could not show that he could have great **self-control** in the classroom.

When he got off the bus and got home, he wanted to be silly and do whatever he wanted. He started making noises and talking in funny voices. Unfortunately, he found that his father had such a terrible headache that he did not go to work, and his older brother was studying for an important history test. They wanted him to stop making so much noise.

1. What is happening in this situation from the point of view of Justin? How does he feel and why? What do you think he would like to happen next?

2. What is happening in the situation from the father's point of view?

____

____

3. What is happening in the situation from the brother's point of view?

____

____

4. What actions can Justin take so he can still do what he wants while also thinking about the point of view of his father and brother?

____

____

A good thing to learn is to know how to ask for what you need from your point of view while also thinking that another person may have a different point of view. These would be important words to say when you are having a **cooperative conversation**. What words can Justin say to ask for what he needs in an **easygoing** way? Could he ask to go for a walk or if he could talk quietly out in the yard or a different place to have fun without disturbing the others?

Justin: ____

____

26.7 Survey the Scene: Birthday Plans Need to Change

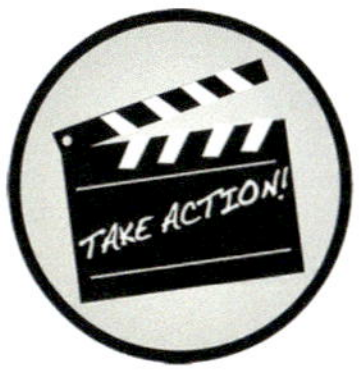

Directions: Survey the scene to see what is happening in the following situation. Underline clues that will *help* you think about the different points of view of the different characters. Use two different colors to underline the point of view clues you find for the two different people.

Ron Salazar has been looking forward to his birthday party for three months. The plan has been to have his friends spend the day at the amusement park in the nearby city. Unfortunately, his father, Mr. Salazar, has just lost his job and does not have enough money to pay for the original plan. Mr. Salazar is hoping to suggest that Ron can have his friends come over to their house to watch movies and have pizza. If Mr. Salazar gets a job within the next year, he can hopefully afford the trip to the amusement park for Ron's next birthday. Ron usually gets upset when plans change, so his father is worried about how Ron will react.

1. What is happening in this situation from the point of view of Ron's father? How does he feel? Why does he feel this way? What do you think he would like to happen next? ______________________________

   ____

2. How does Ron feel about the original birthday plan?

3. How will he feel when his father lets him know about the change of plans?

   ____

4. If his father explains why the plans had to change, how do you think Ron should react? ______________________________

   ____

26.8 G.R.E.E.N. Scene #18: Write Your Own Cooperative Conversation Scene about Changing Birthday Plans

Write Your Own Script: Changing Birthday Plans in a Cooperative Conversation

Let's write the script for the conversation Ron and his father could have in this scene when Ron's father is telling Ron about his need to change plans. What could they both say to show they are thinking about each other's point of view in their **cooperative conversation**?

Ron's father: ____

____

Ron: ____

____

Ron's father: ____

____

Ron: ____

____

Ron's father: ____

____

After writing your own **G.R.E.E.N.** Scene #18, refer to the pages in Sections 12.2 through 12.5 for the directions, rules, warm-ups, and review sheets needed to help you make the best **G.R.E.E.N.** Scene.

26.9 Read and Discuss: Being Easygoing When Receiving Feedback

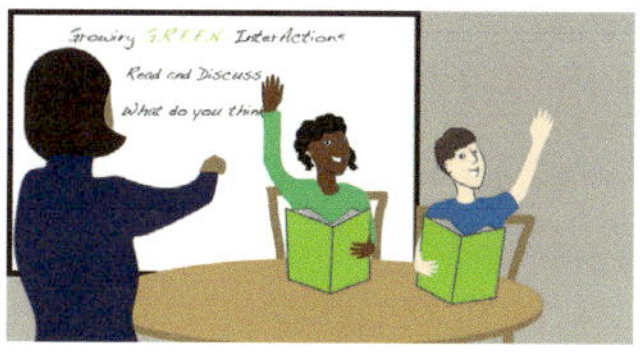

As human beings, we are not always perfect in the things we do or the things we say. That's OK. We all are "works in progress," which means we are always learning and improving.

Circle which one honestly describes you:

I always act perfectly. I am a work in progress.

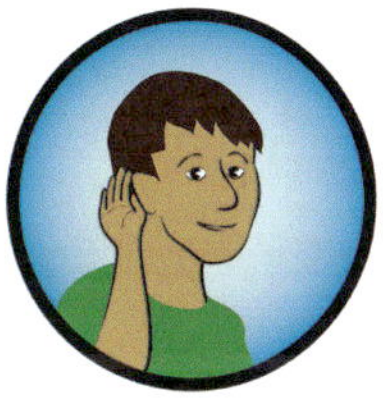

If you understand that you are a work in progress, you know that it is best to be open to getting help from others. One way to get help from others is to get feedback from them. When people give you feedback, they are telling you what you did well and what you can improve. Feedback can be useful, especially when it is constructive. **Constructive feedback** gives you **helpful** ideas so you can improve yourself.

It is important to tell the difference between **constructive** and unhelpful feedback. When you notice what feedback you are receiving, you can respond appropriately to it.

If it is **constructive feedback**, you can say, "Thanks for the **constructive feedback**. It will be good for me to think about that so I can do **better** next time."

If it is *not* **constructive feedback** you can say, "Thanks for the feedback. Next time can you give me feedback that is more constructive? That will help me do **better** the next time."

Think about a time when your teachers give you **constructive feedback** in school. When you are writing, you must reread your work and make edits to it. You often get feedback from your teachers or peers to help you improve your writing. Each time you make **changes** in your written work, your writing gets **better**. This is true for other aspects of your life as well.

True or False: It is useful to be **flexible** enough to accept some **constructive feedback** to improve my life.

true false

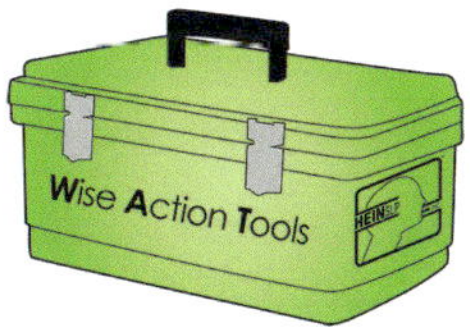

Use the Wise Action Tool on the next page to help you develop your ability to accept and use constructive feedback from others.

I ACCEPT CONSTRUCTIVE FEEDBACK IN THESE AREAS

I show that I am more **easygoing** and **open-minded** when I accept **constructive feedback** in many of these areas. I can add more of these areas as I become more comfortable about accepting feedback from others. Using feedback from others helps me reach my **goals**. As of the date noted below, I accept **constructive feedback** in these areas:

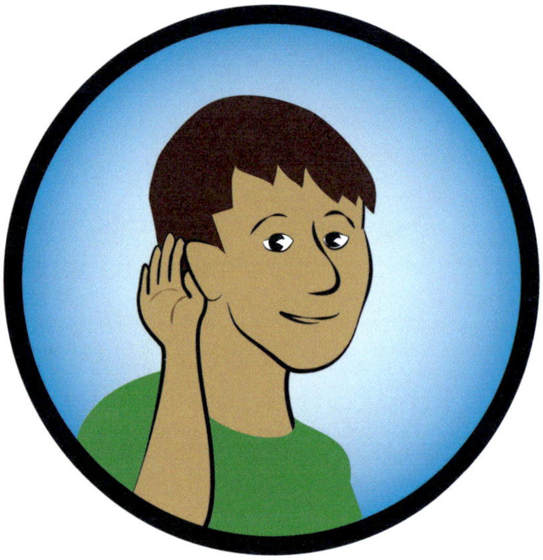

Editing my writing ______________

Playing sports ____________

Getting along with others ________

Managing my time __________

Studying or doing my homework _____

Doing my chores _______________

Taking care of my grooming ____________

Solving problems ____________

Thinking before I act ________

Using the right tone of voice_____________

Choosing the right words ______________

Respectfully asking for help ______________________

Getting along with friends ______________________

Showing empathy for others _____________________

Name _____________________________________ Date _______________________

26.10 Survey the Scene: Seeing Point of View about Following Advice

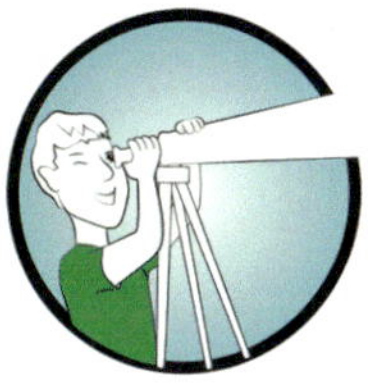

Mr. Calculator, the teacher, shook his head when he saw that Ariel was still racing through her math test without checking any of her work again. She was the first to turn it in, even though every day in class he had given her the same advice: "Take your time and check your work!" Later that night, Mr. Calculator sighed as he graded her paper. The next day, Ariel's eyes filled with tears when she got her test back.

Point of view of person #1: Mr. Calculator

1. What advice did Mr. Calculator give to Ariel? ______________________________

   ____

2. Why did he give Ariel this advice? ______________________________

   ____

3. How do you think Mr. Calculator felt when he saw that Ariel was not accepting his feedback and following his advice? How can you tell?

   ____

   ____

4. What was the consequence of Ariel not accepting his feedback and following his advice? ______________________________

   ____

Point of view of person #2: Ariel

5. Was Ariel thinking about Mr. Calculator's advice when she was taking the test? How can you tell?

   yes   no

   ____

6. What could be the reason for Ariel's choice of rushing through her math test?

   ____

   ____

7. How does Ariel feel now? How can you tell? ____________________

   ____

8. What is the problem in this story? ____________________

   ____

9. What do you think Ariel could say or do now to solve the problem?

   ____

   ____

26.11 Accepting Advice or Not: Help Alan Make the Wisest Choice

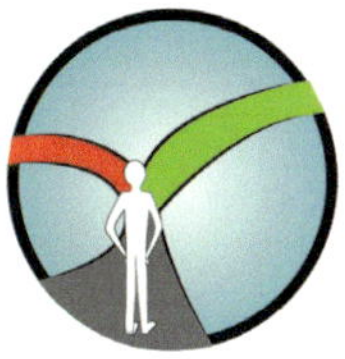

Alan liked to play sports. He was great at baseball and basketball and always did his best to help his team win. He was one of the fastest runners in the school. He really loved going fast. Unfortunately, he also loved going fast when he was doing his assignments in class. He did not check his math work before he turned it in, so he made silly little mistakes that pulled down his grade. When he was writing answers to questions, he tried to write his answers quickly so he could be done and have free time. Sometimes he read the questions too quickly, and, as a result, did not answer them correctly.

One day, right when Alan was looking forward to recess, his teacher came over and handed back the assignment that he had just turned in. His teacher said, "Alan, even though I cannot read the name on this paper, I know it is yours. You skipped the last two questions, probably because you wanted to turn in your paper so fast. Before you go out to recess, I need you to write your name neatly at the top and finish those last two questions."

Think about the point of view of Alan's teacher:

1. Why did Alan's teacher think it was important for him to revise his work before going out to recess? ______________________________

   ____

2. Alan and his teacher are on the same Class Team. What do you think is the **Common Team Goal** for that Team? ______________________________

   ____

3. Help Alan make the wiser choice of the two below. Circle your choice:

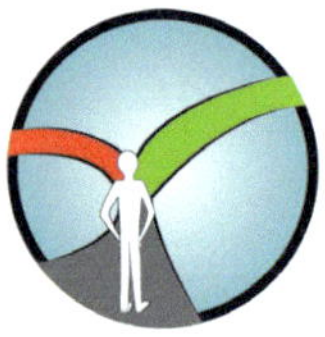

Choice #1 *I Don't Care, It's Good Enough!*	Choice #2 *I'll Do My Best*
Alan could think only about recess. Since his teacher already knew whose paper it was, why did he need to write his name so his teacher could read it? Alan did not want to spend any more time on the assignment. It was good enough.	Alan remembered that his coach and his parents wanted him to get better at doing his schoolwork so that someday he could get a sports scholarship to college. He took the assignment back and did his best to write his name neater and answer the last two questions carefully.

A. Predict what happened next with each choice.

1. What do you think was the consequence of action choice #1?

____

2. What do you think was the consequence of action choice #2?

____

When you accept or reject advice, you are making choices about the consequences that will take place.

4. Use the Choice Checker below to help Alan evaluate these two choices to decide which one wins as the **better** choice:

Evaluating Choices	Choice #1 *I Don't Care. It's Good Enough!*	Choice #2 *Thanks For Helping Me Do My Best*
Does this choice show self-control? (Is Alan navigating challenging situations?)	yes no	yes no
Is this choice logical? (Does it make sense? Is Alan helping himself or hurting himself?)	yes no	yes no
Is this choice considerate and respectful of the teacher?	yes no	yes no
Is Alan challenging himself to accept constructive feedback so he can achieve bigger goals in the future?	yes no	yes no

Which choice wins with more yes answers? ______________________________

What **Guiding G.R.E.E.N. Thought** do you think Alan uses in this situation to help him make a better choice for himself and his Teams?

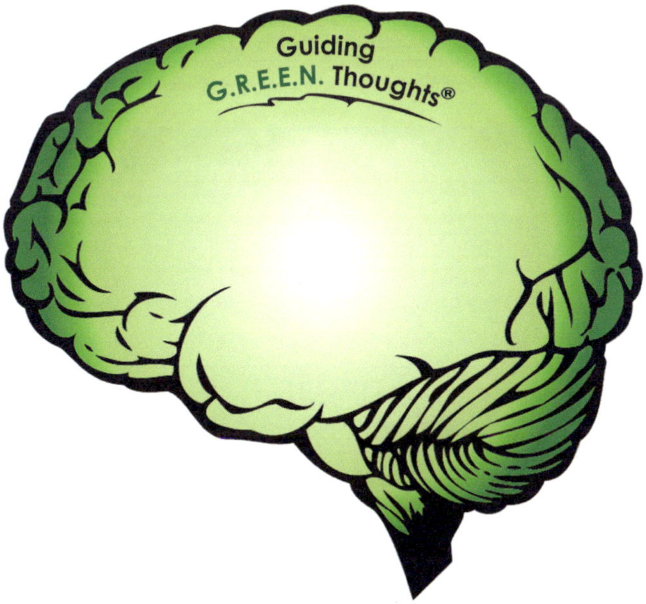

26.12 G.R.E.E.N. Scene #19: Write Your Own Script to Accept Advice

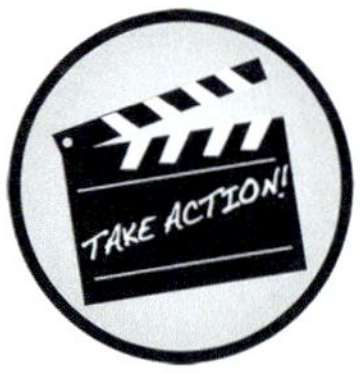

1. What constructive feedback and advice do people give you?

    ____

2. Do you follow the advice? Do you listen to it and change your actions so your situation can get better?

    yes no

3. Do you think it is logical to listen to good advice?

    yes no

4. Choose the character in your life who gives you constructive feedback. Write a scene in which you have a conversation with that person. Write the scene so the person is giving you the advice and you are listening to it and accepting it. After you act this out in your own G.R.E.E.N. Scene, see whether you can act similarly in your real-life scenes. Refer to the pages in Sections 12.2 through 12.5 to help you make the best G.R.E.E.N. Scene.

    Advice giver: ____

    ____

    You: ____

    ____

    Advice giver: ____

    ____

    You: ____

26.13 Change the Scene to Make It G.R.E.E.N.!: Accepting Advice to Go to Bed Earlier

Survey the scene to see whether Paul is accepting advice from his father so he can get up easier in the morning.

At 9:30 on a school night, Paul was watching TV. His father came into his room and said, "Remember, it has been difficult to wake you up in the morning so you are not late for school. I think it would be a good idea for you to get ready for bed now so it will be easier for you to get up in the morning without having to struggle with me to get to school on time."

Paul responded, "I don't know what you are talking about! I don't have any trouble getting up. Besides, I need to watch this next show because it is one of my favorites!"

1. What did Paul do that his father would think was "**R.E.D.**" behavior? In other words, how was Paul acting that showed he was not **grateful**, not **easygoing**, not **navigating** this situations well, and not making a good choice for his Home Team? ______________________________

____

____

2. Help Paul **rewind** the scene: When his father gave him **helpful** advice, what *should* Paul *have said or done instead* to be more **grateful**, **respectful**, **easygoing**, and **navigating**? ______________________________

____

____

26.14 Change the Scene to Make It G.R.E.E.N.: Please Set the Table, Tommy!

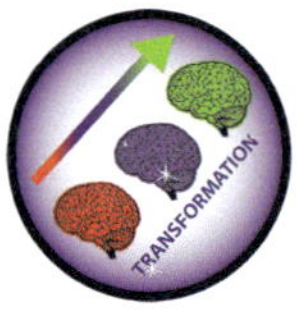

Survey the scene; then choose to pause and **rewind** it!

Change the Scene to Make it **G.R.E.E.N.**!

Directions: Read what Tommy is saying to his friend about the interaction he had with his father. First, with a red pencil, underline any actions or words that you think are R.E.D. behavior. Then please help Tommy think about how he could be more easygoing and navigate the scene better.

Tommy: My father came into my room when I was playing my video game and told me it was time to set the table for dinner. I told him I couldn't stop playing because I would lose all of my points in the game. He said that if I did not come to set the table right away, I would be on restriction from the computer for a week. I told him he wasn't being fair and that he should set the table himself and leave me alone. Boy, did I get in a lot of trouble!

1. Do you think Tommy acted **respectful** and **G.R.E.E.N.** with his dad in this scene?

   yes no

2. Because Tommy said he couldn't stop playing and didn't say anything else in the beginning about helping set the table, what do you think his father might have thought he was saying to him?

   A. I am not going to set the table.

   B. I am going to set the table when I save my points.

   C. I am going to set the table right away, but I must save my points first.

   D. OK, I'll be right there.

3. Help Tommy think about the **Common Team Goal** while thinking of his **Personal Goal** so *both* **goals** can be met, if possible.

   A. What do you think is Tommy's **Personal Goal**? ____________________

   ____

   B. What do you think is the **Common Team Goal** for the family? __________

   ____

4. 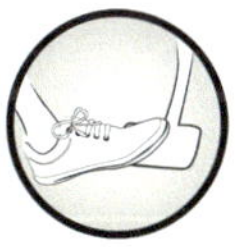

   Help Tommy *step on the brake* to pause and **rewind**: What do you think is the best time and place in this scene to hit the pause button so Tommy can do his best to **change** the rest of the scene and make it **better** for himself and his father? Let's help Tommy **rewind** this scene so it can be more successful and **G.R.E.E.N.**

   With a **purple** pencil or crayon, put a dot at the point in the scene right before it starts to turn **R.E.D.** Then **rewind** the scene to that point and act out a **better G.R.E.E.N.** scene from there.

5. Could Tommy use words to tell what he needs while also using words that show he is thinking of what his father needs, too? Could Tommy **politely** and **respectfully** ask his father whether he could save his points first and then go set the table as quickly as he can?

   yes   no

6. What words could Tommy say to **respectfully** ask for what he needs while also letting his father know that he is also thinking about helping the Home Team?

   ____

   ____

26.15 G.R.E.E.N. Scene #20: Write a Better Scene with Tommy Asking to Quickly Save His Work before Doing a Chore

Narrator: Tommy is in the middle of playing his on-line game *and* does not want to lose the points he has received, but his father is now asking him to set the table.

Help Tommy **rewind** this scene so he can:

- think of his father's point of view while thinking of his own
- think about being more **easygoing** and **cooperative**
- think about being more **navigating**, determining the best way to respond when people ask him to do something
- think about using **respectful** words and a **respectful** tone of voice to ask for time to quickly finish what he's doing before going to do his chore for the Team.

Tommy's father: *It's time to set the table, Tommy.*

Tommy: ____

____

Tommy's father: ____

____

Tommy: ____

____

Tommy's father: ____

____

Tommy: ____

____

Refer to the pages in Sections 12.2 through 12.5 to help you act out the best G.R.E.E.N. Scene after you write it!

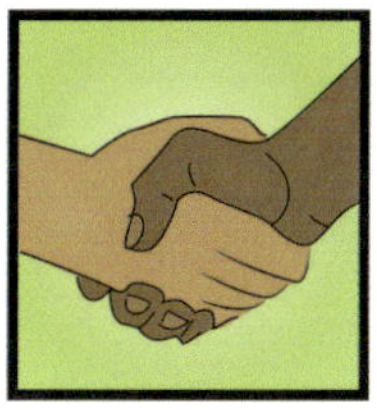

27 Is It Time for a Compromise?

27.1 Read and Discuss: What Does It Mean to Make a Compromise?

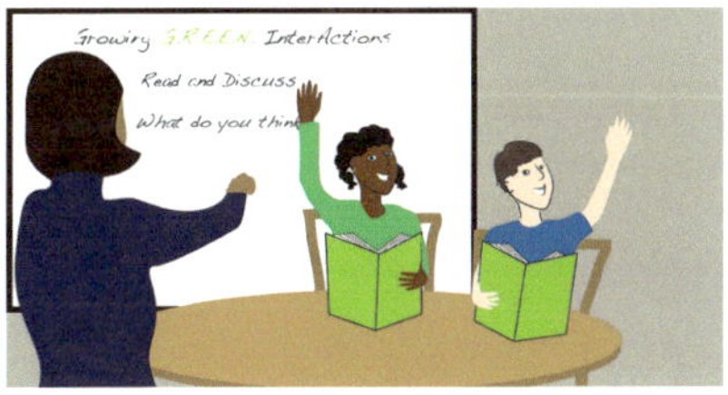

To be **easygoing**, you sometimes need to make a **compromise**.

Sometimes in a real-life scene, people get stuck in their own point of view. The people cannot move **forward** unless they make a **compromise**.

What does it mean to make a **compromise**?

- When you make a **compromise**, you don't get everything you want.
- When you make a **compromise**, you get some of what you want.
- When you make a **compromise**, you make a new plan so that each Team member gets some of what they want and gives some of what the other person wants. Everyone can be satisfied with the new **compromise** plan.

If you have different points of view, you have different ideas about what action to take in a situation. You each may want a different plan. It might seem as if you and your Teammates are on different Teams. But if you work together to determine how to get some of what you want, you can create a new **compromise** plan together.

In order to **compromise**, it is important to understand that you cannot always have everything you want. This is not how things work in the world. It helps our Teams when we act **flexibly** and **generously**.

In order to **connect** with your Team, each side gets to take some ideas from their own plan to put them into a new Team plan so both sides can be satisfied. Both sides give up some parts, but also get to keep some parts they want in the new Team **compromise** plan. Instead of both sides being stuck with two or more plans that don't work, one new **compromise** plan lets the Team work together and move **forward**.

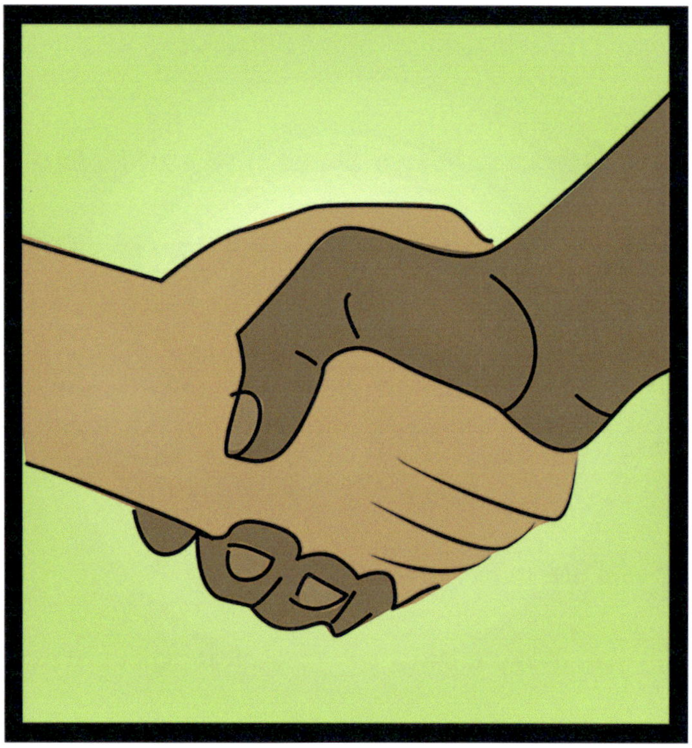

A **compromise** may not be possible in all situations. Sometimes we need to follow the other person's plan or our own plan because one plan might be safer or will meet the Team **goals better**. The following are some situations to think about. Is it a good time for a **compromise**? If it is not a time for a **compromise**, see if you can explain why.

27.2 Survey the Scene: Is this a Time for a Compromise? Late for School

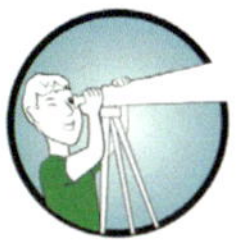

Survey the scene to see if this situation is a time for making a **compromise.**

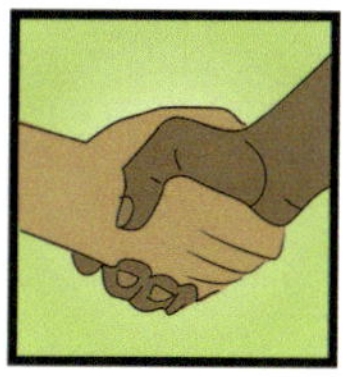

I am playing a video game. My parent calls to me to leave the house right away because I am late for school.

1. Is this a time to make a **compromise**? Decide if this is a time to choose action choice A or B.

   Choice A: This is a time to ask for what I need with one of the following questions:

   Can I play five more minutes longer and then leave?

   Can I play later if I leave now?

   Choice B: This is a time to just listen to what the other person is saying and get up to leave the house immediately!

2. Circle what you think:

   A. This is a time to make a **compromise**.

   B. This is *not* a time to make a **compromise**.

Why or why not? ____

____

27.3 Survey the Scene: Is this a Time for a Compromise? Setting the Table

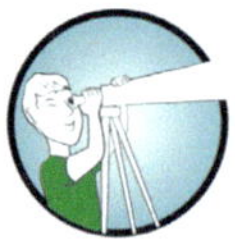

Survey the scene to see if this situation is a time for making a compromise.

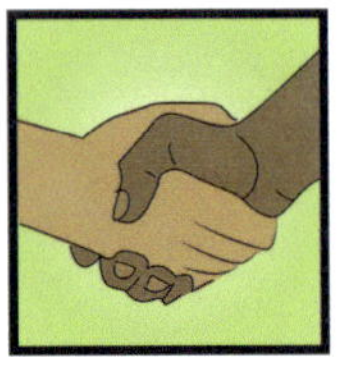

I am playing a video game. My parent calls me to help set the table for dinner. Is this a time to compromise? (Can I ask a question about taking care of my own needs, but also let the other person know that I will be responsible for doing my part to help our Team meet its goals very soon?)

1. Is this a time to make a compromise? Decide if this is a time to choose action choice A or B.

   Choice A: This is a time to ask for what I need with one of the following actions:

   I can say, "Yes, I can help, but could I please finish this level first and then come? It will take only two minutes."

   I can say, "Yes, I can help, but could I please save what I have done and then come? It will take me only one minute."

   Choice B: This is a time to just say and do the following:

   I can say, "Sure, I'll help you right away!" and get up immediately, even though I might lose my points and have to go back to the beginning of the game when I return later.

2. Circle what you think:

   A. This is a time that I could try to make a compromise.

   B. This is *not* a time to make a compromise.

   Why or why not? ____

   ____

27.4 Survey the Scene: Is this a Time for a Compromise? While Watching a Show

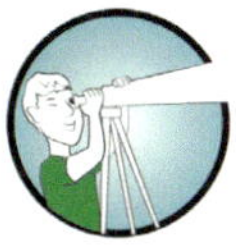

Survey the scene to see if this situation is a time for making a **compromise.**

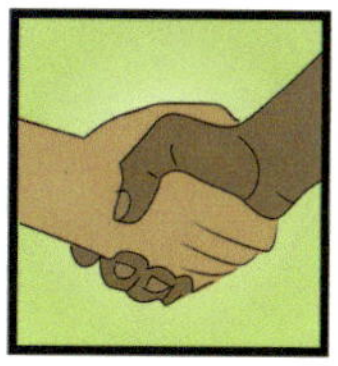

I am watching one of my favorite shows on the computer. My brother asks me, "Can I please get on the computer to check to see what my homework is for tomorrow?"

1. Is this a time to make a compromise? Decide if this is a time to choose action choice A or B.

   Choice A: This is a time to tell what I would like to finish doing and also figure out a good time for the other person to be able to do what they want to do, too.

   I can say, *"I would like to finish watching this and then I will give you a turn on the computer. I will be done in ten minutes."*

   I can say, "I can pause this, but then I'd like to finish watching this in just a few minutes. How long will it take you to check your assignment?"

   Choice B: This is a time to just say and do the following:

   I can say, "Sure, you can get on the computer right away!" and get up immediately, even though you would have to start watching your show again later from the beginning.

2. Circle what you think:

   A. This is a time that I can try to make a compromise.

   B. This is *not* a time to make a compromise.

   Why or why not? ____

   ____

27.5 Guiding G.R.E.E.N. Thoughts for Compromising

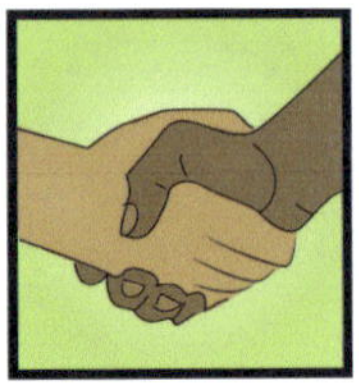

These are some **Guiding G.R.E.E.N. Thoughts** to help you make a **compromise** plan that is good for both sides.

A **compromise** plan means that everyone involved can get *some* of their needs met.

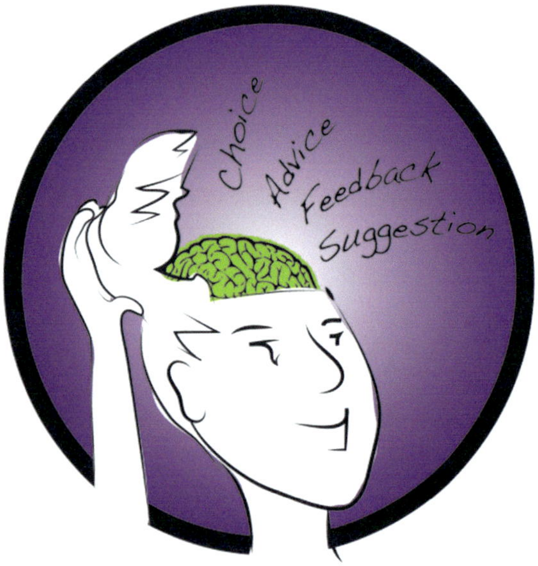

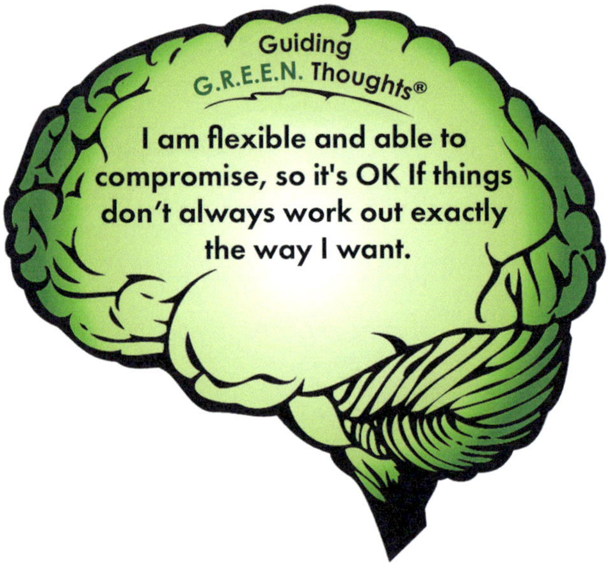

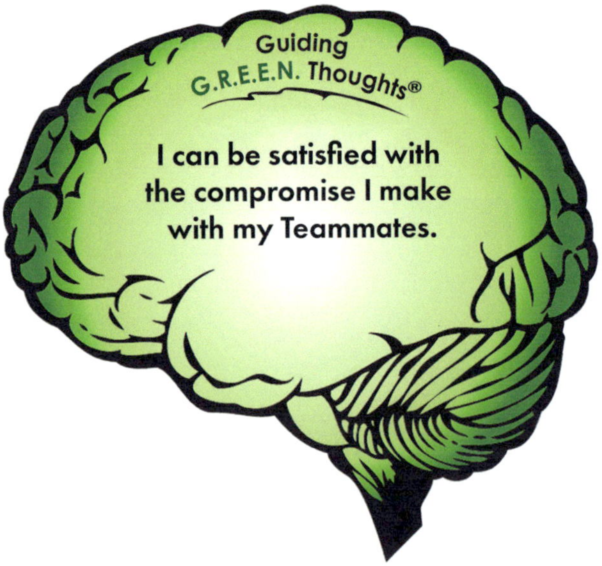

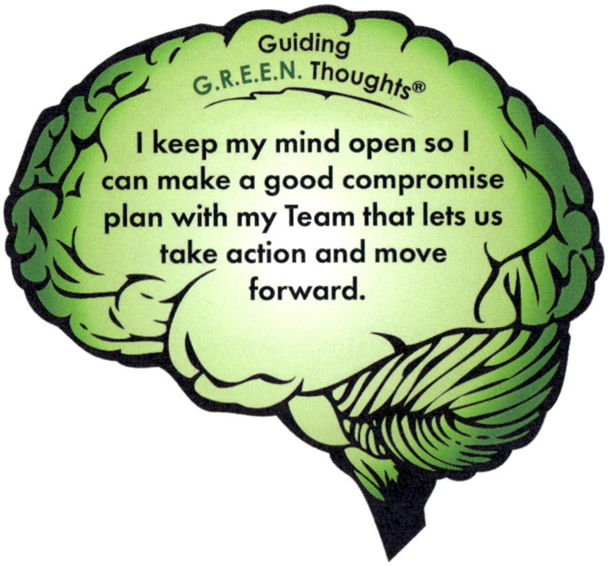

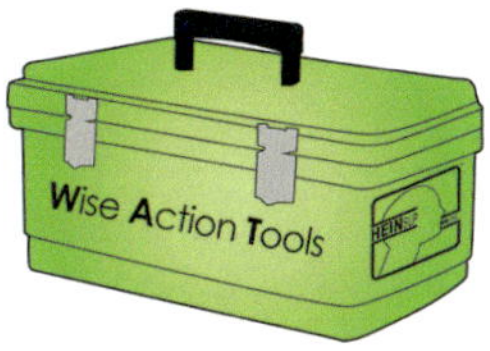

WORKSHEET FOR MAKING A G.R.E.E.N. TEAM COMPROMISE

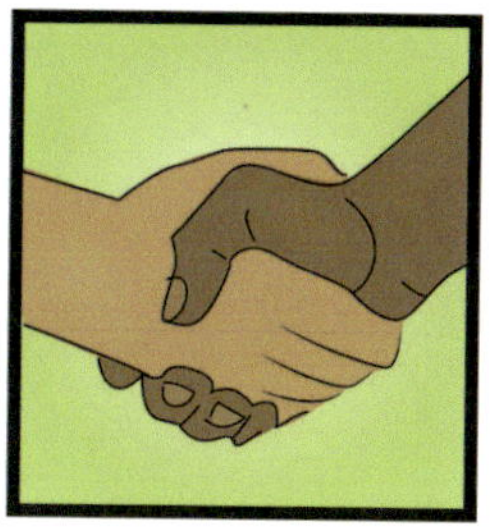

Here is the situation that needs a Team compromise:

____

____

____

Our Shared G.R.E.E.N. Compromise:

This is the G.R.E.E.N. compromise we have made together.

We both get some needs met so we can both move forward.

If I ____

____

then you _______________________________________

____

If you ____

____

then I ____

____

27.6 Survey the Scene: Help Roger and Carlos Make a Compromise

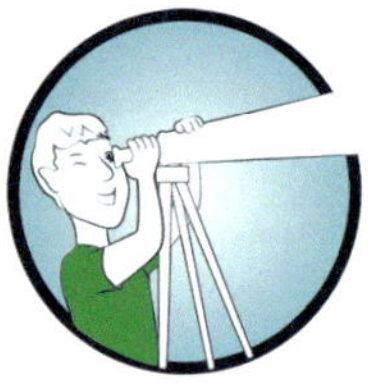

In the next section, draw pictures that show how these two friends develop a compromise plan to navigate their challenging situation.

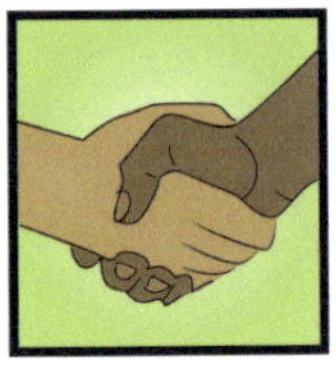

Roger and Carlos are friends and classmates. They sit next to each other in their writing class. Roger likes to tell jokes, but when he is in class, he sometimes blurts out things that disturb the other students when they are trying to focus on their work.

Today, in the middle of class, while everyone is supposed to work on their essays, Roger starts telling Carlos something that he thinks is funny. Carlos tells Roger that he is trying to get his work done and cannot pay attention to Roger now. Carlos still really wants to tell Roger what he thinks is so funny.

What can Roger and Carlos do so they both get their needs met?

If Roger stops ______________________ now, Carlos promises that he will ______________________________ later.

Both people must do what they say they will do for the compromise to be a true compromise.

27.7 Drawing the Steps of the Compromise Plan: Please Wait to Tell Me after Class

1. Draw what is happening in the situation that shows that a compromise plan is needed (show that Roger and Carlos are wanting to do different things because they have different needs):

2. Write what Carlos says to Roger. Carlos says to Roger, "If you will ________

____

then I will ______________________________________

____

3. Show Carlos talking to Roger in class, and Roger agreeing to the plan. This is the first action step of the **compromise** so both friends can get their needs met:

4. Show Roger listening to Carlos after class. This is the second action step of the **compromise** that the two friends follow so they can both get their needs met.

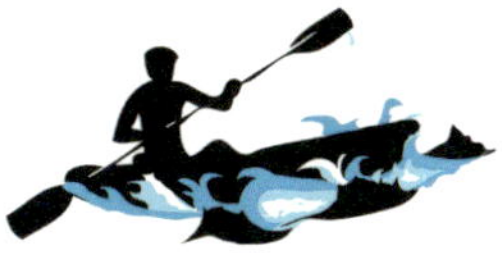

28 What Does It Mean to Be Navigating?

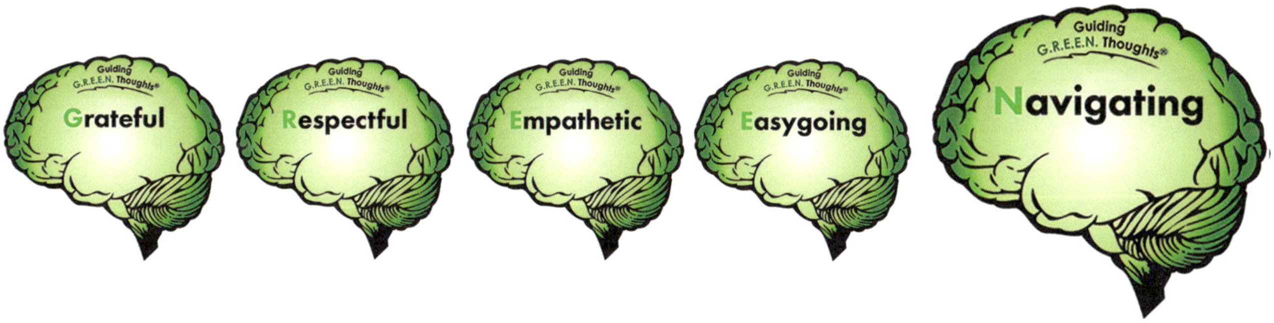

When you are living your life, obstacles may get in your way. People and things may cause you to go in a different way than you had planned. These obstacles can cause you to get stuck. But if you want to reach your **goals**, you will want to move around these obstacles safely and carefully. When you act in a **navigating** way, you stay in control and discover how to move around obstacles and continue toward achieving your **Personal Goals** and **Common Team Goals**.

Learning how to **self-calm** allows you to be a strong navigator with a solid foundation. Can you picture that when you interact with others, you are similar to a strong tree with your branches reaching out to others on your Teams? Your **navigating** skills are the roots that hold you solidly in the ground. Your ability to stay calm helps you stand tall and secure without falling over. Acting **G.R.E.E.N.** is built on this strong foundation of successfully **navigating** the challenges in your world.

28.1 Guiding G.R.E.E.N. Thoughts to Help You Navigate Successfully

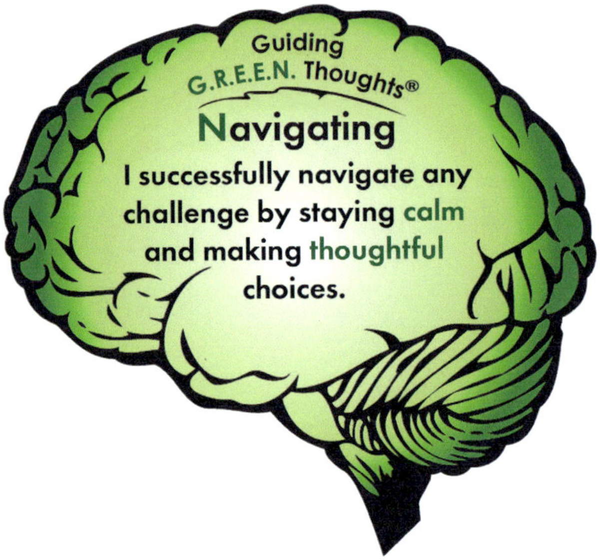

Here are some **Guiding G.R.E.E.N. Thoughts** that can help you develop your **navigating** skills. The lessons in this program can guide you to use these thoughts successfully.

- I am open to new thoughts and accept feedback from other people.
- I use **self-control** to make the best choices.
- I wait for the best time to act.
- I understand and accept when someone tells me "no."
- I ask for help when I need it.
- I allow myself to be **flexible** and **change** my actions to **better** ones.
- I can adjust to changes.

29 Wait for the Best Time to Act

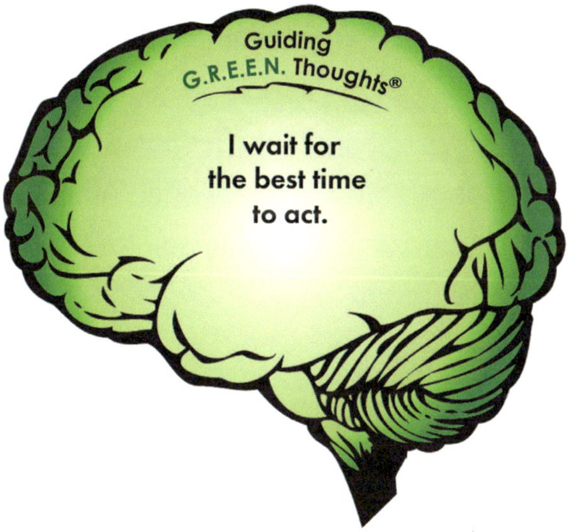

When you are in your real-life scenes you often must wait before you can do what you want to do. You may not want to wait, especially if you really like that activity and are excited about doing it:

- You may want to eat those chips right away.
- You might want to have your turn with the video game right away.
- You may want to play with your new basketball right away.
- You may want to say something right away.
- You may want to go outside right away.

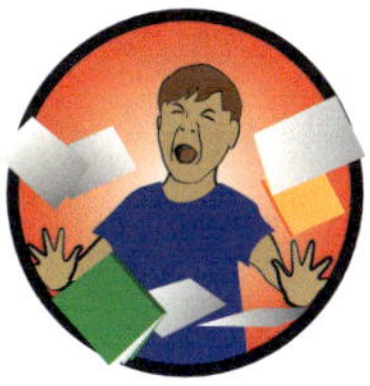

Your first impulsive thought may be to just do whatever you want to do right away. But you may encounter negative consequences if you do not Think First and wait until the best time to act.

Instead of acting impulsively, you can choose to use **self-control** and wait. There are usually **positive** consequences when you do this. You also can feel pride that you can have control over yourself and your actions.

Once you realize you can use **self-control**, it gets easier to do it the next time and the next.

In the next scene, you practice choosing to wait until the other actor tells you to go. You can feel the **self-control** that comes from waiting for this other person to give you directions. In other **G.R.E.E.N.** Scenes and in your real-life scenes, you may have to wait even longer than in this scene. When you use **self-control** and know *why* you must wait, you can coach yourself to wait for the best time to act for yourself and the rest of the Team.

29.1 It Helps to Know Why You Must Wait

Why must you wait? It helps you to wait if you know *why* you must wait.

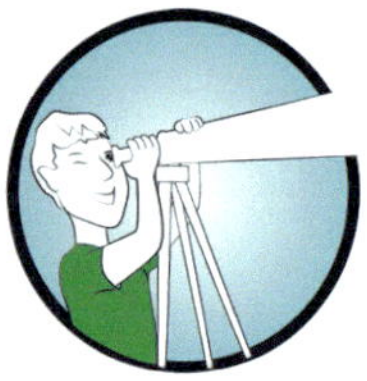

1. The first thing you can do is to **survey the scene** to see *why* you might have to wait.
   A. *Who* else is in the scene? Do they need to go first?
   B. *What* do they want or need? Is their need more important than what you need right now?
   C. Is it not the right time for you to have what you want?

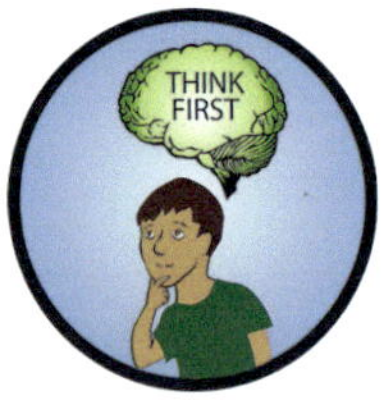

2. If you can think of a reason you might have to wait, it will be easier to wait without having to ask *why*.

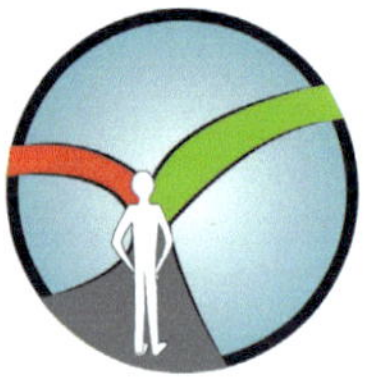

3. In some scenes, you may be unable to determine why you must wait. If you can't figure it out, you may want to ask someone. After the other person in your scene gives you an answer that you can understand, you can choose to wait **patiently**.

29.2 I Can Think of Why I Must Wait

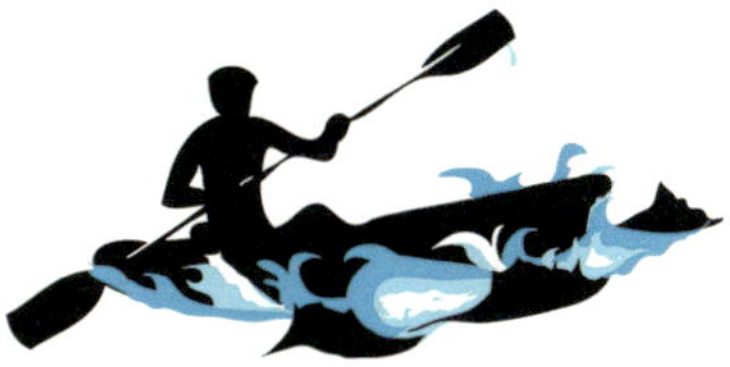

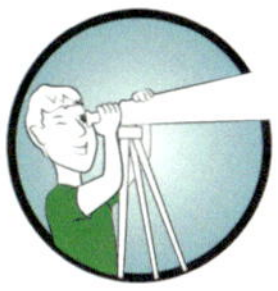

These are some situations in my life when I am asked to wait. These are some usual reasons why I must wait.

1. This is one situation when I usually have to wait. ______________________

   ____

   This is the usual reason I must wait in this situation. ______________________

   ____

2. This is another situation when I usually have to wait. ______________________

   ____

   This is the usual reason I must wait in this situation. ______________________

   ____

3. Here is another situation when I must wait and the usual reason I must wait.

   ____

   ____

After I act in G.R.E.E.N. Scene #21, I can act in my own G.R.E.E.N. Scene using a situation from my own life. It helps me stay **calm** and **patient** in my real life after I have practiced **calmly** waiting in G.R.E.E.N. Scenes.

29.3 G.R.E.E.N. Scene #21: I Wait for the Best Time to Act

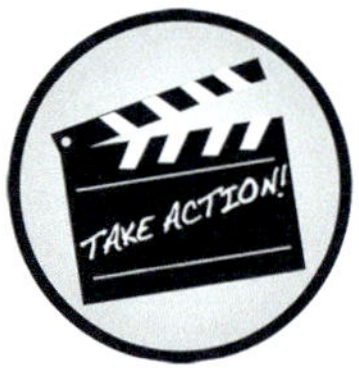

Reasons for Acting in This Scene

1. Acting in this scene lets me practice being **patient**.
2. Acting in this scene helps me choose to wait, like choosing to wait for a red light signal to turn **green** when I am driving or riding or walking safely.

***Directions for this* Scene:**

1. Refer to the pages in Sections 12.2 through 12.5 for the directions, rules, warm-ups, and review sheets needed to help you make the best G.R.E.E.N. Scene.
2. The Director puts a real (or imaginary) backpack for the Navigator on the other side of the room. The Signal Controller puts a line on the floor in the middle of the room and stands in front of the line.
3. The Director gets the clapboard and says, "Quiet on the set. G.R.E.E.N. Scene #21. Take one! Action!" If the scene gets repeated with the same set of actors, the Director will say, "Quiet on the set! G.R.E.E.N. Scene #21, Take two. Action!"

29.4 The Scene: I Wait for the Best Time to Act!

Navigator: (The Navigator walks up to the Signal Controller.): *I must get over to the shelf to get my backpack.*

Signal controller: *Please stop right here and wait until I tell you to go.*

Navigator: *May I ask why I must stop here?*

Signal controller: *Yes. You must wait because many other people are already getting their backpacks. You will be in the next group of people. I'll let you know when it will be your turn to go.*

Navigator: *Thanks. I will wait.*

Signal controller: (The signal controller waits about 20 seconds before letting the Navigator move forward.) *OK, you can go now. Thanks for waiting* ***patiently***.

Navigator: *No problem!* (The Navigator walks over to get the backpack.)

29.5 Guiding G.R.E.E.N. Thought Choices for G.R.E.E.N. Scene #21

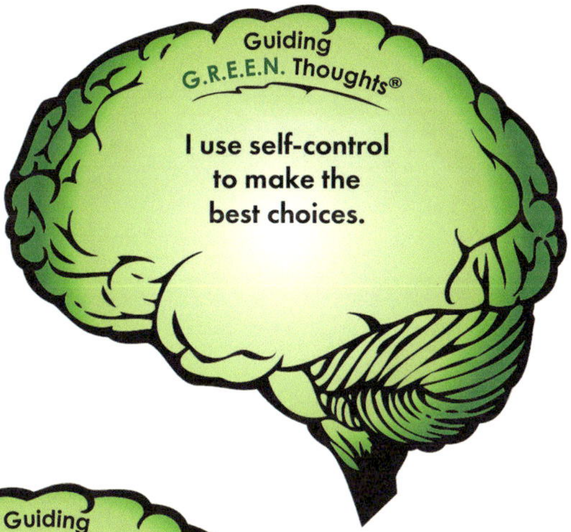

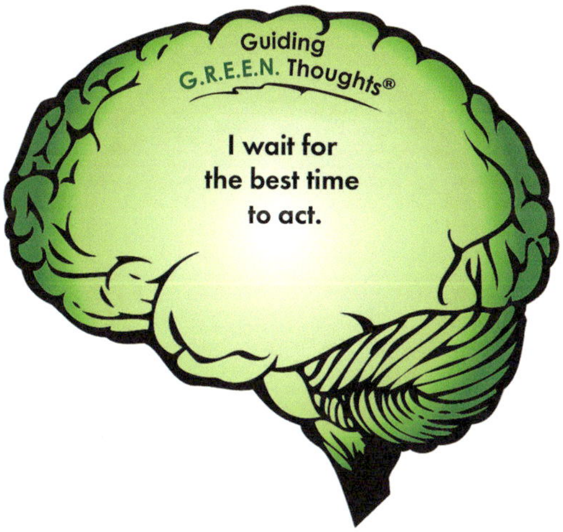

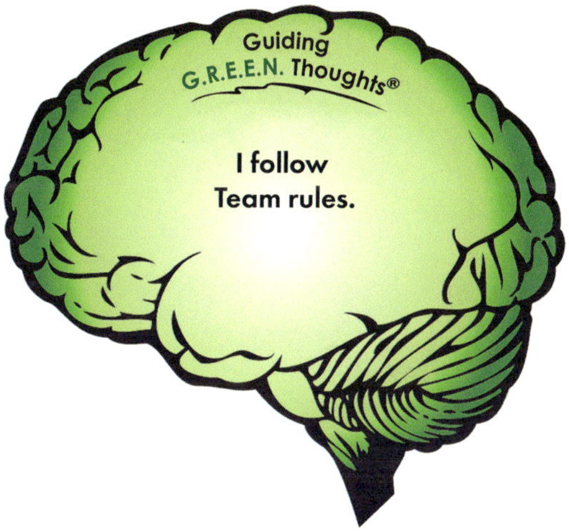

My own Guiding G.R.E.E.N. Thought for this scene:

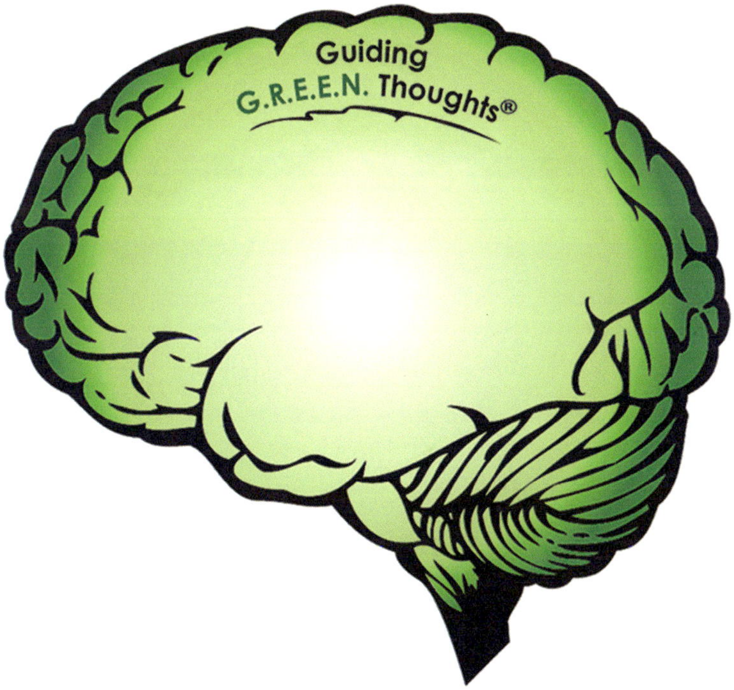

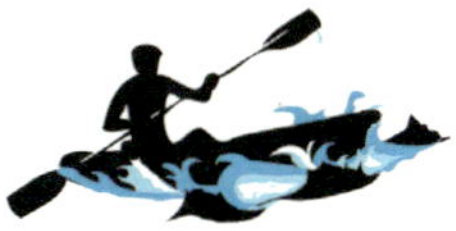

30 Ask for Help When You Need It

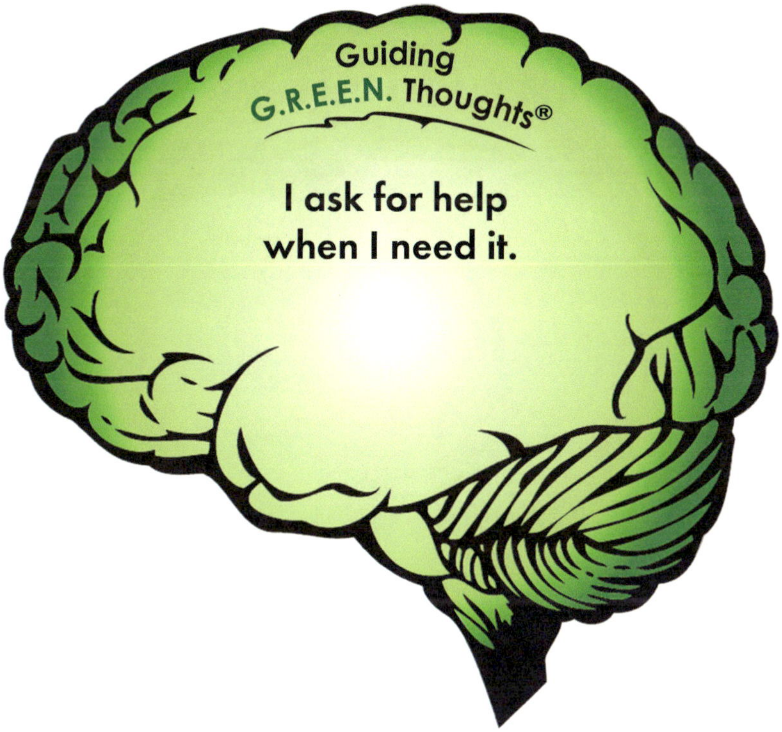

30.1 Asking for Help Can Be Helpful!

As you get older, you can learn to do many things. Sometimes you can learn to do things by yourself; however, you often need someone to help you learn new things.

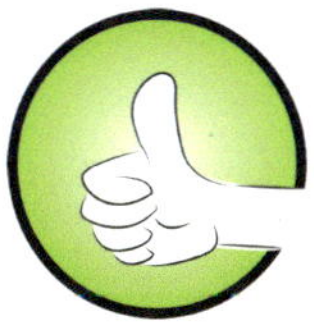

When you are in school, some things you learn must be taught to you by someone else. At home, you can learn from people older than yourself. You can learn new things from a grandparent or parent or older sibling. You also can learn how to do things better from coaches and from **helpful** friends.

You can ask for help in many ways:

- You can ask for someone to repeat instructions.
- You can ask for the other person to show you how to do something.
- You can ask another person to watch how you are doing something so you can get some advice on how to do it better the next time.

30.2 Being Open-Minded to Ask for Help

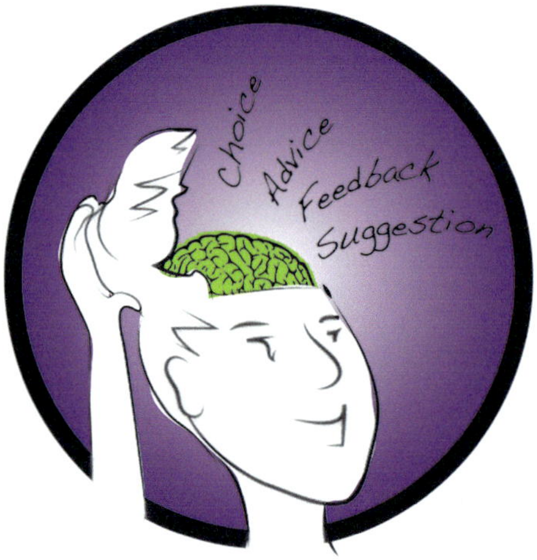

When you are asking for help, you want to be **open-minded**. This will help you **pay attention** to what the other person is saying to you or showing you. When you are **open-minded**, you can hear or see details that you did not notice before.

You must be open to feedback if you are trying to learn something new. Sometimes you might not do the job as others think it should be done. You might need help learning how to do it in a better way. When you are **open-minded**, you become better at learning how to do new things.

Once you know how to do something, you won't need to ask for help in doing it. You will be able to proudly do that activity successfully on your own consistently. You can add it to the list of things you know how to do by yourself!

30.3 How Much Help Do You Need?

#1: Skills That Can Be Performed Independently

This list helps you realize what you can do independently, which means you can do these things without needing help from anyone. For a skill to be on this list, you should be able to do it consistently, meaning that you can do it independently every time it needs to be done.

I can do these things by myself at home:

____ Get up on time for school

____ Do my homework

____ Get ready for school

____ Help make dinner

____ Pack what I need to take

____ Set the table

____ Water plants

____ Clear the table

____ Feed pets

____ Get ready for bed

____ Set my alarm

I can do these things by myself at school:

____ Greet people I know

____ Start my work on time

____ Follow classroom rules

____ Complete my work

____ Understand directions

____ Use **self-control** strategies

#2: Skills I Can Perform with Some Help

The skills on this list are harder for you to do right now. They are the things you cannot do without some help. When something is hard to understand or do, you can let someone know that you need some help. When you learn to ask for help, you will find that your scene gets **better**. You will learn to do these things independently after you have some practice doing them with help. Then these skills can be moved to the Independent list.

I can do these things with some help at home:

____ Get up on time for school

____ Do my homework

____ Get ready for school

____ Help make dinner

____ Pack what I need to take

____ Set the table

____ Water plants

____ Clear the table

____ Feed pets

____ Get ready for bed

____ Set my alarm

I can do these things with some help at school:

____ Greet people I know

____ Start my work on time

____ Follow classroom rules

____ Complete my work

____ Understand directions

____ Use **self-control** strategies

Ask for help if you need it!

#3: Things I Cannot Do Now Even with Help

Some things are too difficult to do now even if you get help. You may not be old enough to do them, or may not be able to do them safely even with help. You can ask people to do these things for you. You might say something like, "I can't do this myself. Can you do this for me?"

I can't do these things right now even with help:

____ Use the stove

____ Do Laundry

____ Use power tools

____ Take medicine

____ Drive a car

____ Budget my money

When you get older or when you learn to take the time to pay attention in order to make logical, wise choices consistently, you may learn to do some of these things with help. You may then show yourself and others on your Teams that you can do these on your own in the future.

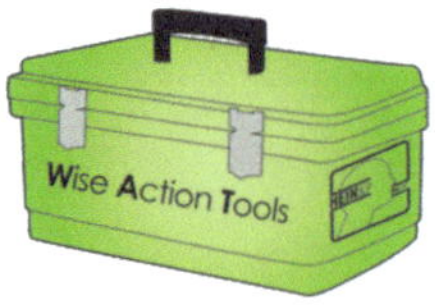

CHARTING HOW MUCH HELP I NEED TODAY

____

TODAY'S DATE

I Keep track of how much help I need to do things. This helps me and others know what I can do by myself and what things I can do with help. I can have **Personal Goals** to build my skills and work hard to move things over to the left on this chart. I can work to move things from the list of things I can't do, to the list of things I can do with help, and then to the list of things I can do by myself. First, I will write on this chart how much help I need doing things today! Then I will see how much progress I have made the next time I fill out this chart.

Things I can do well **by myself**	Things I can do well **if I get some help**	Things I **can't do** right now

My name ____

30.4 Change the Scene to Make It G.R.E.E.N.: Tommy Doesn't Understand the Directions!

Let's **survey the scene** to see what is happening with Tommy. Tommy sometimes has trouble paying attention to his teacher. Understanding is a challenge for him when she gives more than one direction at a time. Tommy does not do anything to help himself when someone is giving him information that he does not understand. He doesn't tell the teacher if he missed what she said. He doesn't ask for repeats or any other kind of help. Instead, Tommy gets frustrated and mad whenever someone gives him too many directions at once. Then he stops listening! He interrupts the teacher by making loud noises. He distracts his classmates.

1. With a red pencil, circle any action in the paragraph above that you think is not **helpful** to Tommy or his Team. This action can look like **Rude**, **Egocentric**, and **Disruptive** (**R.E.D.**) behavior to other people in his classroom.

Directions for Questions 2–4: Circle the best answer for each question:

2. Tommy asks for what he needs in the classroom.

   yes   no

3. Tommy gets mad and starts making noises when he does not understand his teacher. Is this **helping** or hurting the Classroom Team?

   helping   hurting

4. Tommy gets mad and starts making noises when he does not understand his teacher. Is this helping him reach his **Personal Goal** of getting good grades in his class?

   yes   no

5. What is a **Guiding G.R.E.E.N. Thought** that Tommy can use to help him make a **transformation** and make the classroom scene **better**? As you read and act out the next **G.R.E.E.N.** scene, think about how these **Guiding G.R.E.E.N. Thoughts** are helping Tommy successfully **navigate** this situation.

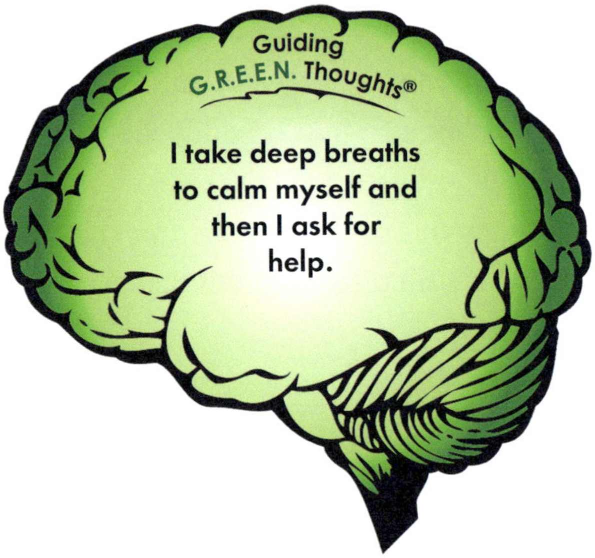

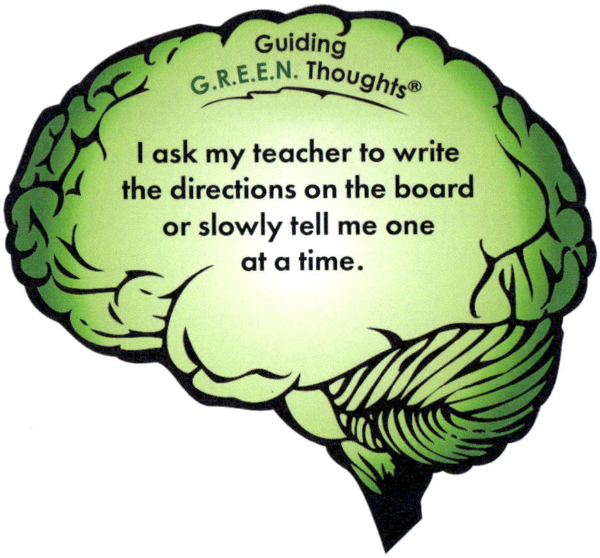

Here is something else Tommy can think about to help him in this scene:

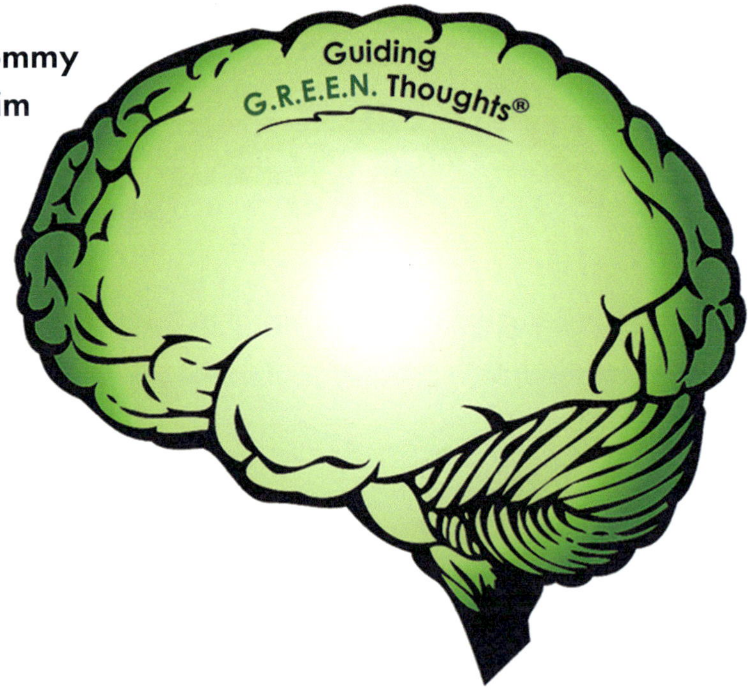

30.5 G.R.E.E.N. Scene #22: I Get Calm and Ask for Help

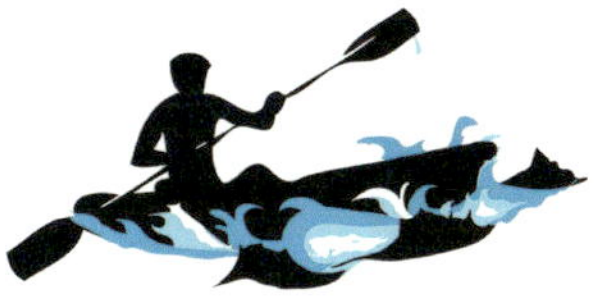

Directions for G.R.E.E.N. SCENE #22:

1. Think First to **survey the scene** and choose **Guiding G.R.E.E.N. Thoughts**:

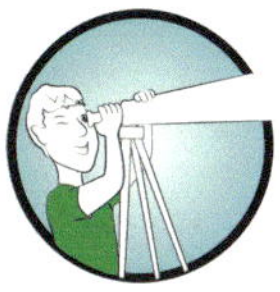

A. Before acting, read Section 30.4 and complete the "**Surveying the Scene** Before Taking Action" sheet (this way you will learn what all of the characters need and what the **Common Team Goal** may be).

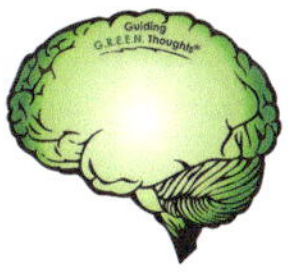

B. Choose or write out the **Guiding G.R.E.E.N. Thoughts** that Tommy could use to help him **navigate** this scene.

2. Set up for a successful G.R.E.E.N. Scene:

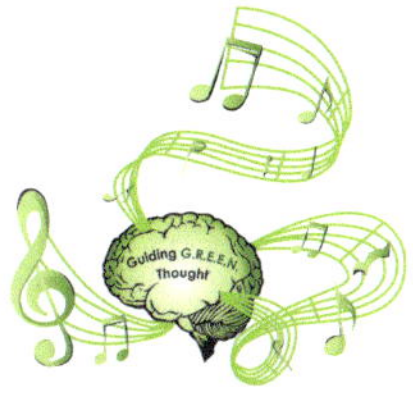

A. Give Tommy the instruction sheet to help him "Brake to Take a 5 Break" (Section 13.4). At an appropriate time during instruction, play the "**Brake to Take a 5 Break"** song on the "**Songs for Guiding G.R.E.E.N. Thoughts"** album. Decide whether this song should be played during the G.R.E.E.N. scene to help Tommy get calm with his controlled breathing.

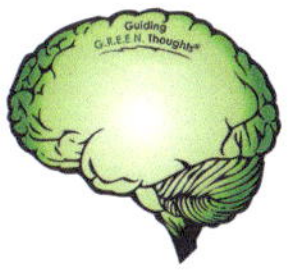

B. Give Tommy the **Guiding G.R.E.E.N. Thoughts** that were chosen to help him remember to:

- "Brake to take a 5 Break" to get calm and
- ask a teacher to repeat the directions if he did not hear them

C. Give Tommy a blank piece of paper so he can follow the directions with it once he understands what they are.

D. The Director gets the clapboard and says:

"Quiet on the set. G.R.E.E.N. *Scene #22. Take one. Action!"* If the scene gets repeated with the same set of actors, the Director will say, *"Quiet on the set.* G.R.E.E.N. *Scene #22. Take two. Action!"*

E. If there are audience members, they may be asked to fill out the G.R.E.E.N. Scene Review Sheet to give the actors constructive feedback. (Section 12.4–12.5)

The Scene: I Get Calm and *Ask for* Help

Narrator: Tommy's teacher gives the class a direction, but Tommy does not pay attention to it.

Teacher: *Class, I want you to write your name* and *date on the paper in the top right corner* and *then write one thing you like to do in the summer.*

Narrator: Tommy realizes he did not hear what the teacher said. He starts to get frustrated, but then remembers **Guiding** G.R.E.E.N. **Thoughts** that he can use to help him in this scene. Tommy then chooses the best **Guiding** G.R.E.E.N. **Thoughts** so he can take the best action in this scene.

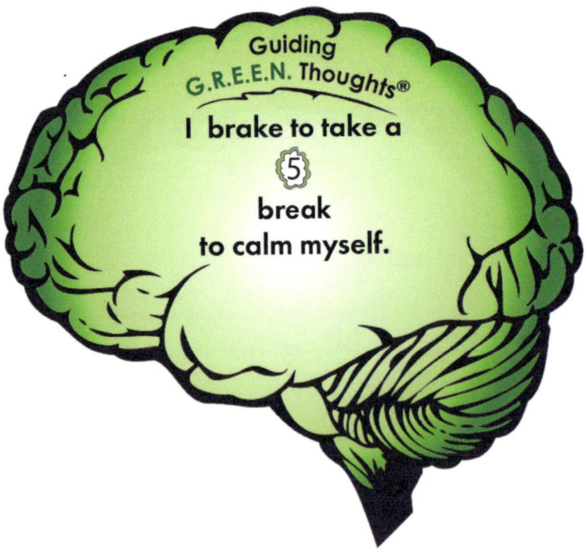

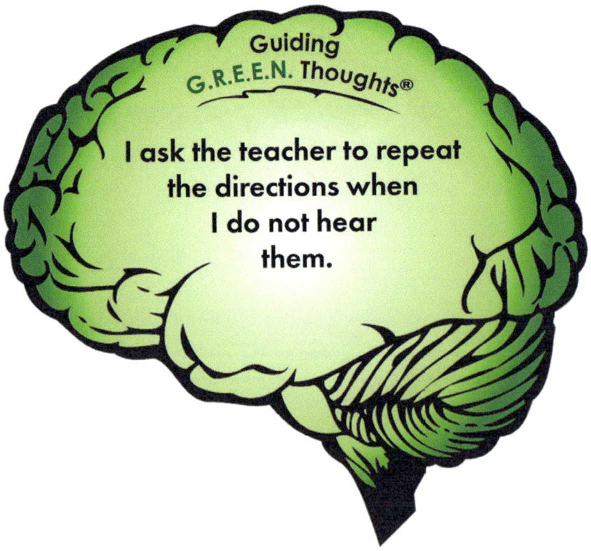

Narrator: Tommy starts to "Brake to take a 5 Break." He slowly breathes in and out five times to help himself get calm again. Tommy tracks his controlled breathing by counting on his fingers. (The narrator waits for Tommy to finish his controlled breathing.) When he is calm, he then reaches for another **Guiding G.R.E.E.N. Thought** to remind himself to ask the teacher to repeat the directions.

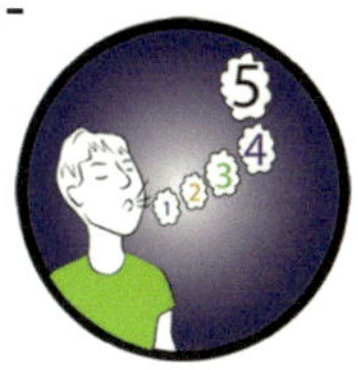

Tommy (says this *after* his 5 Break): *"I'm sorry, I did not hear what you told us to do. Can you please repeat the directions slowly?"*

Teacher: *Yes, thank you for asking so politely. Now get ready to listen to the directions.*

Narrator: The teacher then says the directions somewhat slower and very distinctly.

Teacher: *I want you to write your name and date on the paper in the top right corner and then write one thing you like doing in the summer.*

Tommy: *OK, I will. Thanks for repeating the directions.*

Narrator: Tommy follows the directions and asks for the teacher for more help if he still does not know what to do.

31 Accepting When Someone Tells Me "No"

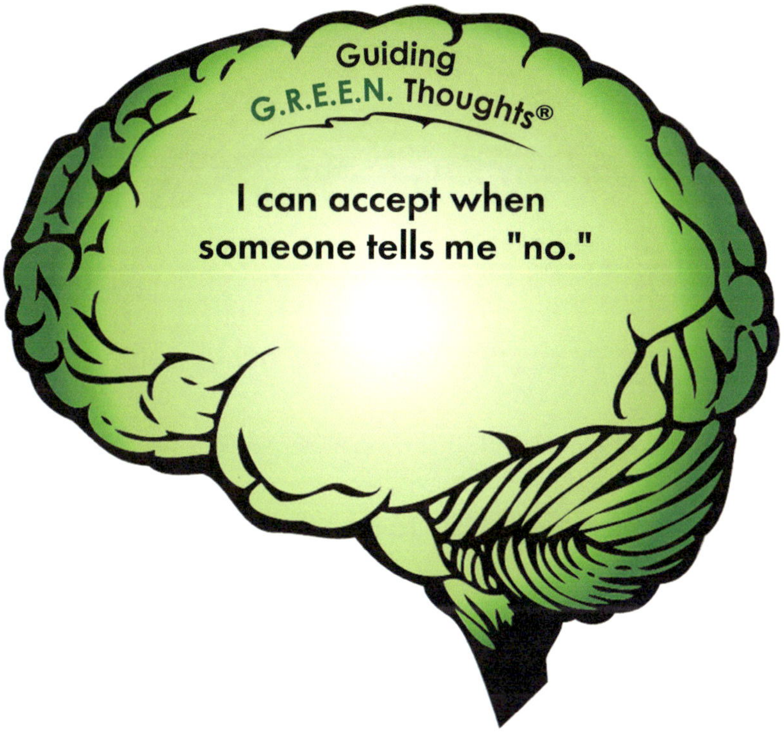

31.1 You Can Accept When Someone Tells You "No" When You Know Why

Many times in life you can't get what you want when you want it. Someone may tell you, "No, you can't have it!" or "No, you can't do it!" There is usually a good reason that will make it easier for you to accept that the person is saying "no." It is easier to accept the word "no" if you understand why the other person said "No!"

If someone tells you "no," you can ask *why*:

"Why are you saying 'no'?"

"What is the reason you are saying 'no'?"

"Can you please tell me why you are saying 'no'?"

When the other person tells you the answer, you can begin understanding why that person is saying "no."

You can then use **self-calming** strategies and other **navigating** tools so you can be OK with **changing** to another choice instead.

31.2 Thinking of Reasons Why People Say "No"

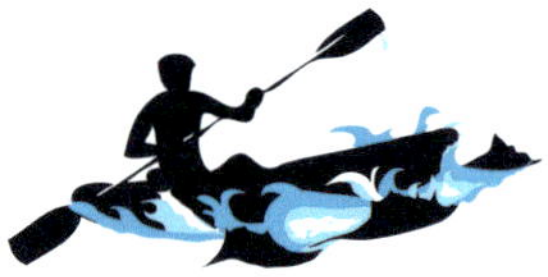

People may say "no" to you for many reasons.

- The action or activity you want to do may not be safe.
- What you want to do might hurt or bother others on your Team.
- There might not be enough time to do what you want to do.
- It might not be your turn.
- You might have to share with others.
- You might have enough already.

Can you think of other reasons why people might say "no" to you?

____

____

____

____

31.3 G.R.E.E.N. Scene #23: Why Did Kevin's Parents Say "No"?

Change the Scene to *Make It* G.R.E.E.N.: *The Scene before* Transformation

Kevin wants to spend the night at a friend's house. He says, "I want to stay over at Mike's house tonight!" His parents say, "No, not tonight!" Kevin stomps up the stairs and slams the door.

1. With a red pencil, underline Kevin's behavior that you think others on his Home Team would think is **R.E.D.** (**R**ude, **E**gocentric, and **D**isruptive).

2. Why do you think Kevin's parents said "No"?

____

3. Did Kevin *ask* permission to spend the night at Mike's house?

yes no

4. Did he demand to sleep over?

yes no

(Read the lesson in Section 19.10 to help you understand the difference between "asking" and "demanding.")

5. Did Kevin ask why he couldn't go to his friend's house?

yes no

Let's **rewind** the scene so Kevin can ask "why." Asking for the reason may help Kevin do a **better** job of **navigating** and acting **G.R.E.E.N.** with his Home Team.

***The Scene after* Transformation**

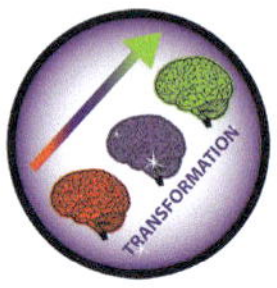

Kevin wants to spend the night at a friend's house.

Kevin: *Can I stay over at Mike's house tonight?*

Kevin's father: *No, not tonight!*

Kevin: *Why can't I go tonight?*

Kevin's father: *You can't go tonight because you must go to school tomorrow morning.*

Kevin: *Could I go to his house on Saturday night?*

Kevin's father: *That should be OK. We will check with his parents to make sure it is OK with them.*

Kevin: *Thanks, Dad.*

Because the Scene Is Now "G.R.E.E.N. for the Team," You Can Act It Out!

Refer to the pages in Sections 12.2 through 12.5 for the directions, rules, warm-ups, and review sheets needed to help you make the best **G.R.E.E.N.** Scene.

Show Kevin's **transformation** on the **Thought Transformation Scene Changer**. What **Guiding G.R.E.E.N. Thoughts** do *you* think helped him make the **transformation** so the new scene was **better** for everyone? Here are some possible **thoughts**:

I use **self-calming** strategies when I am with my Team.

I can accept when someone tells me "no."

I ask "why" so I can understand if someone tells me "no."

Thought Transformation Scene Changer

Name ______________________________ Date ____________________

1. The Scene at first, *before* G.R.E.E.N. Thought Transformation.

a. Write or draw how I am acting with other people in this scene *before* the G.R.E.E.N. Thought **Transformation**.

b. What feedback am I getting from others about my actions? ____________________

____

c. How are all the people in this scene feeling, including me? ____________________

____

2. Get the Power!

Change the scene!

Be **open-minded** to make a **Transformation**.

Think of Guiding **G.R.E.E.N.** Thoughts to make it happen!

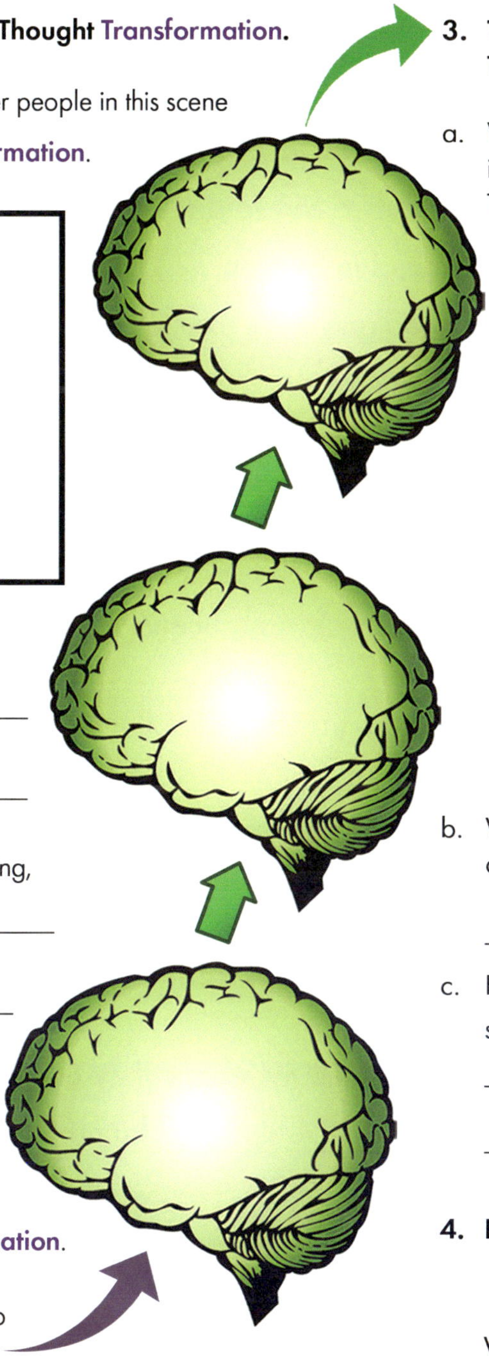

3. The new scene *after* G.R.E.E.N. Thought Transformation.

a. Write or draw what is happening in this scene *after* **G.R.E.E.N.** Thought **Transformation**.

b. What feedback am I getting from others about my actions? __________

____

c. How are all the people in this scene feeling now, including me?

____

____

4. Is this new scene better?

yes no

Why? ____________________

____

5. This page shows a powerful Transformation from ____________________ **to** ____________________.

31.4 G.R.E.E.N. Scene #24: Let's Navigate Past the Word "No"

Directions

1. Think First to **survey the scene** & choose **Guiding G.R.E.E.N. Thoughts**

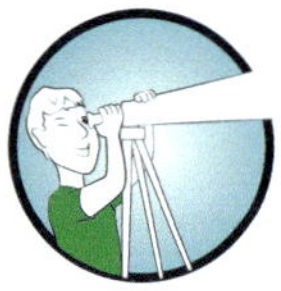

   A. Before acting, read over the **G.R.E.E.N.** Scene in the next section and complete a **Surveying the Scene before Taking Action** sheet (found in Section 12.2). This way you learn what the characters need and what the **Common Team Goal** may be.

   B. Write out the **Guiding G.R.E.E.N. Thoughts** that Carl could use to help him **navigate** this scene (Section 31.7).

2. Set Up for a Great **G.R.E.E.N.** Scene

   A. Carl has the writing assignment sheet in front of him.

   B. Carl has the **Guiding G.R.E.E.N. Thoughts** he could use to help him **navigate** successfully through this scene.

   C. Review **G.R.E.E.N.** Scene Warm-Ups! (Section 12.5)

   D. If there are audience members, they can be given the **G.R.E.E.N.** Scene Review Sheet. (Wise Action Tool found in Section 12.5)

   E. The Director gets the clapboard and says:

   "Quiet on the set! **G.R.E.E.N.** Scene #24. Take one. Action!"

   If the scene gets repeated with the same set of actors, the Director will say: "Quiet on the set! Scene #24. Take two. Action!"

3. Act Out the Scene.

4. G.R.E.E.N. Scene Review:

   Audience members can complete their G.R.E.E.N. Scene Review Sheets and provide constructive feedback to the actors (see Section 12.5).

31.5 The Scene: Let's Navigate Past the Word "No"

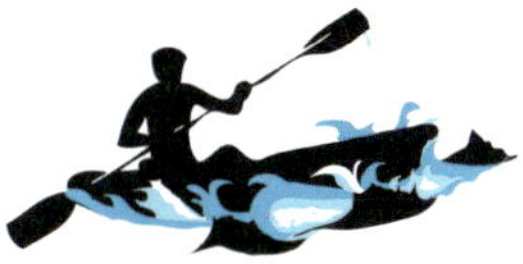

Narrator: Carl is in his writing class. He has been having a hard time focusing on his assignment. He is supposed to be describing the picture in front of him, but he can't stop thinking about his favorite video game. His teacher says it is time for recess. The classroom rule is that students must write three complete sentences before they can go out for recess. The teacher, Ms. Gold, is going from desk to desk to see if each student has written at least three sentences. She comes to Carl's desk.

Carl: *Can I go to recess?*

Ms. Gold: *Let me see how much you have written. No, Carl. I'm sorry, but you have only written one sentence. You need to write two more sentences about that picture before you can go out.*

Narrator: Carl does not like to hear the word "no." Actually, there have been some times that he has been so frustrated in hearing the word "no" that he has shouted and thrown down his pencil.

But Carl has learned to have **powerful G.R.E.E.N. Transformations**!

He is learning to use **self-calming** strategies. He is also learning to reach up to give himself **Guiding G.R.E.E.N. Thoughts** to help him **navigate** successfully, and act **safely** and **logically**, even if he hears the word "no." Instead of becoming frustrated, he uses his **self-calming** strategies and words to problem solve with his teacher.

Carl: *Why do I need to write two more sentences, Ms. Gold?*

Ms. Gold: (Ms. Gold takes a deep breath so she can be **patient** and **supportive**, while using a **respectful** tone of voice to answer.) *Carl, you are in this class to learn to write. I cannot help you unless you put in some effort. Everyone in this class has been working on writing one paragraph about this picture. You have written only one sentence. I know you can write two more. I know you can do it.*

Carl: *Can you* help *me think of something to say?*

Ms. Gold: *OK, Carl. Look* carefully *at this picture. You wrote that a man is carrying three dogs on a surfboard. That is a great start. Now make your best guess about how the man feels. Look at his* face *and guess how he is feeling and why he is feeling that way. Write a sentence about that.*

Then, look at the dogs and *guess how they feel* and *why they feel that way. Write a sentence about that. After you write those two sentences, you can then go outside for recess. Next time you can ask for* help *during* class *so you won't miss any recess.*

Carl: *Thanks for* helping *me, Ms. Gold. I will get this done so that we can both have a break.*

Ms. Gold: *I will* **appreciate** *that, Carl.*

31.6 The Writing Assignment That Needs to Be Finished

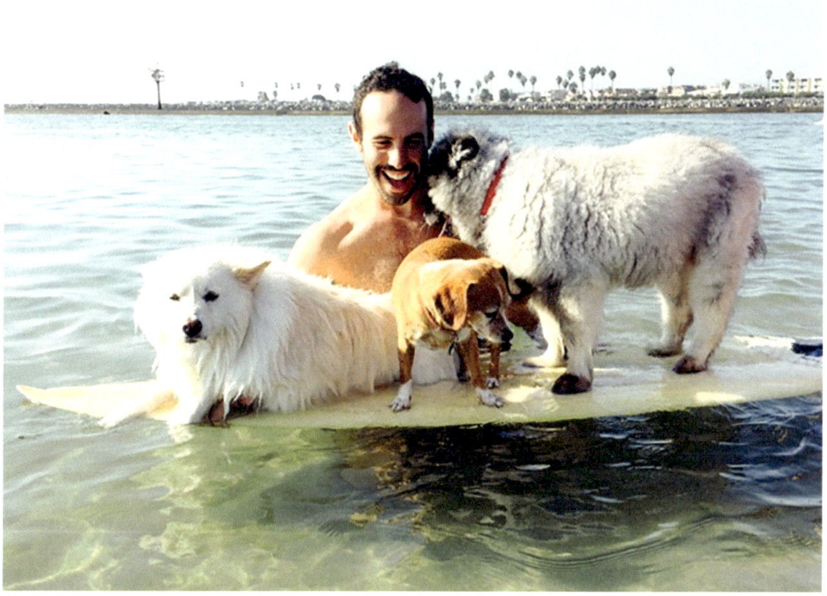

This is the picture that Carl has to write about before he goes to recess.

Help him write the other two sentences:

A man is carrying three dogs on a surfboard.

31.7 Write Guiding G.R.E.E.N. Thoughts You Think Carl Chose to Make a Transformation

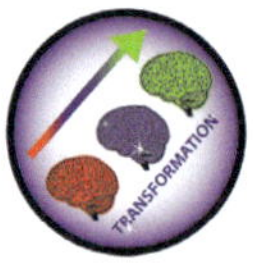

Carl used **Guiding G.R.E.E.N. Thoughts** to make a **transformation** in his actions. He might have acted in an old way, but he chose to act **better** for himself and his Team.

On this page you can write some **Guiding G.R.E.E.N. Thoughts** that you think Carl used to help him **change** his actions to make them **better**. Review Carl's story to help you think about what strategies he may have used and some thoughts he gave to himself.

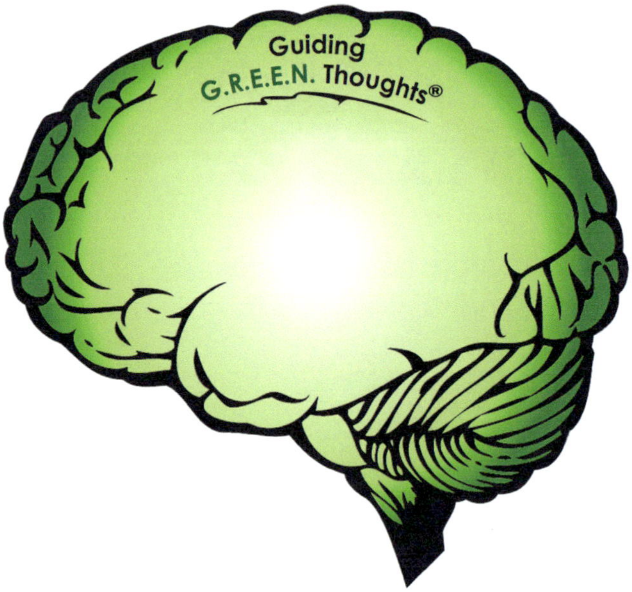

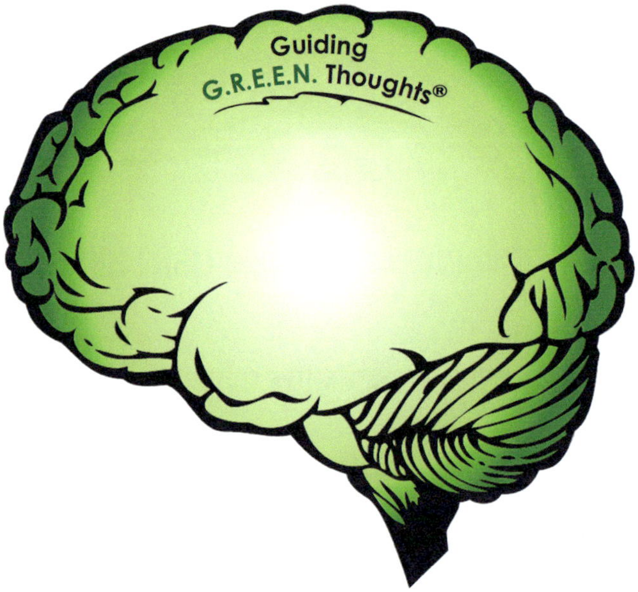

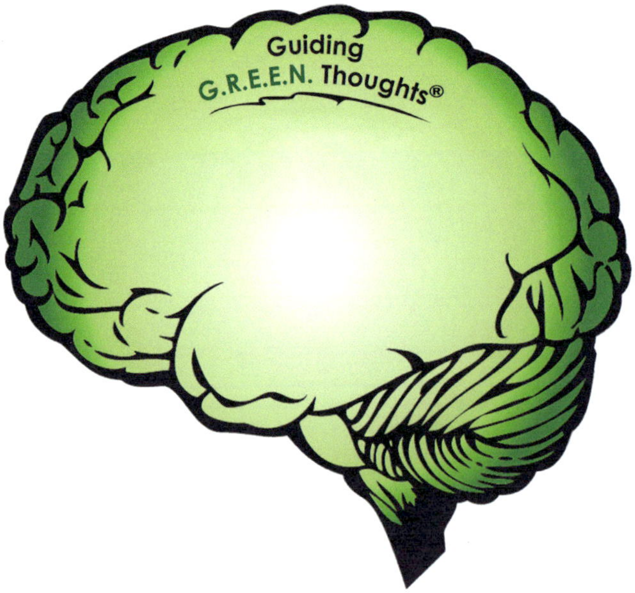

You may also fill in the **Thought Transformation Scene Changer** to show how Carl may have acted before, what **Guiding G.R.E.E.N. Thoughts** he used to **change the scene**, and how he is acting now. (Find the **Thought Transformation Scene Changer** in Section 15.5.)

32 Adjusting to Changes

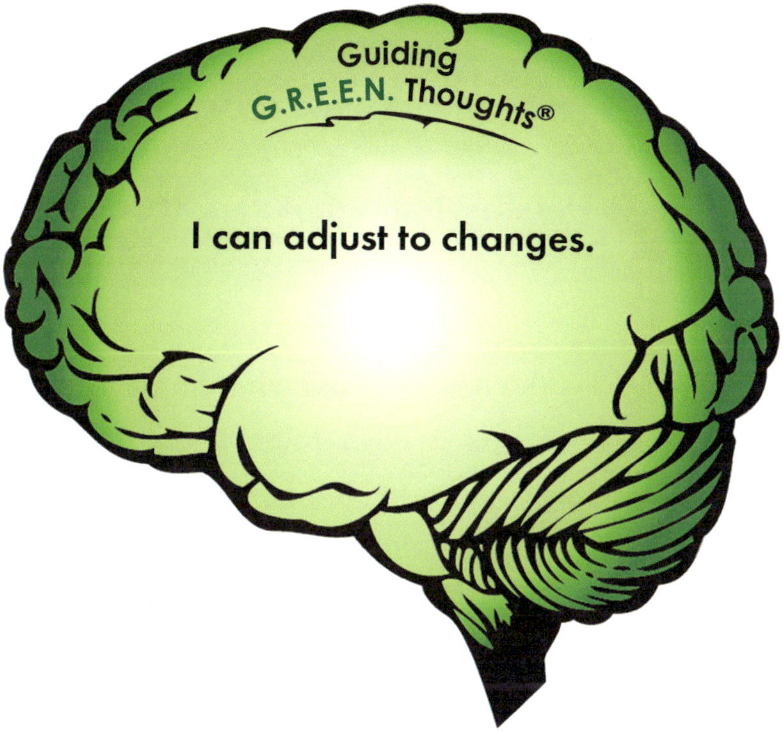

32.1 Adjusting to Changes by Being Open-Minded

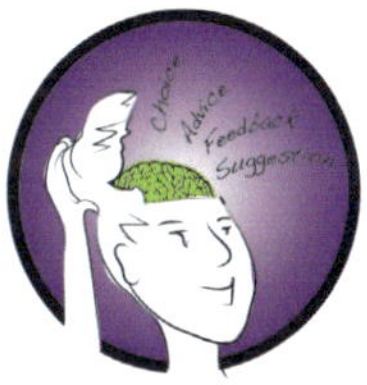

Most people experience changes in their lives. It is almost impossible for things to stay the same from year to year. Since changes will happen in your life, it is best to **accept** them. In fact, as changes are made in your life, they can help you grow and help you learn new things. It does require that you are **open-minded** and that you can learn to **adjust** to the changes.

In school, you get to learn to **accept** changes in who is in your class, who is teaching your class and what class or what school you are in.

At home you may also need to **accept** changes about who is in your family and where your family is living. You may also need to **accept** changes about what kinds of activities happen in your home and in your family on different days. People will think you are acting maturely if you can **accept** changes and **adjust** to new situations.

The next section is a story about Nathan. Help him **adjust** to the changes he needs to make in school.

32.2 Survey the Scene: Helping Nathan Adjust to Changes at School

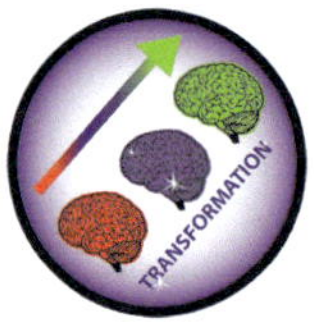

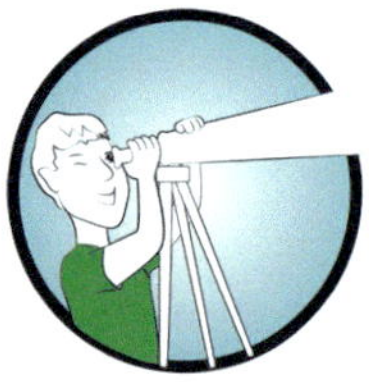

Directions: Survey the Scene to see what happened to Nathan last year and what his challenge is now. Think about what Guiding G.R.E.E.N. Thoughts you might suggest to Nathan to help him make a transformation to begin navigating successfully in his new life situation.

New things make Nathan uncomfortable. Last year he started at a new school. He had a hard time **adjusting** to being at the school and being in his new classroom. At first, he did not want to listen to the teacher and did not want to follow any directions. He often found himself yelling and getting into trouble for not helping out his teacher and his classmates who were trying hard to get their work done. He felt all alone and did not know what to do. Happily, he got some guidance in the first two months of school to learn some strategies to help himself **adjust** to his new school, classroom, teacher, and classmates. He learned some **self-calming** strategies and learned strategies to **listen better** to his new teacher. By the end of the year, he was acting successfully in his classroom and was proud of himself for learning how to get along easily with his teacher and his classmates.

Unfortunately for Nathan, that school year ended, and he had to move up to a new grade and a new class with a new teacher and many new classmates. On his first day of the new school year, as soon as he had to line up with his new class, he started to feel like he did at the beginning of the previous year. He was starting to feel as if he did not want to listen to this new teacher because she was different than the one he had last year. He started to feel uncomfortable, but...he did Think First to remember that he could choose **Guiding G.R.E.E.N. Thoughts** to help him make a **transformation**. They would help him **navigate** successfully through his new challenges.

Help Nathan think of **Guiding G.R.E.E.N. Thoughts** to help him have a successful **transformation** so he can be ready to **navigate** his new challenging situation. After that, fill out the **Thought Transformation Scene Changer**. Show Nathan's **transformation** and what **Guiding G.R.E.E.N. Thoughts** you think he used successfully to make a **better** scene for himself and his new School Team.

32.3 Guiding G.R.E.E.N. Thoughts for Nathan to Choose

Nathan can make a **transformation** in his actions. He might have acted in an old way, but he is choosing to act **better** for himself and his new Team.

On the next page you can write in some **Guiding G.R.E.E.N. Thoughts** that you think Nathan may use to help him make the best choices in his actions. Review Nathan's story to help you think about what strategies he might use and some **Guiding G.R.E.E.N. Thoughts** he can give himself.

Write in some **Guiding G.R.E.E.N. Thoughts** that Nathan can use to help him **adjust** to changes and choose the best actions for himself and his new Team.

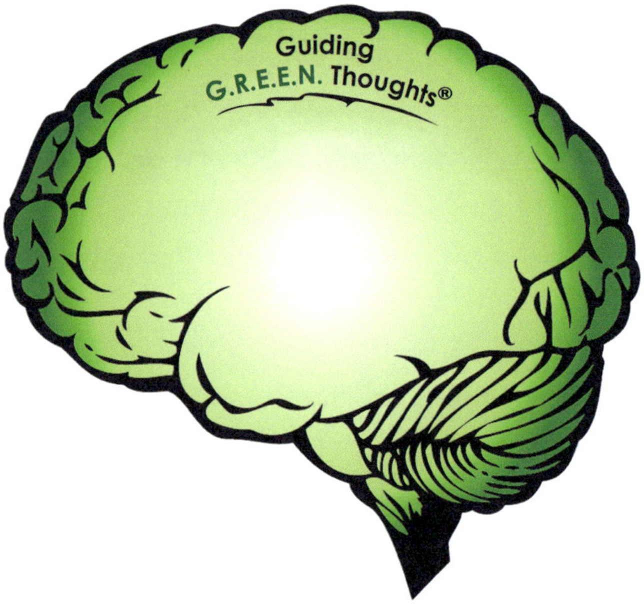

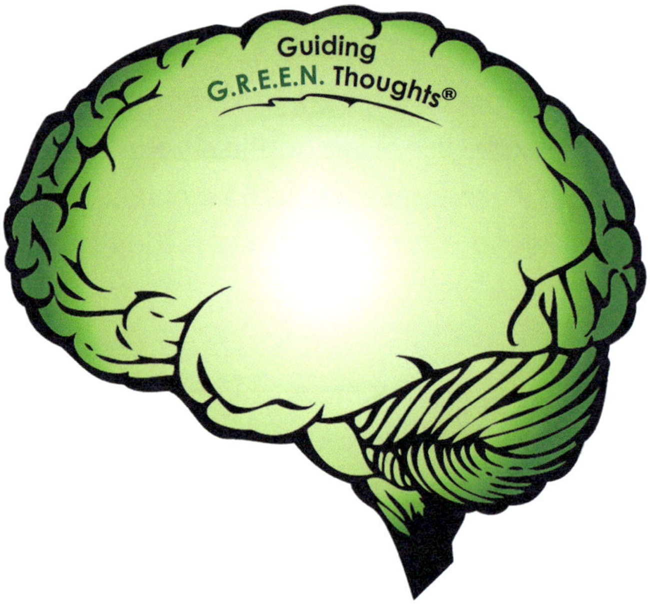

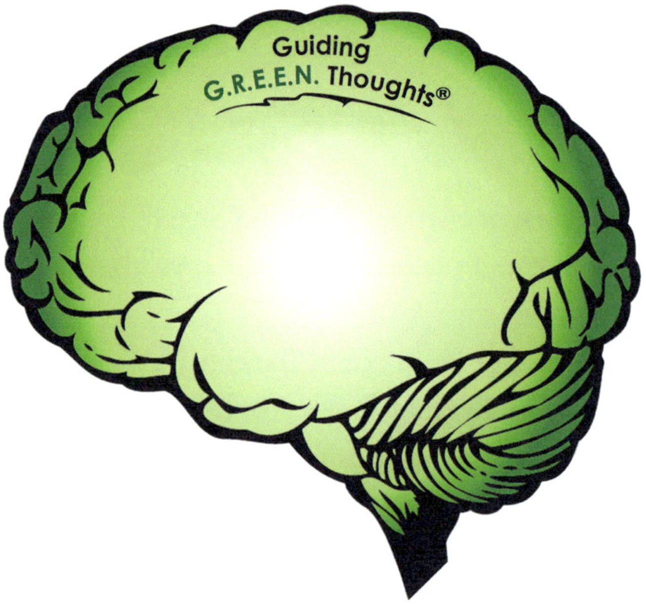

32.4 Thought Transformation Scene Changer for Nathan

Using a **Thought Transformation Scene Changer,** show how Nathan used your suggested **Guiding G.R.E.E.N. Thoughts** to make a **trans-formation**, making **changes** for a **better** scene for himself and his Class Team.

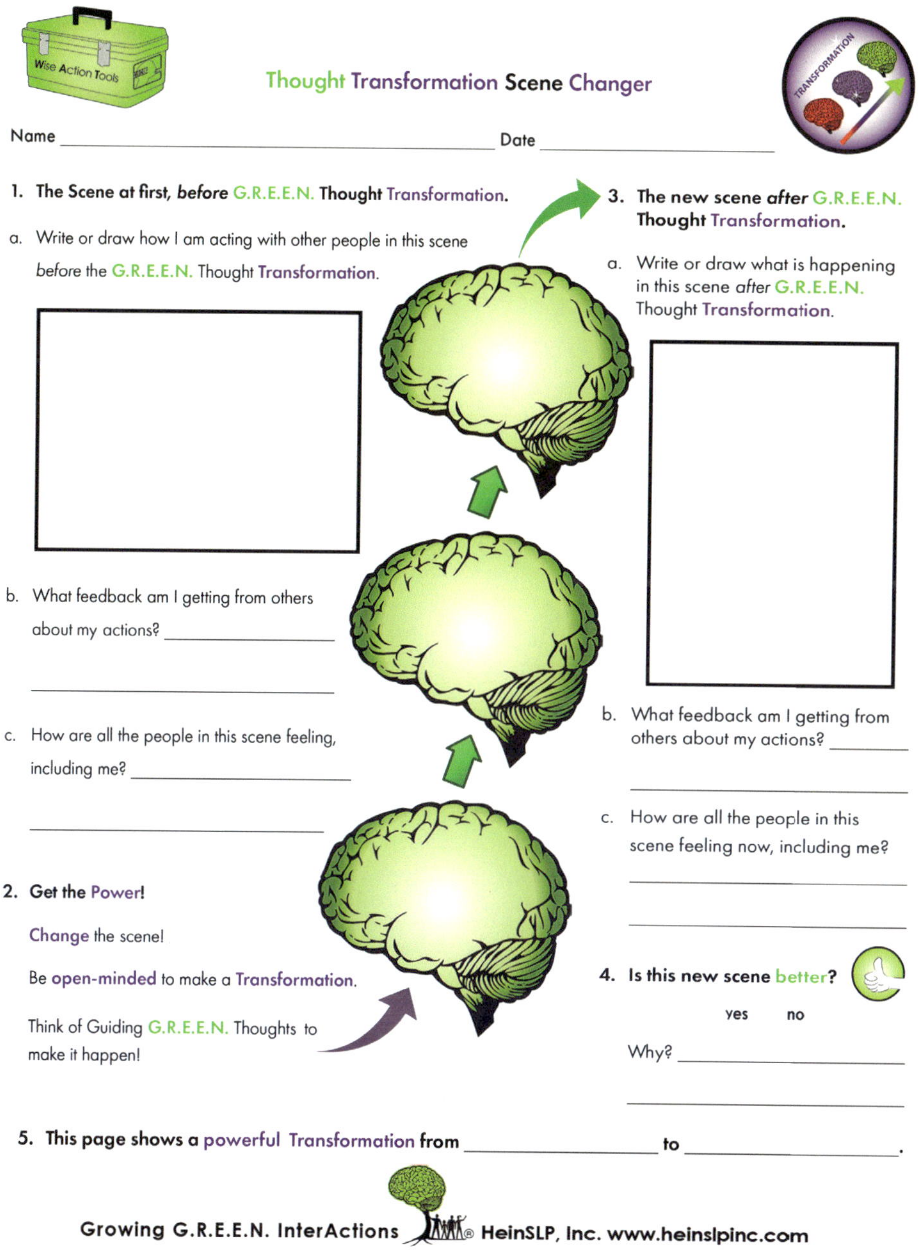

Thought Transformation Scene Changer

Name ______________________ Date ______________

1. The Scene at first, *before* G.R.E.E.N. Thought Transformation.

a. Write or draw how I am acting with other people in this scene *before* the G.R.E.E.N. Thought Transformation.

b. What feedback am I getting from others about my actions? ______________

c. How are all the people in this scene feeling, including me? ______________

2. Get the Power!

Change the scene!

Be open-minded to make a Transformation.

Think of Guiding G.R.E.E.N. Thoughts to make it happen!

3. The new scene *after* G.R.E.E.N. Thought Transformation.

a. Write or draw what is happening in this scene *after* G.R.E.E.N. Thought Transformation.

b. What feedback am I getting from others about my actions? ______________

c. How are all the people in this scene feeling now, including me? ______________

4. Is this new scene better?

yes no

Why? ______________

5. This page shows a powerful Transformation from ______________ to ______________.

Growing G.R.E.E.N. InterActions® HeinSLP, Inc. www.heinslpinc.com

32.5 Stating What Is Being Learned

A good check of how **G.R.E.E.N.** you are acting is to "name" the main idea being taught. By doing so, it becomes more likely that the concept, skill, or strategy you have learned will be remembered in the next session and in less structured activities.

32.6 Positive Reinforcement for Acting G.R.E.E.N.

Positive, **G.R.E.E.N.** behavior can be rewarded with the **Growing G.R.E.E.N. Certificate.** The certificate can be given to an individual or a whole group when they act especially **G.R.E.E.N.**

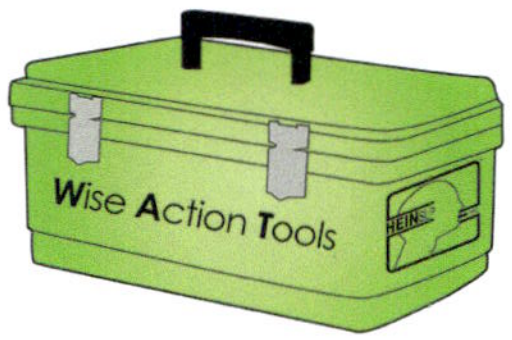

LESSON LOG FOR WHAT I AM LEARNING

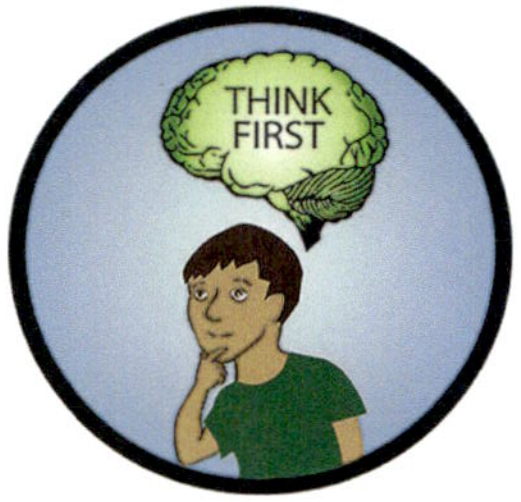

Date	Main Idea of What I Did and Learned Today

Growing G.R.E.E.N. Certificate

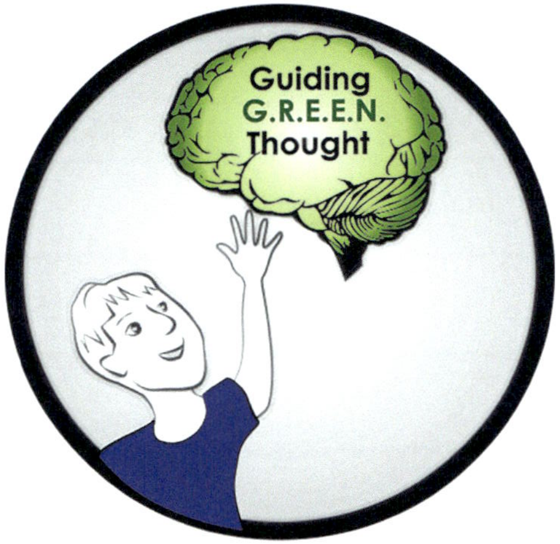

______________________________ has been:

- ☐ Thoughtful
- ☐ Positive
- ☐ Open-Minded
- ☐ Respectful
- ☐ Kind
- ☐ Cooperative

Presented by ____________________ Date ______________

GLOSSARY

The page where each word is first used in this Lesson Book is noted in this glossary.

accomplish (page 29)—achieve, what you are able to get done or complete

achieve (page 7)—to do something or accomplish something successfully

acronym (page 2)—a word that is made up of the first letter of other words that relate to each other

adjust (page 394)—being able to get used to something that is different than what you have been experiencing before

advice (page 61)—ideas someone on your Team gives you so you can do a better job at something the next time you try

appreciate (page 3)—having the feeling and awareness that you are lucky and grateful that you have someone or something in your life

arrogant (page 306)—acting in a way in which a person thinks they are better and more important than anyone else

bad sportsmanship (page 305)—acting in a negative way toward the opposing team before, during, or after a game whether you win or lose

baseline (page 34)—starting point, a description of how you are acting at first before you start focusing on doing things to help yourself act better with your Teams

benefit (page 35)—have a better situation; have something positive happen

bitter (page 306)—a feeling a person has when they feel strong disappointment, resentment and anger about a situation in which they feel they were not treated fairly

boastful (page 306)—acting in a way in which a person talks about how great they are

brain chemicals (page 105)—neurotransmitters that are released by one neuron and received by another to pass information through the brain. Some essential neurotransmitters include glutamate, GABA, serotonin, dopamine, endorphins, and noradrenaline.

briefly (page 309)—for a short period of time

caring voice (page 285)—a tone of voice that shows you care about the other person

challenging (page 3)—a description of a situation in which it is difficult to figure out what to do

civil, civilized (page 5)—acting in a polite and cooperative way with others so the group can move forward safely and successfully, following the group rules

civilization (page 2)—the complex and useful ways that people can live, work, and build great things together; a culture that has achieved an advanced level

coach yourself (page 137)—guide yourself to make the best action choices

combative (page 253)—having a tone of voice and/or using words that show that the person wants to argue or have a fight

comment (page 228)—a statement you can make that shows you are listening to someone by expressing your opinion about what they said, stating how you think they might feel about what they are saying and/or showing support; G.R.E.E.N. comments help connect you to your Team

common (page 3)—something that is shared with others

Common Team Goals (page 3)—goals that everyone on a Team would like to accomplish; these are goals that the whole group would like to achieve together

complain (page 100)—say negative things about something that happened

complicationcomplicated (page 126)—a problem or something that is happening that is keeping things from working and moving forward

compromise (page 317)—a settlement of a disagreement in which each side gives up something so both can move forward with a shared plan

connecting (page 25)—to join or link together so things can work better

consequences (page 95)—good things or bad things that happen because of an action

considerate (page 209)—aware and concerned about how you treat someone or something, making people feel like their needs are as important as yours

constructive feedback (page 168)—supportive feedback that provides you with useful ideas about how you might do something better than you did it before

content (page 292)—a feeling a person has when they are happy and satisfied

continuing (page 156)—doing something without stopping

controlled breathing (page 138)—a strategy in which you pay close attention to how you slowly breathe in and breathe out several times to help you focus inward to calm yourself

conversational (page 255)—related to people talking to each other for different purposes

cooperative, cooperate (page 3)—willing and able to work well together

cooperative conversation (page 90)—people taking turns listening to each other and telling each what they are thinking so they can then work together to solve any problems

coping strategies (page 33)—things you can do or things you can tell yourself that help you stay calm and move forward in doing what is expected of you

courteous (page 306)—acting in a way that is polite and shows good manners

Dark Ages (page 17)—a long period of tiime in Europe when people stopped focusing on learning how to work together to make a great civilization

decide (page 29)—choosing to do one thing or another

demanding (page 241)—acting in a way to force someone to do something

destination (page 103)—a place people want to get to

disappointed (page 258)—a feeling that a person has when something they hoped would happen does not happen

disconnect (page 25)—to break off or stop the connection between people or things

discouraged (page 298)—a feeling a person has when they feel like they will not be able to be successful even though they tried

disrespectful (page 261)—not showing respectful behavior

Disruptive (page 99)—a description of action that is disturbing what other people are trying to do, causing some trouble that keeps the group from smoothly moving forward successfully or safely

distract (page 47)—the way a person acts when they do something that pulls another person's attention away from what they want or need to pay attention to

distracting (page 99)—a description of actions that draw people away from what they are supposed to be paying attention to so they have more trouble getting their job done

Easygoing (page 2)—cooperative, working easily and peacefully with others

editing (page 191)—making changes to written work so it can be better

Egocentric (page 98)—concerned only with yourself, thinking only about yourself and how things affect you and no one else

egotistic (page 306)—acting in a way in which a person thinks only of themselves, acting self-centered

Empathetic (page 2)—showing you care about another person's feelings

empathetic conversation (page 309)—a conversation in which you listen to find how someone is feeling about something that is happening to them and then share your supportive thoughts

envious (page 306)—a feeling a person has when they would prefer to be in another person's situation

essential (page 79)—necessary; something that is needed for something else to happen

expensive (page 295)—high in price

experiences (page 105)—different things that happen to us in our life from which we learn

eye contact (page 123)—looking at a person when you are talking or listening to them

features (page 109)—ways to describe something to help it be compared with something else

feedback (page 58)—information you can get *from people around* you to let you know how they think you are acting with them; information you can get *from your own body* to let you know how you are feeling about how you are acting

fidget (page 133)—a calming tool to hold and squeeze to help get out extra body energy while you focus on something that someone else is asking you to pay attention to and do

Five Break (page 123)—a controlled breathing, calming strategy that lasts for five breaths after which you guide yourself to think about what you can do next to help your Team meet its goal

flexible (page 91)—having the ability to change how you think or act when necessary

flipping the switch (page 151)—changing how you are thinking so you can change your actions to get calm and navigate through a situation

frustrated (page 64)—feeling uncomfortable because something does not seem to be working out right

G-rated conversation (page 256)—a conversation that is on-topic and is pleasant and appropriate for anyone to hear

generous (page 306)—acting in a way in which a person is willing to give more of something than is necessary or expected

gloating (page 306)—expressing great pleasure about your own success and someone else's failure

goals (page 3)—important things you keep focusing upon because you want to achieve them through your words and actions; ways you want to act or things you want to accomplish

good sportsmanship (page 305)—acting in a positive way toward the players on both sides of a game before, during, and after a game no matter whether your side wins *or* loses

gracious (page 306)—acting in a way that is kind, polite, well-mannered, and civil

Grateful (page 2)—saying and doing things that show you are thankful for what you have and appreciate the people around you

greedy (page 99)—not wanting to share what you have

G.R.E.E.N. (page 2)—an acronym that stands for the words **Grateful, Respecful, Empathetic, Easygoing,** and **Navigating,** which are the ways to act when we want to do our best for ourselves and the people in our lives

Guiding G.R.E.E.N. Thoughts (page 57)—powerful words that you can read, think about, and find in your own brain to use for guiding yourself to make your best action choices

humiliated (page 306)—a feeling a person has when someone has made them feel like something is wrong with them and they are worth less than a full person

ignore (page 21)—to pay no attention to something or someone

illogical (page 111)—a way of thinking or a way of acting that does not make sense to do because it will make things get worse

impulsive (page 2)—a description of action that occurs quickly without thinking or planning, so there is not thought of the consequences

independently (page 403)—able to be performed by yourself without any help from others

inhibit (page 106)—hold back or stop something

inspired (page 23)—encouraged and stimulated to do something by getting someone to feel strongly about doing it

installation (page 173)—putting something in place so it can be used; putting something into action

insult (page 261)—to say something negative about someone else

InterActions (page 1)—actions that people take with each other; communication that occurs between two or more people

interrupt (page 76)—to say or do something without waiting for someone else to be finished saying or doing something else, so it interferes with or stops the other person from finishing what they were doing

irresponsible (page 259)—a person acting in a way in which they cannot be trusted to act in a safe and dependable way

irritated (page 238)—to be bothered

jealous (page 295)—a feeling a person has when they want what someone else has

key words (page 182)—the most important words within a sentence that help tell the main idea

liberation (page 173)—letting something out so it can be free

logical (page 7)—ideas fit together, things makes sense, the idea or action leads to something working better

magnanimous (page 306)—acting in a way that is very kind and generous toward an opposing team that you defeated

making an inference (page 271)—making your best guess about someone or about a situation by finding clues that can help you figure things out

motive (page 224)—the reason for someone to act in a certain way

mutually beneficial (page 94)—a kind of action in which everyone benefits in some way because of the action

Navigating (page 2)—finding ways to manage any challenges so you can keep moving forward without getting upset

navigator (page 393)—someone who can navigate through a challenging situation successfully

necessities (page 114)—things that you need; this does not include all the things that you want

negative (page 7)—having an attitude that things will not work out well; acting in a way that makes things worse instead of better

negative consequences (page 95)—bad things that happen when choices are not made that will help the Team

neglect (page 98)—ignoring a person or a thing and acting like it is not even there

neurons (page 105)—brain cells

neutral tone of voice (page 238)—a tone of voice that does not show how a person is feeling

obstacles (page 83)—things that get in the way to stop forward movement or progress

offend (page 256)—to upset or cause someone discomfort, anger, or concern

off-topic (page 228)—talking about something that the group is not talking about at the moment

on-topic (page 228)—talking about the same thing as other people in a conversation instead of talking about something that is unrelated

open-minded (page 2)—willing to consider and act upon new ideas

opportunity (page 79)—a chance for something to happen

patience (page 109)—the ability to stay calm and wait for something to happen; the way a person acts when they can wait calmly for something

Personal Goals (page 3)—things you want to accomplish so your life can get better

perspective (page 245)—a point of view, the way someone looks at something

point of view (page 126)—the way a person looks at something or thinks about it

polite (page 3)—to act in a kind way in which you choose to carefully use words and a tone of voice with someone to show that you respect them and think they are important

positive attitude (page 90)—having an attitude that things will work out well and acting in a way that helps make things better

positive consequences (page 95)—good things that happen because one makes choices that help the Team

positive outside (page 349)—the feelings and actions you can choose to show to other people by having the self-control to *not* act upon the negative feelings you also might have on the "inside"

potential (page 27)—the powerful ability that someone or something can have even though it has not yet been shown

powerful (page 2)—full of strong force

predict (page 34)—to guess what will happen next based on what is happening now and what kinds of related things have happened in the past

preferred topic (page 231)—a topic that someone likes to talk about

pride (page 396)—a feeling a person has when they feel good about themselves for what they are and/or what they did

range of feelings (page 291)—a large group of different emotions that human beings have

rationalizing (page 258)—thinking of an incorrect reason why something happened which becomes an excuse for a related negative action

realistically (page 59)—realistic thinking about something in a way so it is as true as possible and can really happen in the way you are thinking about it; being honest with yourself about what you can accomplish

realize (page 102)—to become aware of something by noticing it or thinking about it

R.E.D. action (page 7)—**R**ude, **E**gocentric, and **D**isruptive action that does not help the Team move forward

regulate (page 104)—control

relevant (page 253)—related to the topic or situation

relieved (page 295)—no longer having to worry about something you worried about before

resentful (page 306)—feeling angry about something negative that has happened because of someone else's action

resilient (page 306)—withstanding and recovering quickly from difficulty

resist (page 172)—to fight against or oppose

Respectful (page 2)—polite and considerate of others

responsibility (page 240)—tasks and duties that others can trust you will do in a correct, thorough, and dependable manner; people can depend upon you to get a job done

restriction (page 380)—something that is not allowed

rewind the scene (page 181)—start over so people can act differently to make the scene better for everyone involved

Rude (page 98)—showing poor manners; not polite or respectful

sarcastic (page 212)—a tone of voice and/or words that are the opposite of what you are really saying to make fun of someone or hurt their feelings

see the details (page 177)—to pay attention closely and find one piece of information that you can remember and talk about when a lot of information has been presented

self-aware (page 168)—paying attention and noticing what you are feeling, what you are needing, and how you are acting so you can take the best action

self-calming (page 64)—knowing how to calm yourself down

self-control (page 5)—having the power to control your own feelings or behavior

selfish (page 98)—wanting everything for yourself

self-regulate (page 106)—to control yourself; the ability to control yourself

serious (page 228)—not joking, wanting to get a job done without wasting time

show your gratitude (page 193)—act in a way that shows you are thankful about what someone has done for you or for what someone has given you

sincere (page 239)—honest and truthful

solitary (page 169)—standing alone

step on the brakes (page 136)—stop what you are doing so you can think and change directions if needed

strategies (page 2)—plans or series of actions that are followed to make things easier to successfully achieve a goal

strive (page 68)—to work as hard as you can to accomplish something

suggest (page 102)—to present an idea to someone

support, supportive (page 29)—providing help or encouragement

survey the scene (page 7)—use your eyes to carefully look and your ears to carefully listen to find out who is with you and what is going on around you so you can make the best action choices

synapses (page 105)—connections between brain cells

take responsibility (page 240)—to own your actions and know you are the one in charge of taking those actions; accepting that things have happened because of the actions you took or the actions you did not take

thoughtful (page 2)—action taken with thought about what the action is and how it will affect the situation and the people involved

tone of voice (page 181)—the way that you speak that tells how you are feeling or shows your attitude when you are talking; respectful or rude; positive or negative, pleasant or irritated; sincere, truthful or sarcastic

transformation (page 7)—a change in how someone behaves or acts or the change in a scene or situation because of how the people are acting with each other

trust (page 47)—know that someone will do what they say they will do

visualize, visualization (page 138)—to form a picture in your mind; a picture in your mind

Musical Transcriptions

Keep the Civil in Civilization

Herb Hein

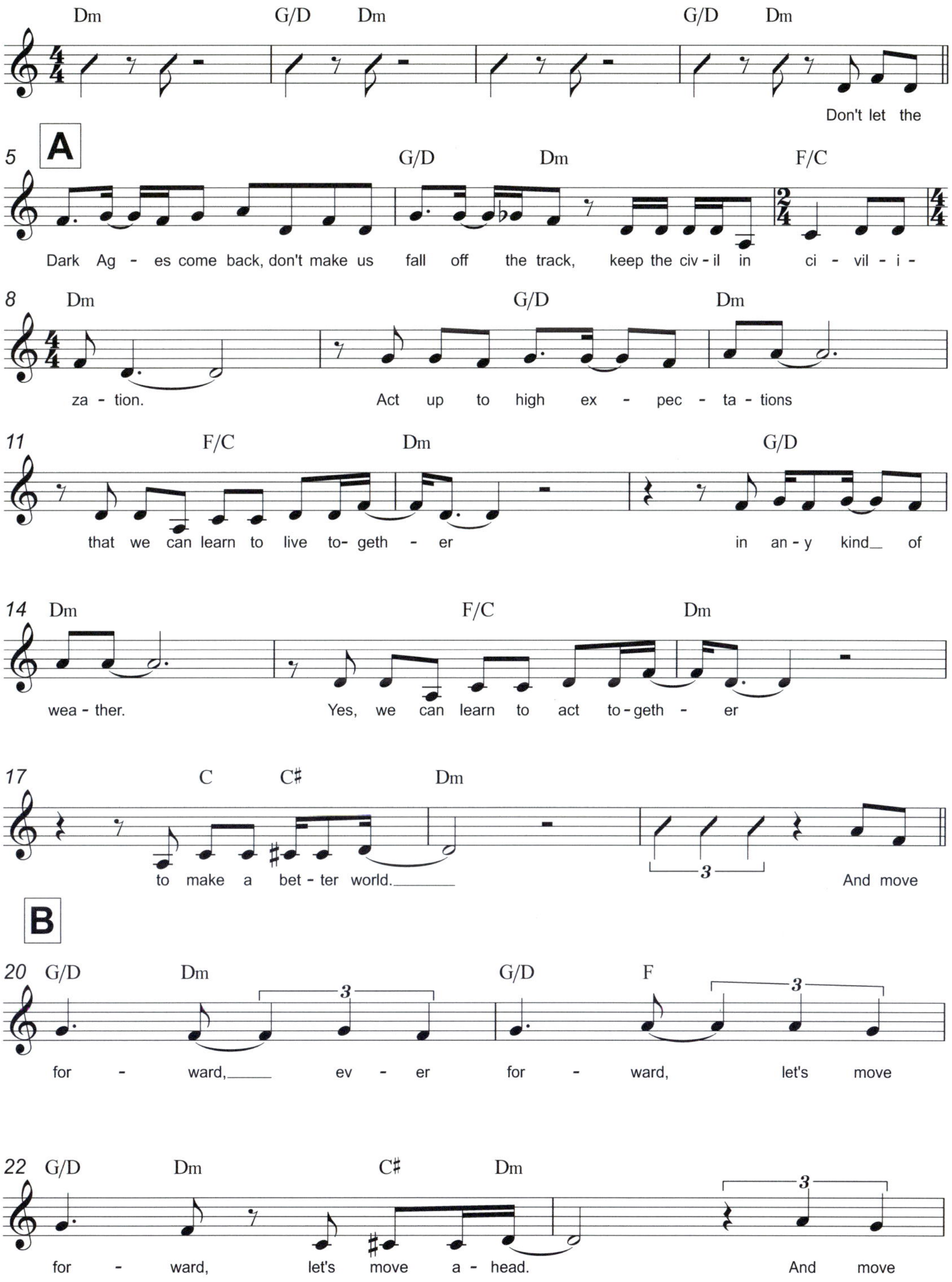

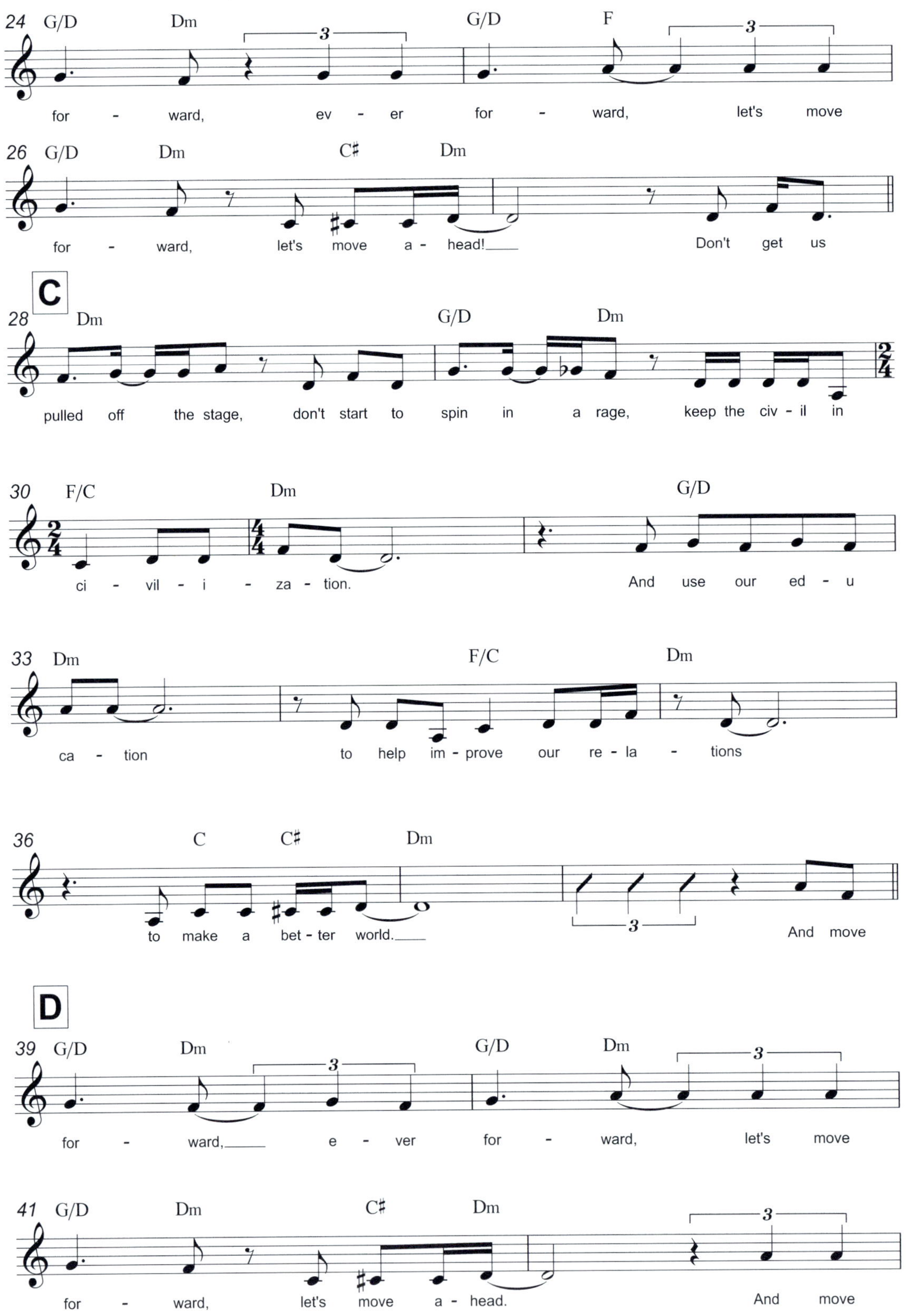
24 G/D Dm G/D F
for - ward, ev - er for - ward, let's move
26 G/D Dm C♯ Dm
for - ward, let's move a - head!___ Don't get us
C
28 Dm G/D Dm
pulled off the stage, don't start to spin in a rage, keep the civ - il in
30 F/C Dm G/D
ci - vil - i - za - tion. And use our ed - u
33 Dm F/C Dm
ca - tion to help im - prove our re - la - tions
36 C C♯ Dm
to make a bet - ter world.___ And move
D
39 G/D Dm G/D Dm
for - ward,___ e - ver for - ward, let's move
41 G/D Dm C♯ Dm
for - ward, let's move a - head. And move

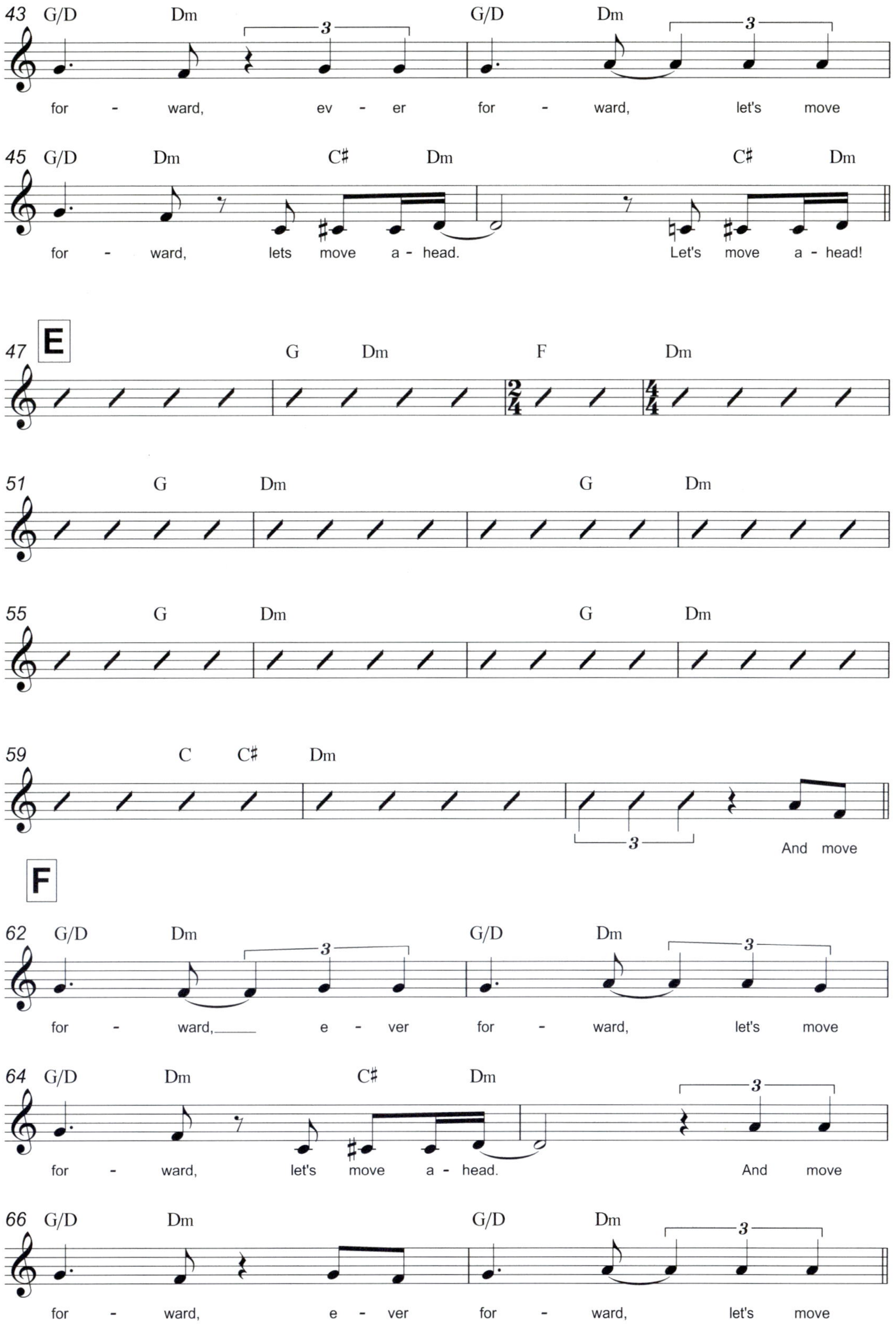
43 G/D Dm G/D Dm
for - ward, ev - er for - ward, let's move
45 G/D Dm C♯ Dm C♯ Dm
for - ward, lets move a - head. Let's move a - head!
E
47 G Dm F Dm
51 G Dm G Dm
55 G Dm G Dm
59 C C♯ Dm
And move
F
62 G/D Dm G/D Dm
for - ward, e - ver for - ward, let's move
64 G/D Dm C♯ Dm
for - ward, let's move a - head. And move
66 G/D Dm G/D Dm
for - ward, e - ver for - ward, let's move

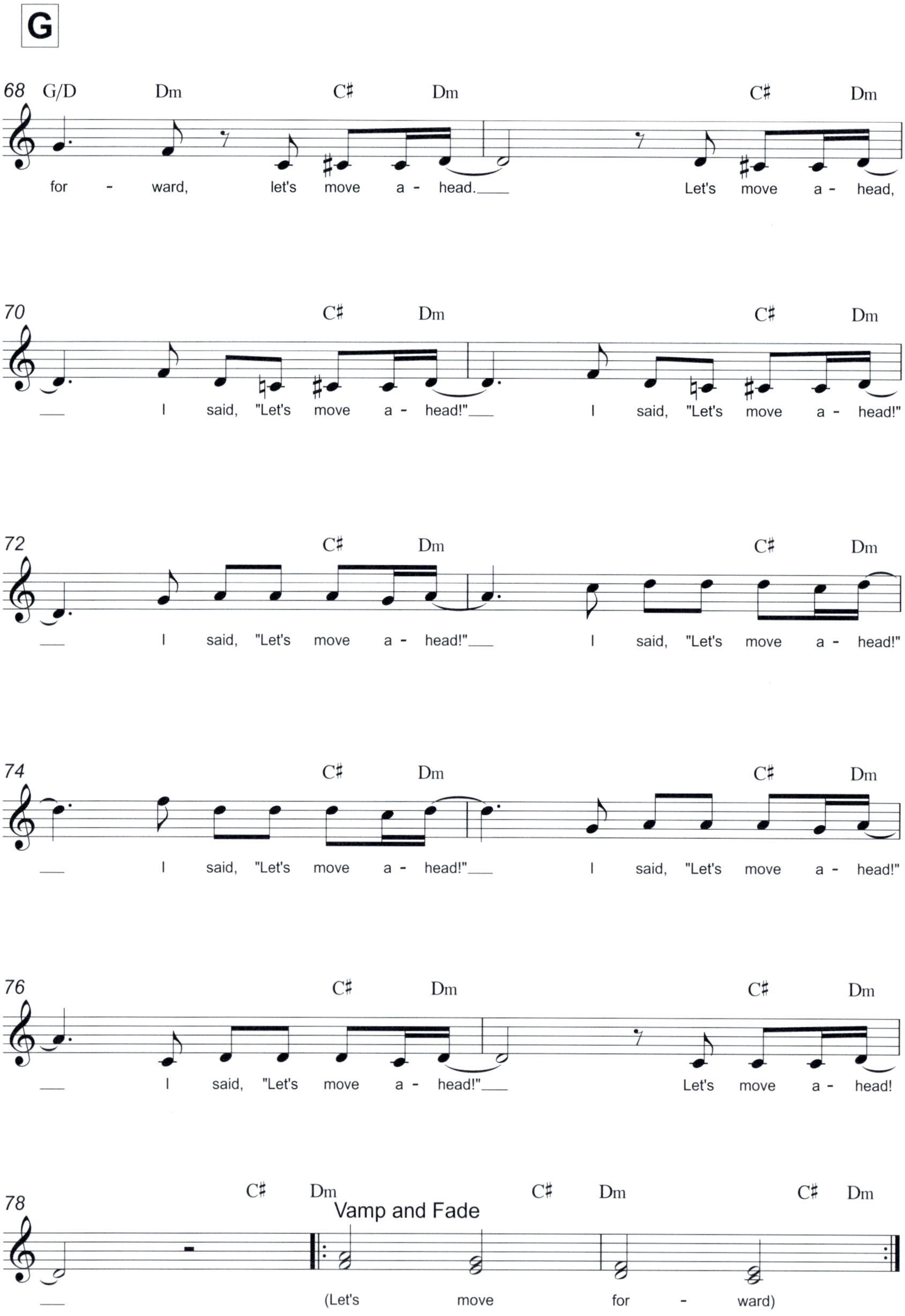
G
68 G/D Dm C♯ Dm C♯ Dm
for - ward, let's move a - head.___ Let's move a - head,
70 C♯ Dm C♯ Dm
___ I said, "Let's move a - head!"___ I said, "Let's move a - head!"
72 C♯ Dm C♯ Dm
___ I said, "Let's move a - head!"___ I said, "Let's move a - head!"
74 C♯ Dm C♯ Dm
___ I said, "Let's move a - head!"___ I said, "Let's move a - head!"
76 C♯ Dm C♯ Dm
___ I said, "Let's move a - head!"___ Let's move a - head!
78 C♯ Dm C♯ Dm C♯ Dm
Vamp and Fade
___ (Let's move for - ward)

Wake Up

Herb Hein

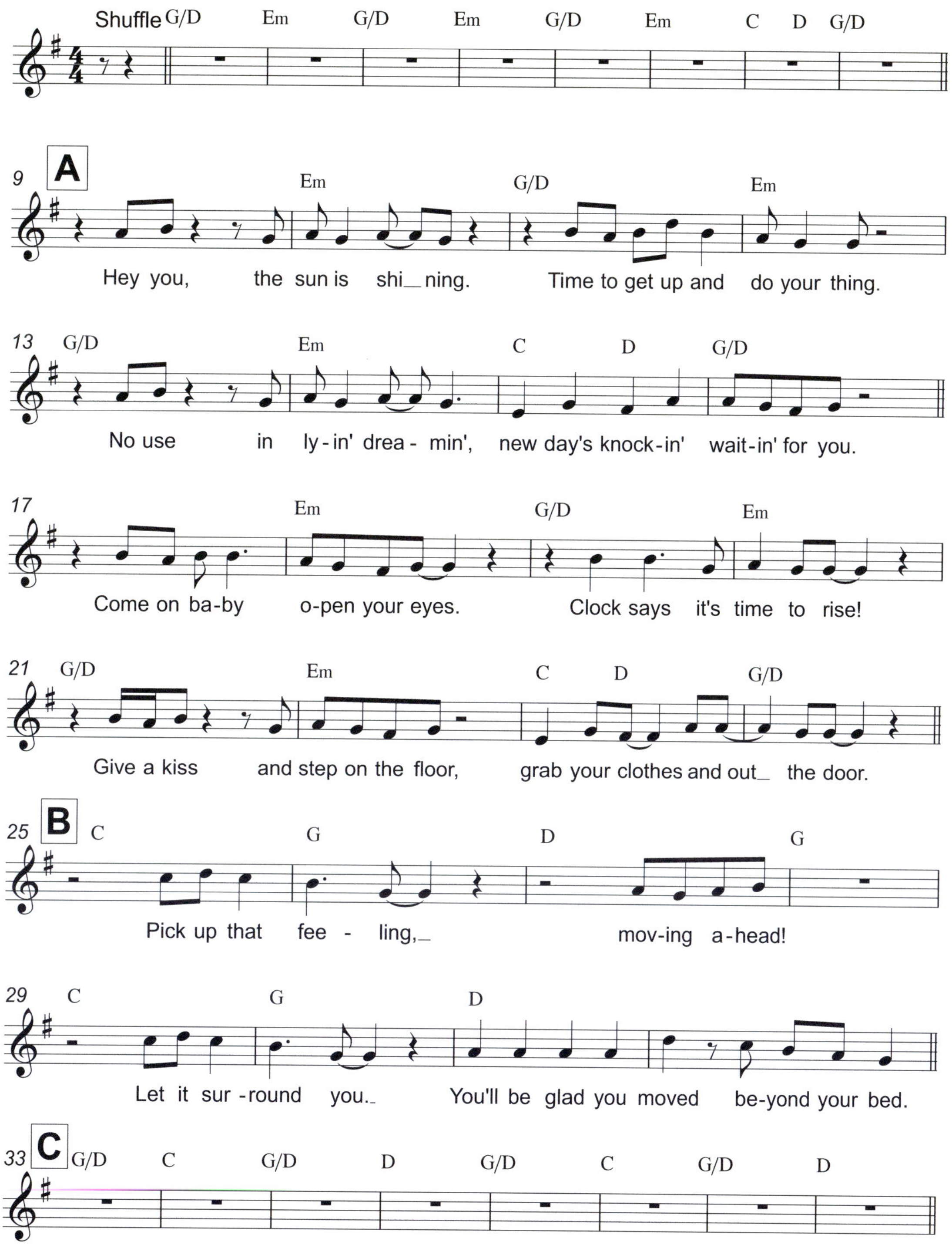

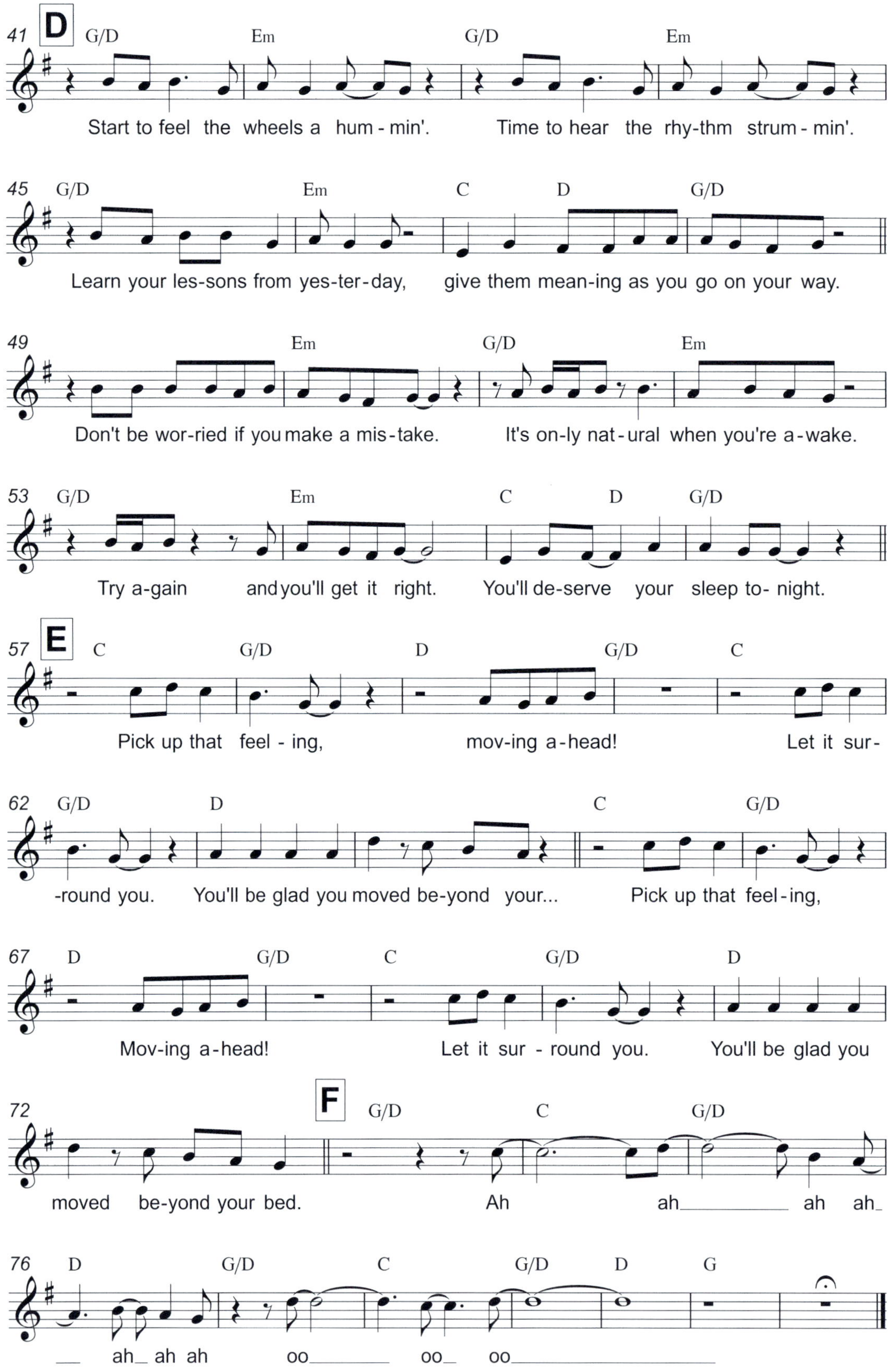
41 D G/D Em G/D Em
Start to feel the wheels a hum - min'. Time to hear the rhy-thm strum - min'.
45 G/D Em C D G/D
Learn your les-sons from yes-ter-day, give them mean-ing as you go on your way.
49 Em G/D Em
Don't be wor-ried if you make a mis-take. It's on-ly nat-ural when you're a-wake.
53 G/D Em C D G/D
Try a-gain and you'll get it right. You'll de-serve your sleep to- night.
57 E C G/D D G/D C
Pick up that feel - ing, mov-ing a-head! Let it sur-
62 G/D D C G/D
-round you. You'll be glad you moved be-yond your... Pick up that feel-ing,
67 D G/D C G/D D
Mov-ing a-head! Let it sur - round you. You'll be glad you
72 F G/D C G/D
moved be-yond your bed. Ah ah ah ah
76 D G/D C G/D D G
ah ah ah oo oo oo

Guiding G.R.E.E.N. Thought Song

Herb Hein

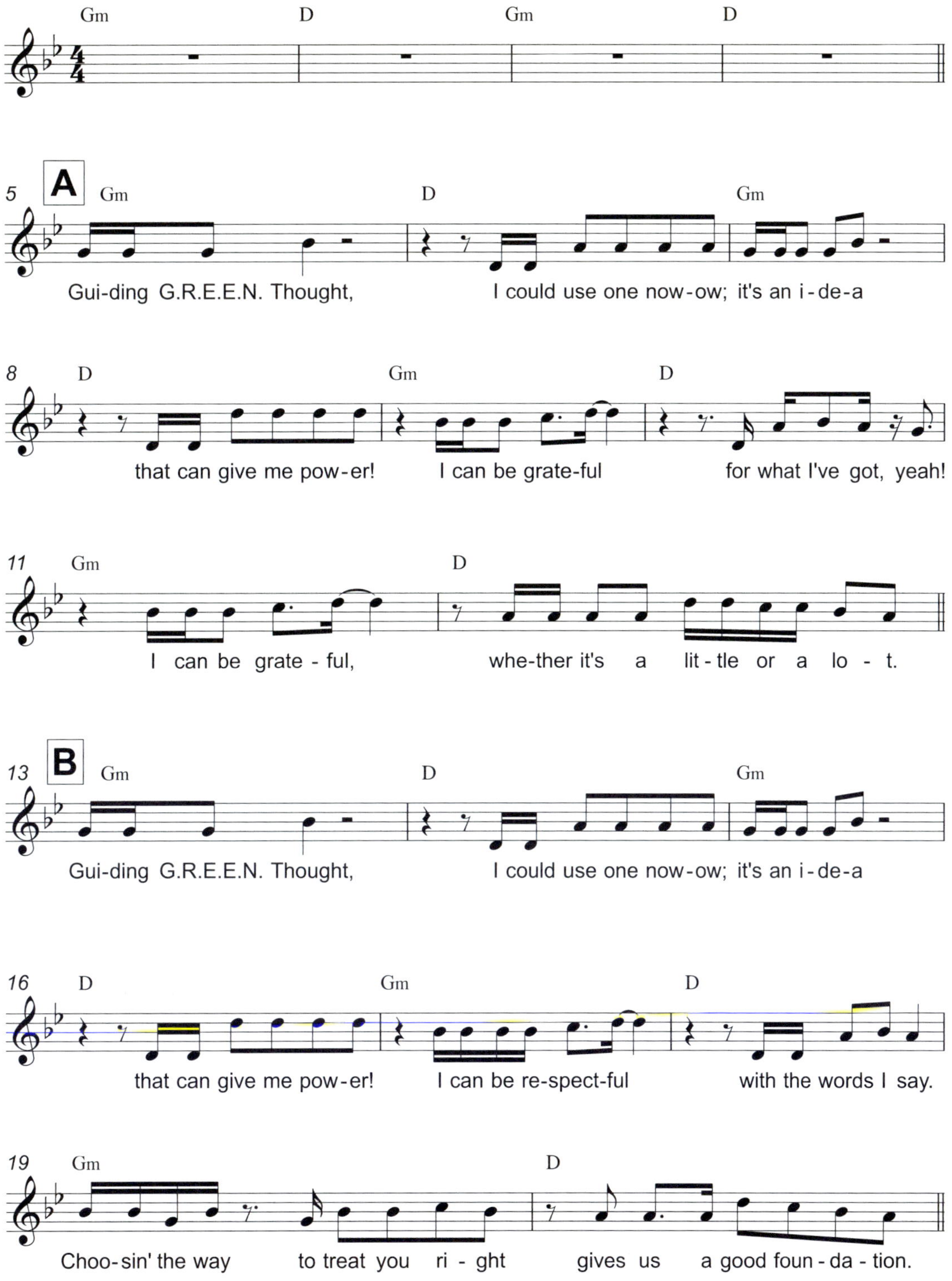

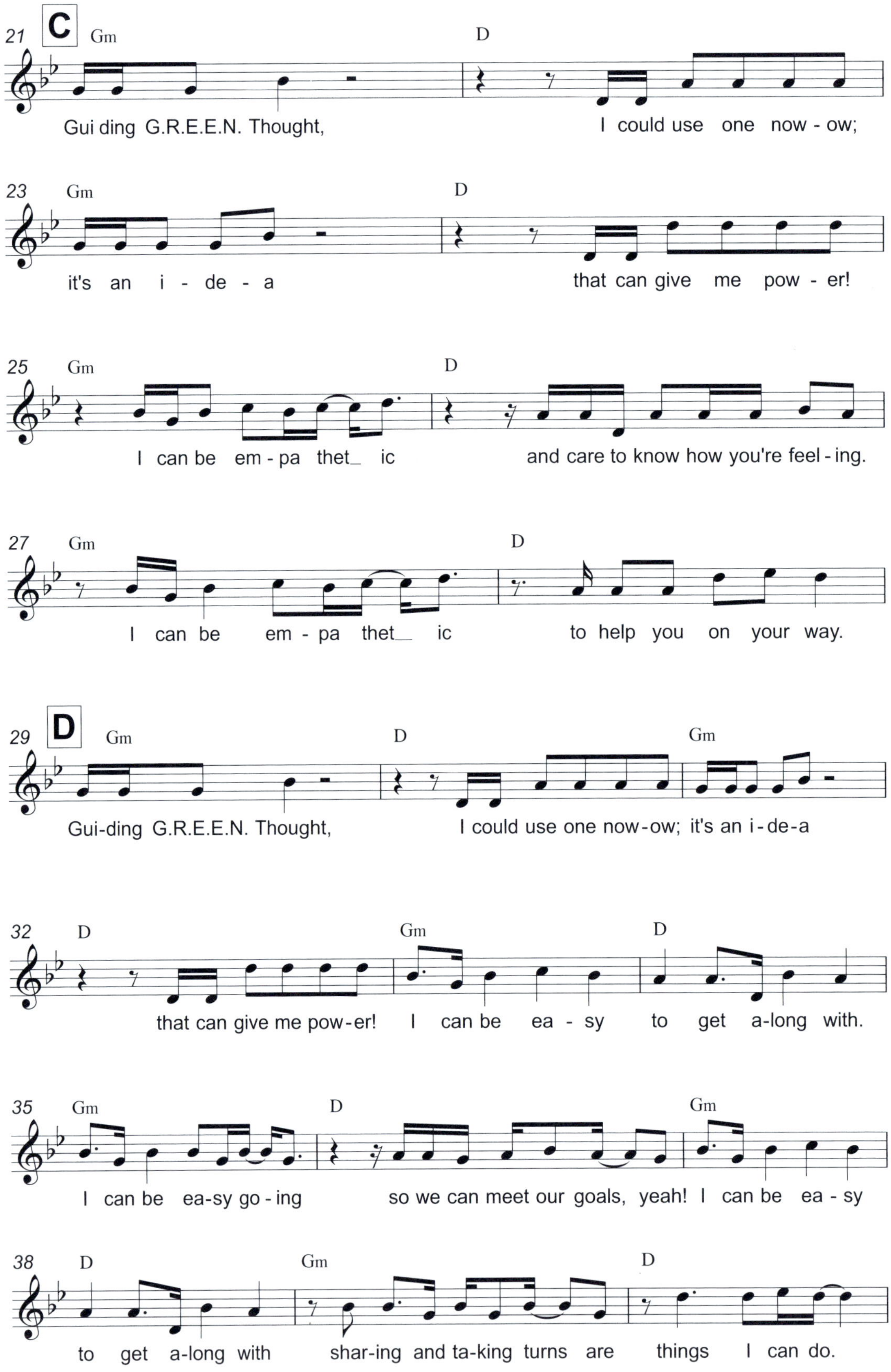
21 C Gm D
Gui ding G.R.E.E.N. Thought, I could use one now - ow;
23 Gm D
it's an i - de - a that can give me pow - er!
25 Gm D
I can be em - pa thet_ ic and care to know how you're feel - ing.
27 Gm D
I can be em - pa thet_ ic to help you on your way.
29 D Gm D Gm
Gui-ding G.R.E.E.N. Thought, I could use one now-ow; it's an i-de-a
32 D Gm D
that can give me pow-er! I can be ea - sy to get a-long with.
35 Gm D Gm
I can be ea-sy go-ing so we can meet our goals, yeah! I can be ea - sy
38 D Gm D
to get a-long with shar-ing and ta-king turns are things I can do.

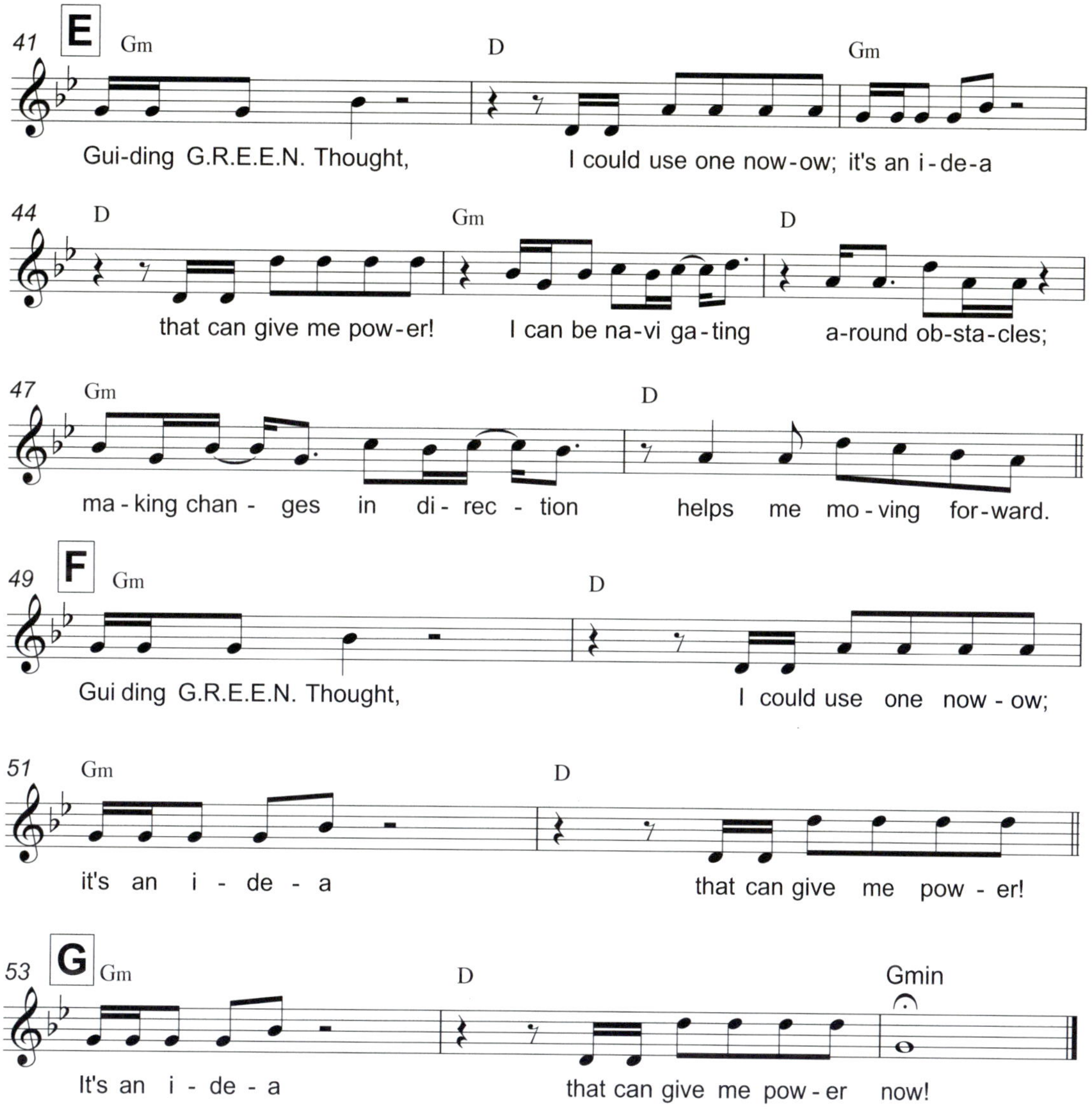
41 E Gm D Gm
Gui-ding G.R.E.E.N. Thought, I could use one now-ow; it's an i-de-a
44 D Gm D
that can give me pow-er! I can be na-vi ga-ting a-round ob-sta-cles;
47 Gm D
ma-king chan-ges in di-rec-tion helps me mo-ving for-ward.
49 F Gm D
Gui ding G.R.E.E.N. Thought, I could use one now-ow;
51 Gm D
it's an i-de-a that can give me pow-er!
53 G Gm D Gmin
It's an i-de-a that can give me pow-er now!

What's Best For The TEAM

Herb Hein

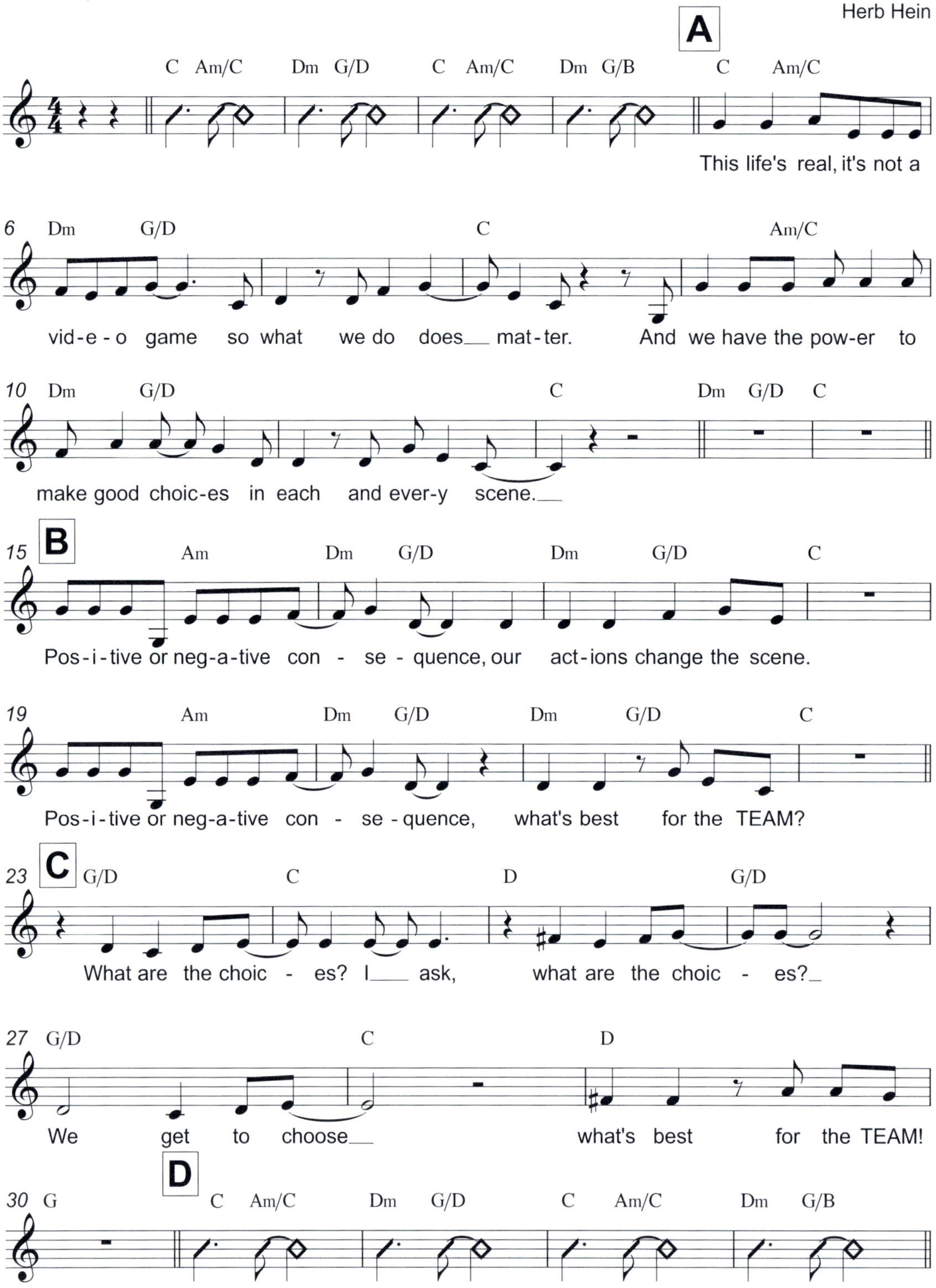

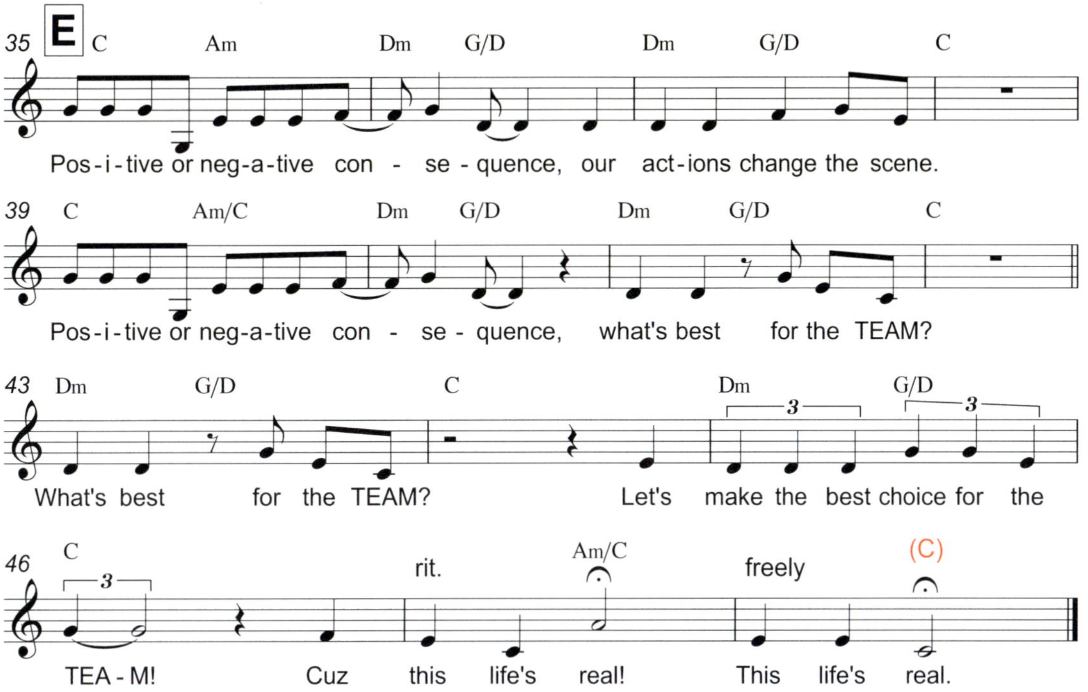
35 E C Am Dm G/D Dm G/D C
Pos-i-tive or neg-a-tive con - se - quence, our act-ions change the scene.
39 C Am/C Dm G/D Dm G/D C
Pos-i-tive or neg-a-tive con - se - quence, what's best for the TEAM?
43 Dm G/D C Dm G/D
What's best for the TEAM? Let's make the best choice for the
46 C rit. Am/C freely (C)
TEA - M! Cuz this life's real! This life's real.

Brake To Take a 5 Break

Herb Hein

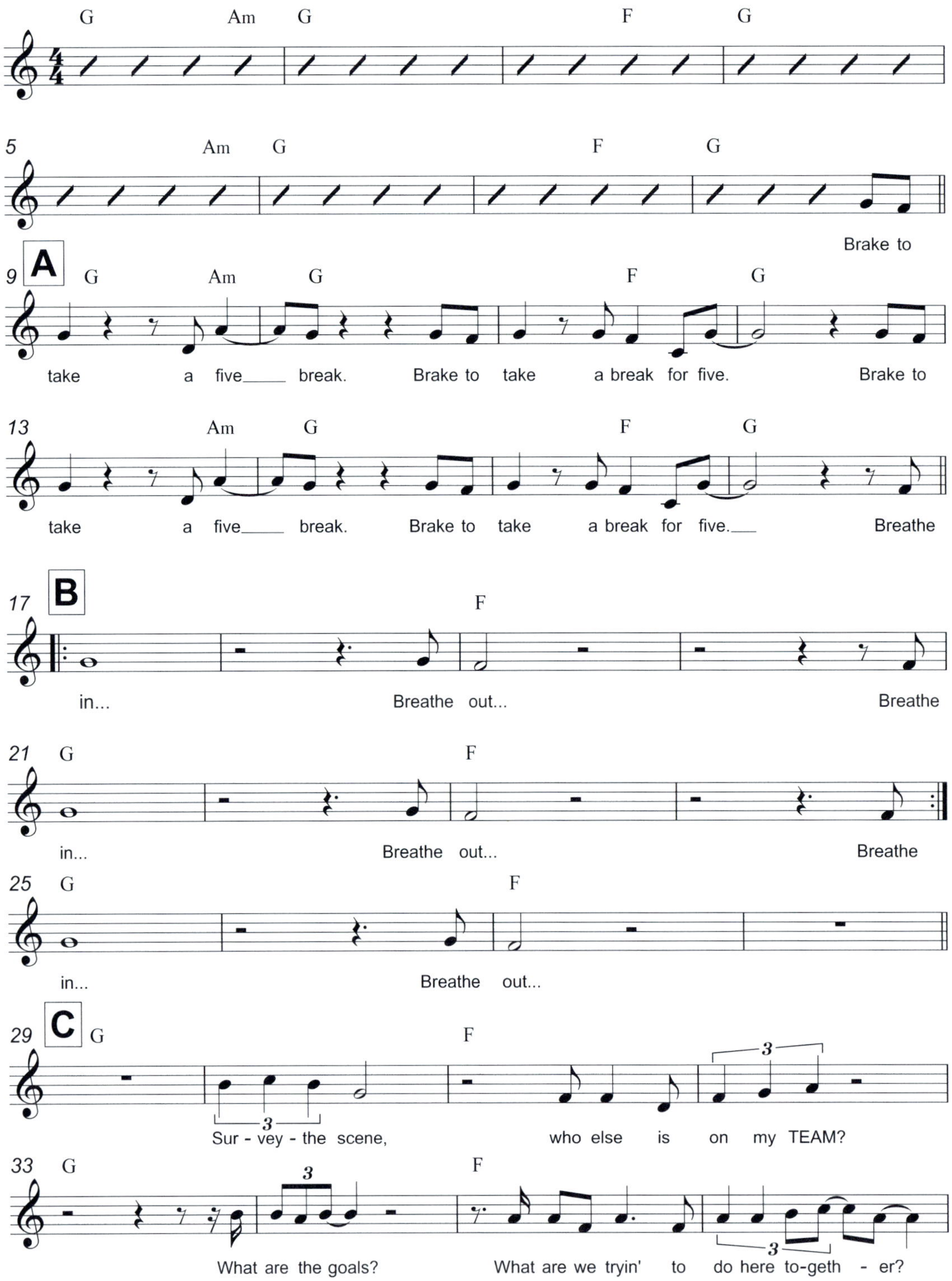

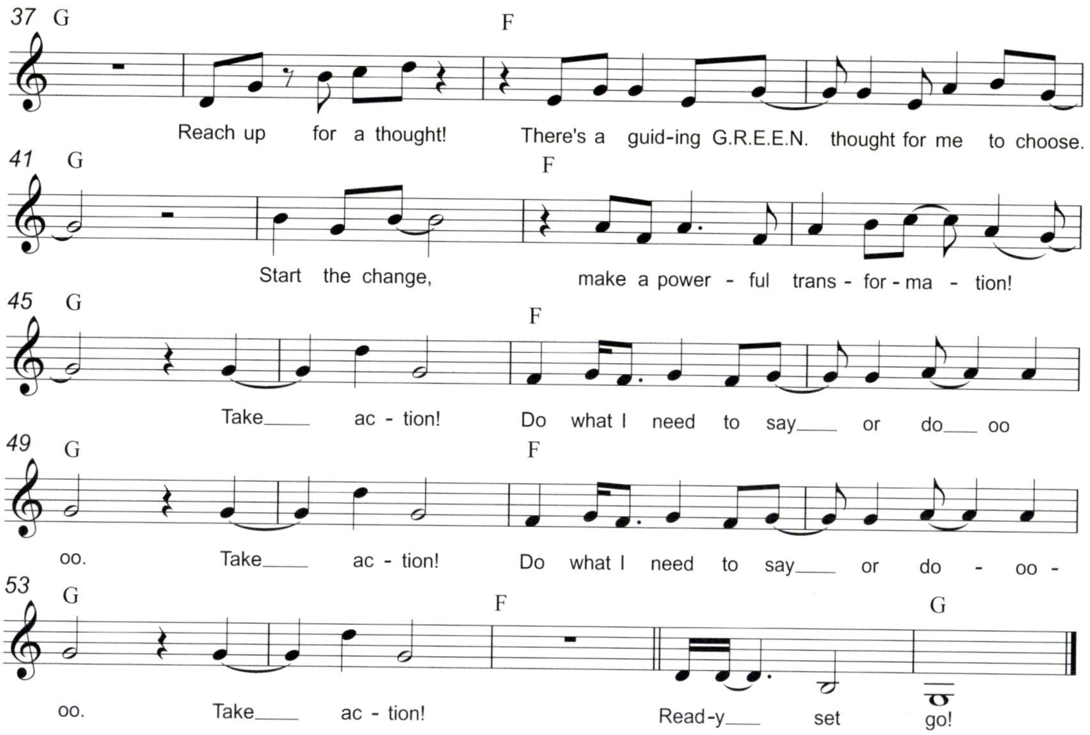
37 G
F
Reach up for a thought! There's a guid-ing G.R.E.E.N. thought for me to choose.
41 G
F
Start the change, make a power - ful trans - for - ma - tion!
45 G
F
Take ac - tion! Do what I need to say or do oo
49 G
F
oo. Take ac - tion! Do what I need to say or do - oo -
53 G
F
G
oo. Take ac - tion! Read-y set go!

Don't Listen To The Moon

Herb Hein

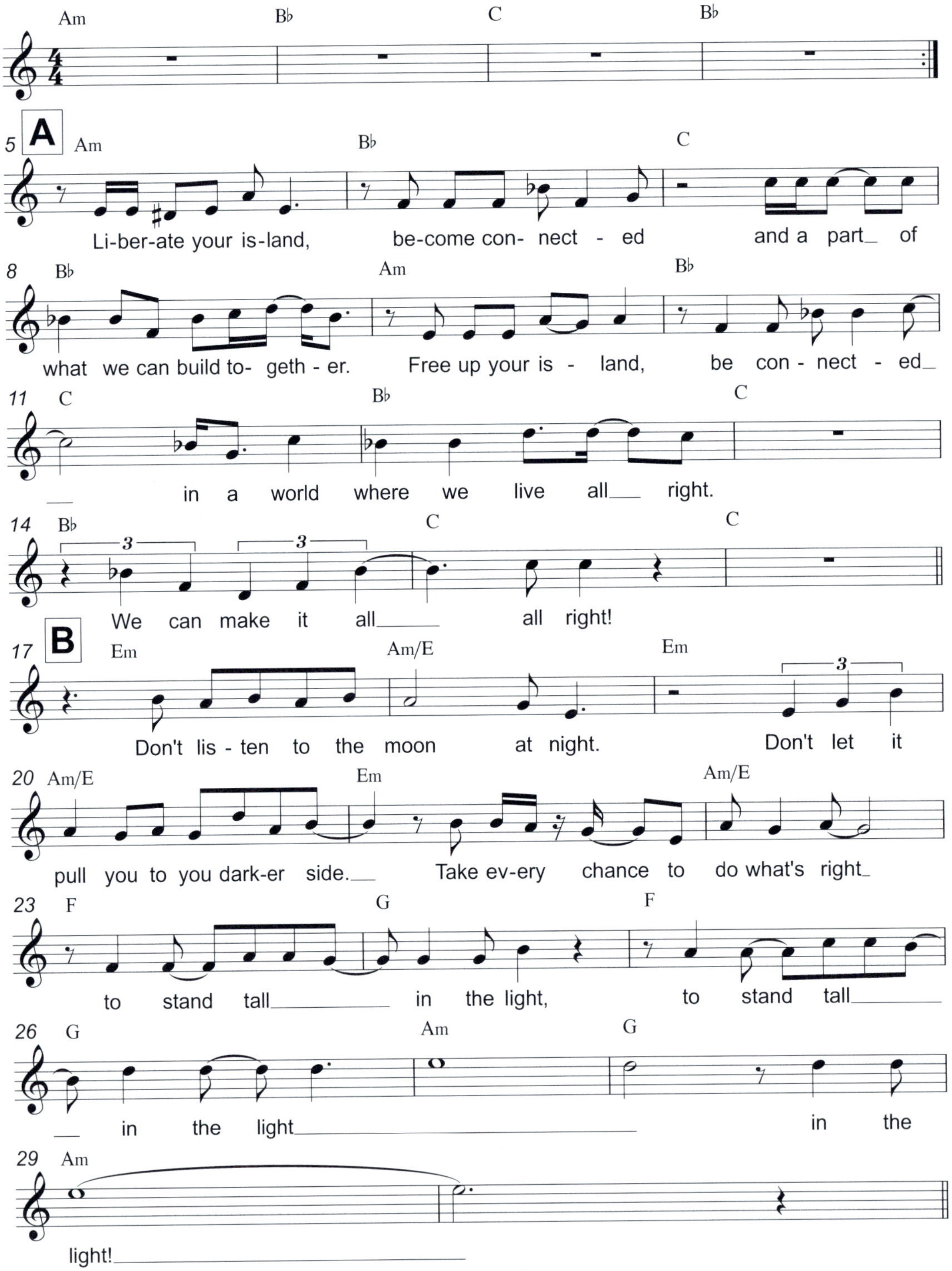

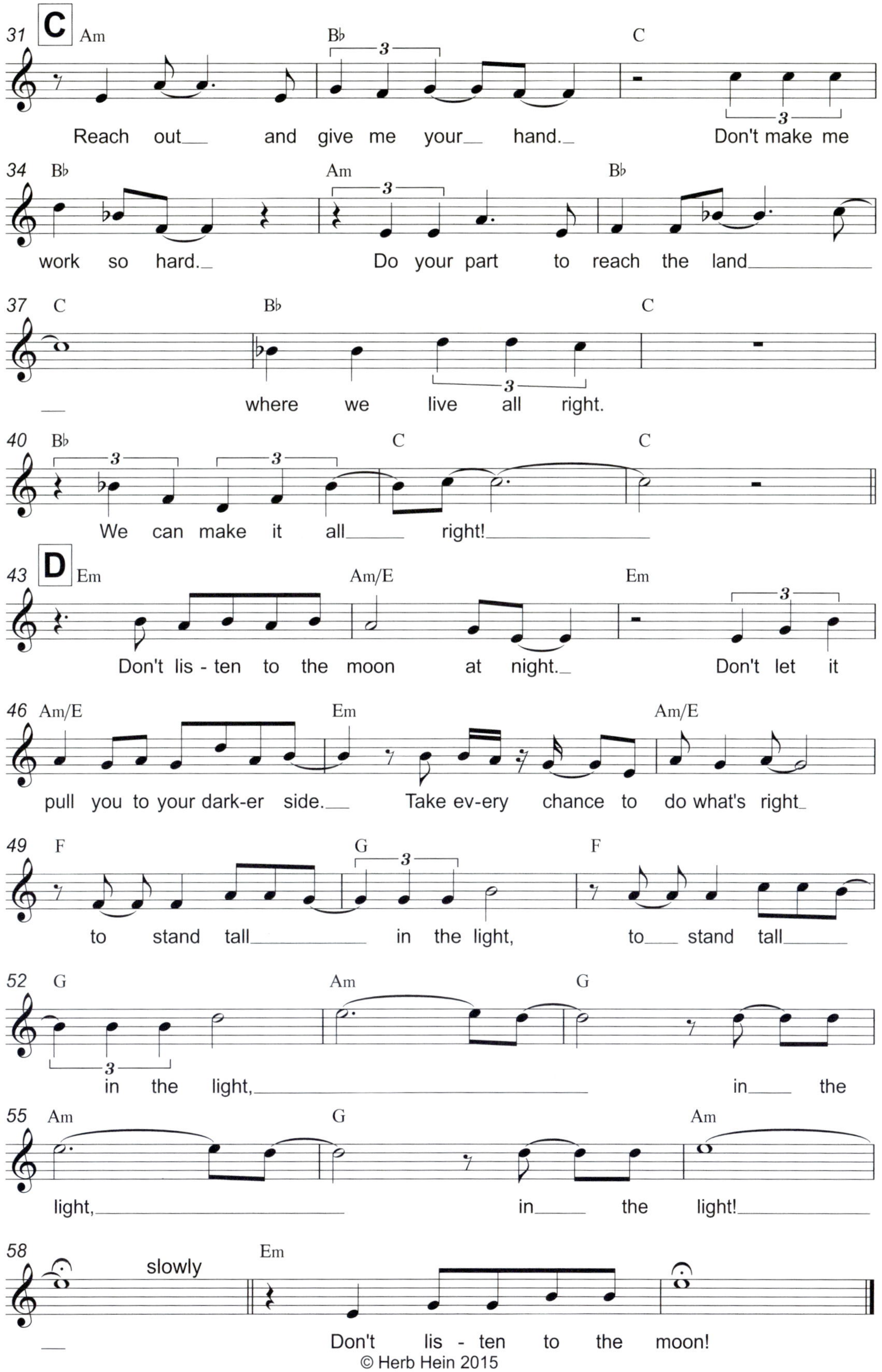
C
Am Bb C
Reach out and give me your hand. Don't make me
Bb Am Bb
work so hard. Do your part to reach the land
C Bb C
where we live all right.
Bb C C
We can make it all right!
D
Em Am/E Em
Don't lis - ten to the moon at night. Don't let it
Am/E Em Am/E
pull you to your dark-er side. Take ev-ery chance to do what's right
F G F
to stand tall in the light, to stand tall
G Am G
in the light, in the
Am G Am
light, in the light!
slowly
Em
Don't lis - ten to the moon!

Transformation Song

Herb Hein

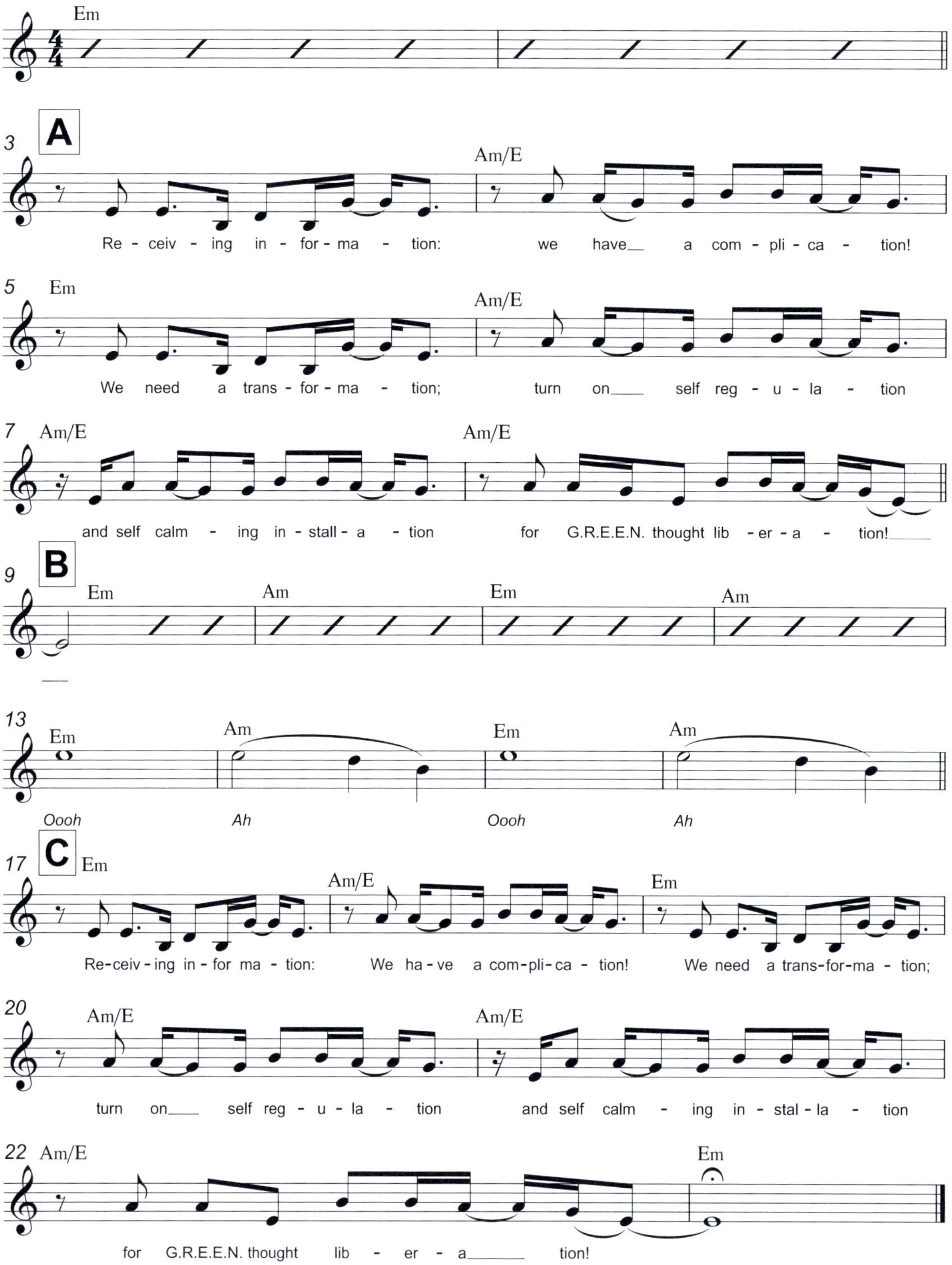

I Appreciate

Herb Hein

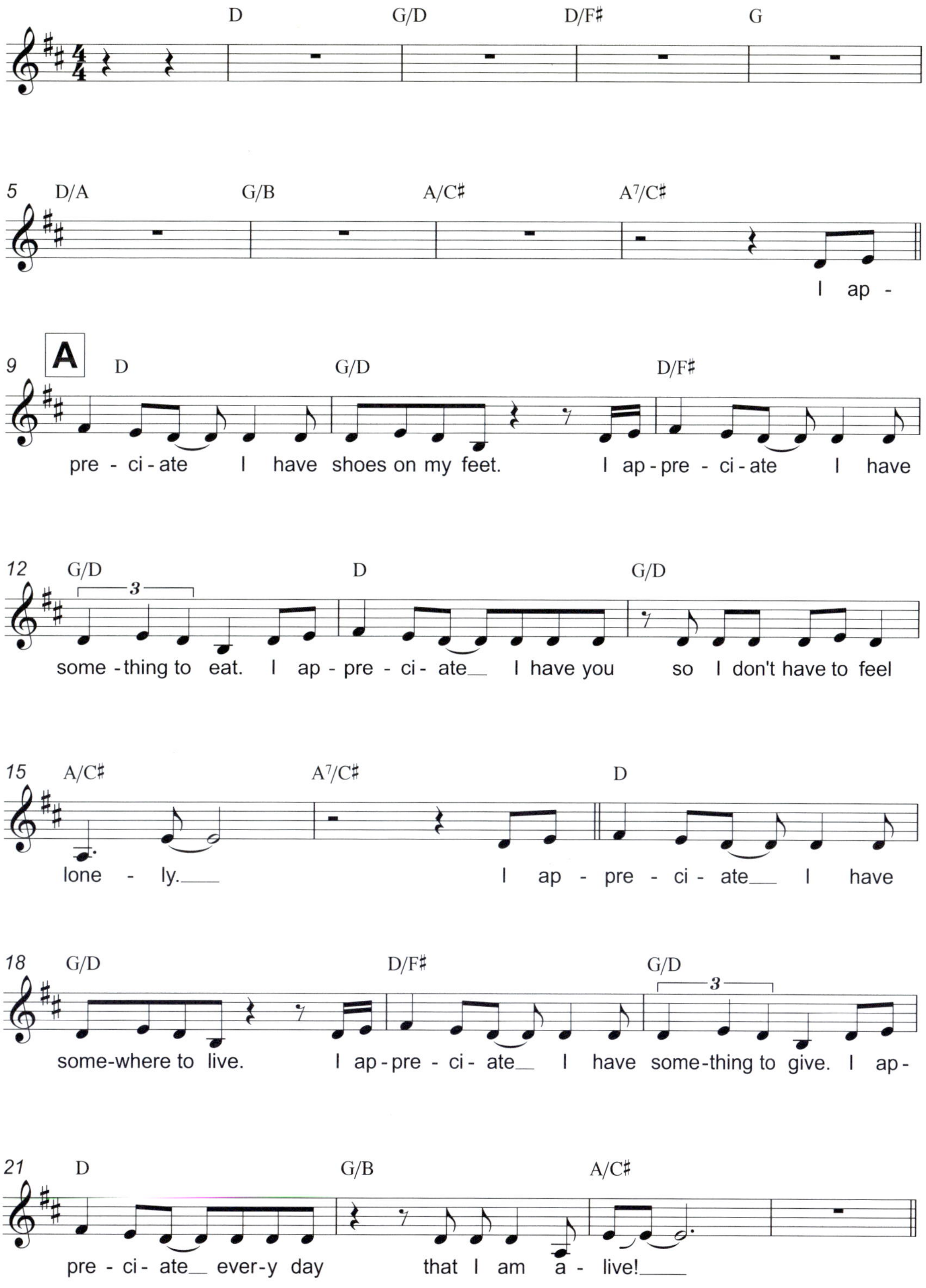

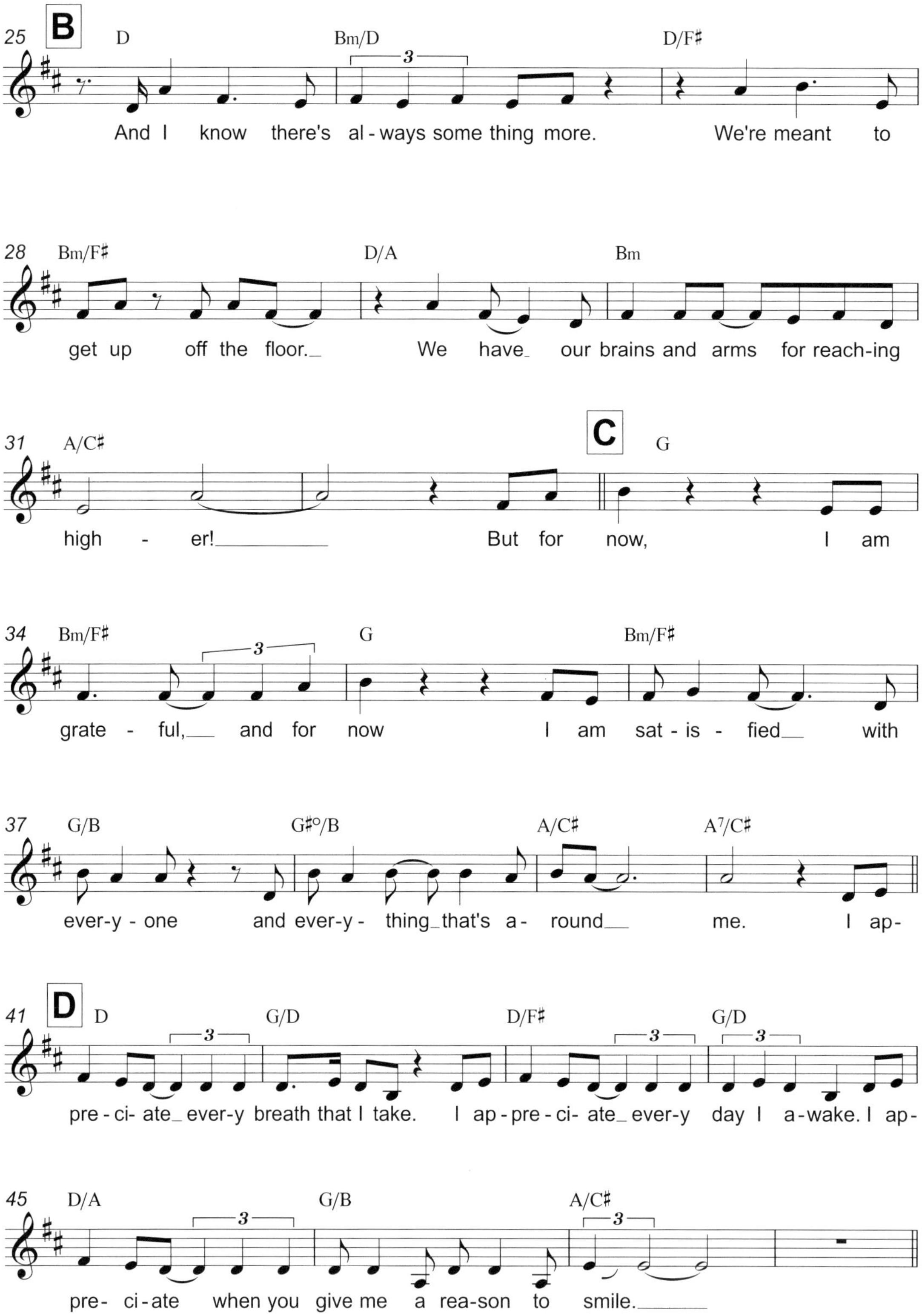
25 B D Bm/D D/F♯
And I know there's al - ways some thing more. We're meant to
28 Bm/F♯ D/A Bm
get up off the floor. We have our brains and arms for reach-ing
31 A/C♯ C G
high - er! But for now, I am
34 Bm/F♯ G Bm/F♯
grate - ful, and for now I am sat - is - fied with
37 G/B G♯o/B A/C♯ A7/C♯
ev-er-y - one and ev-er-y - thing that's a - round me. I ap-
41 D D G/D D/F♯ G/D
pre - ci- ate ev-er-y breath that I take. I ap - pre - ci- ate ev-er-y day I a-wake. I ap-
45 D/A G/B A/C♯
pre- ci-ate when you give me a rea-son to smile.

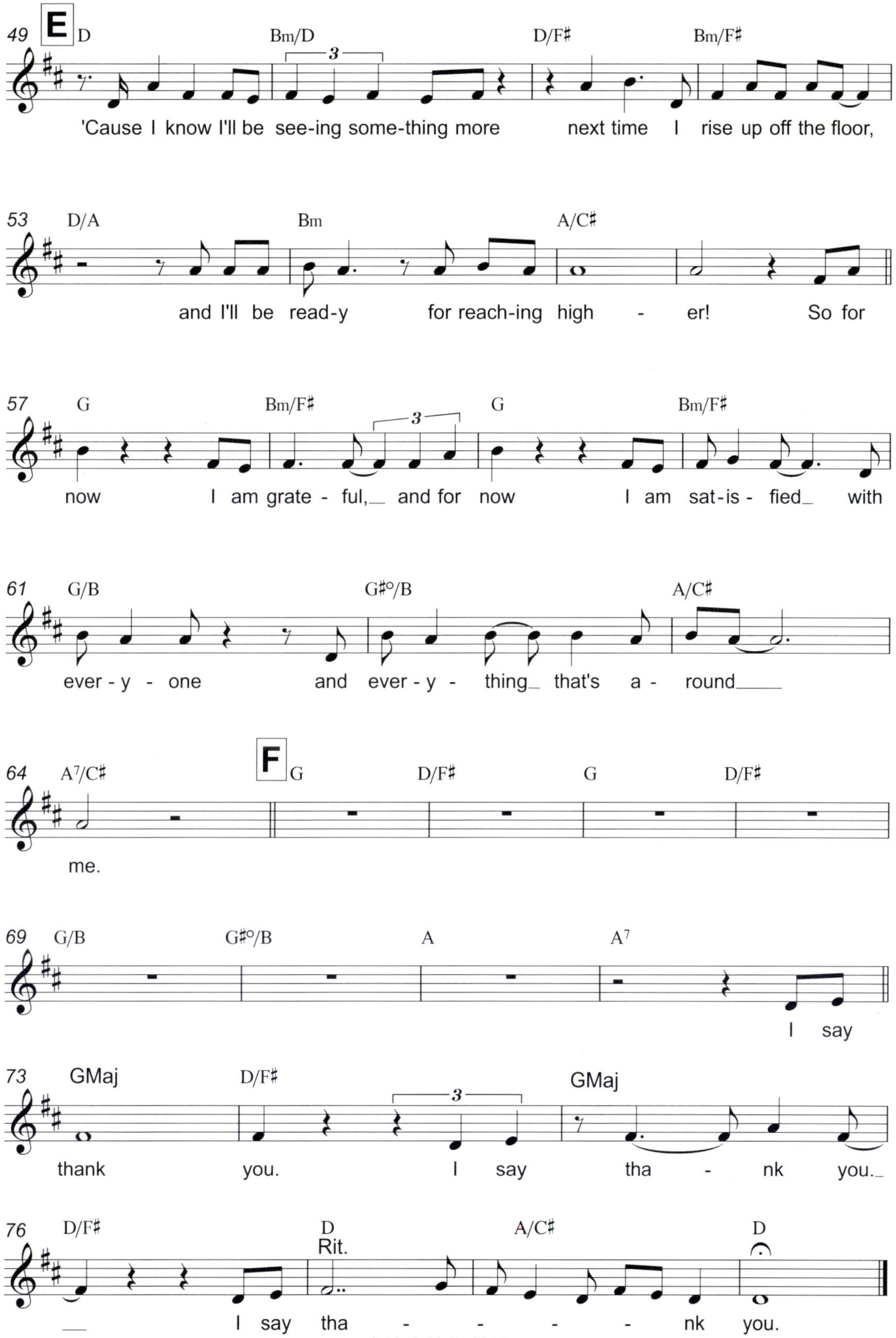

E
49 D Bm/D D/F♯ Bm/F♯
'Cause I know I'll be see-ing some-thing more next time I rise up off the floor,
53 D/A Bm A/C♯
and I'll be read-y for reach-ing high - er! So for
57 G Bm/F♯ G Bm/F♯
now I am grate - ful,_ and for now I am sat-is - fied_ with
61 G/B G♯°/B A/C♯
ever - y - one and ever - y - thing_ that's a - round____
64 A7/C♯
F
G D/F♯ G D/F♯
me.
69 G/B G♯°/B A A7
I say
73 GMaj D/F♯ GMaj
thank you. I say tha - nk you._
76 D/F♯ D A/C♯ D
Rit.
__ I say tha - - - - nk you.

I Don't Ignore You

Herb Hein

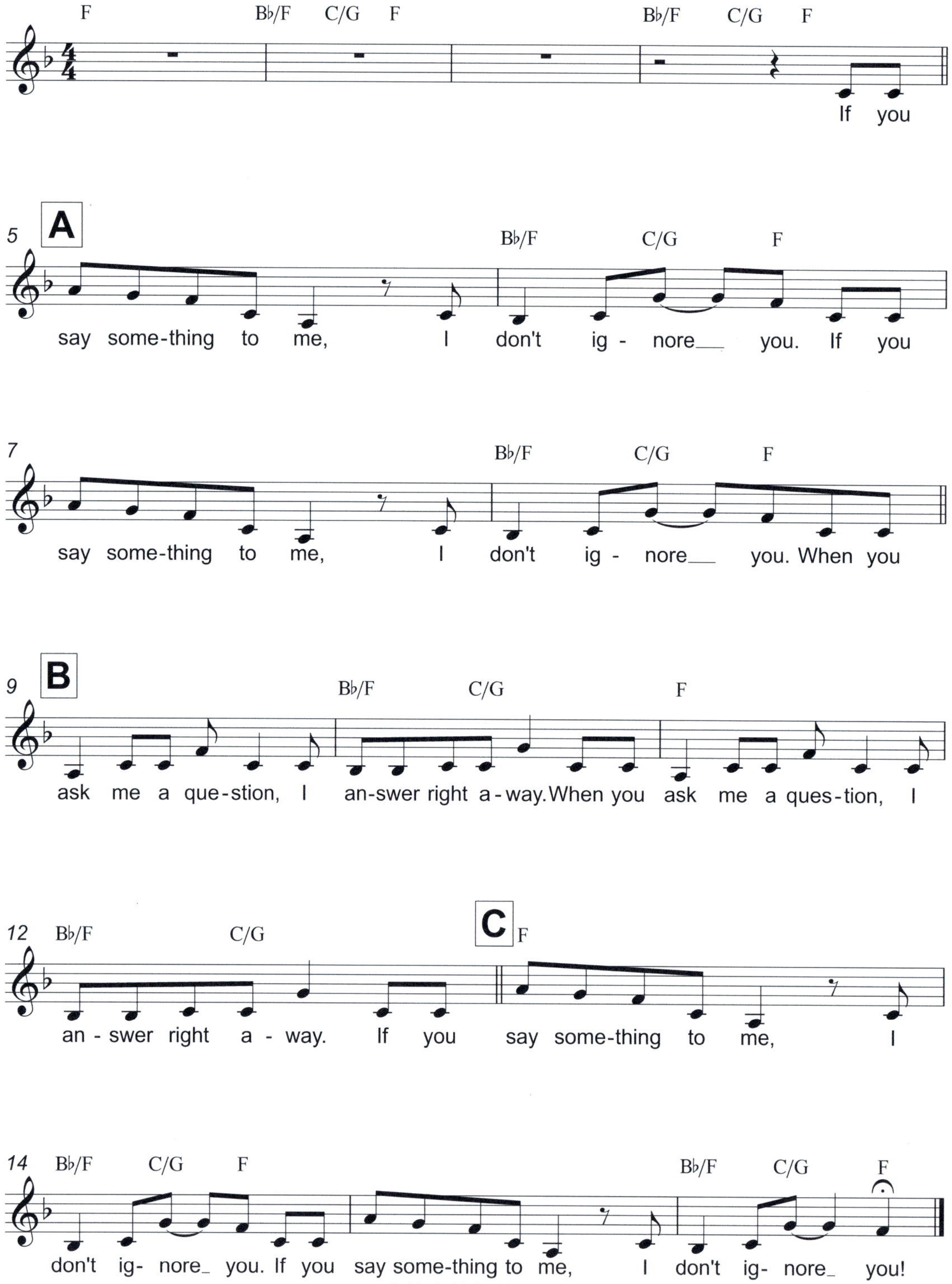

It's Not All About Me

Herb Hein

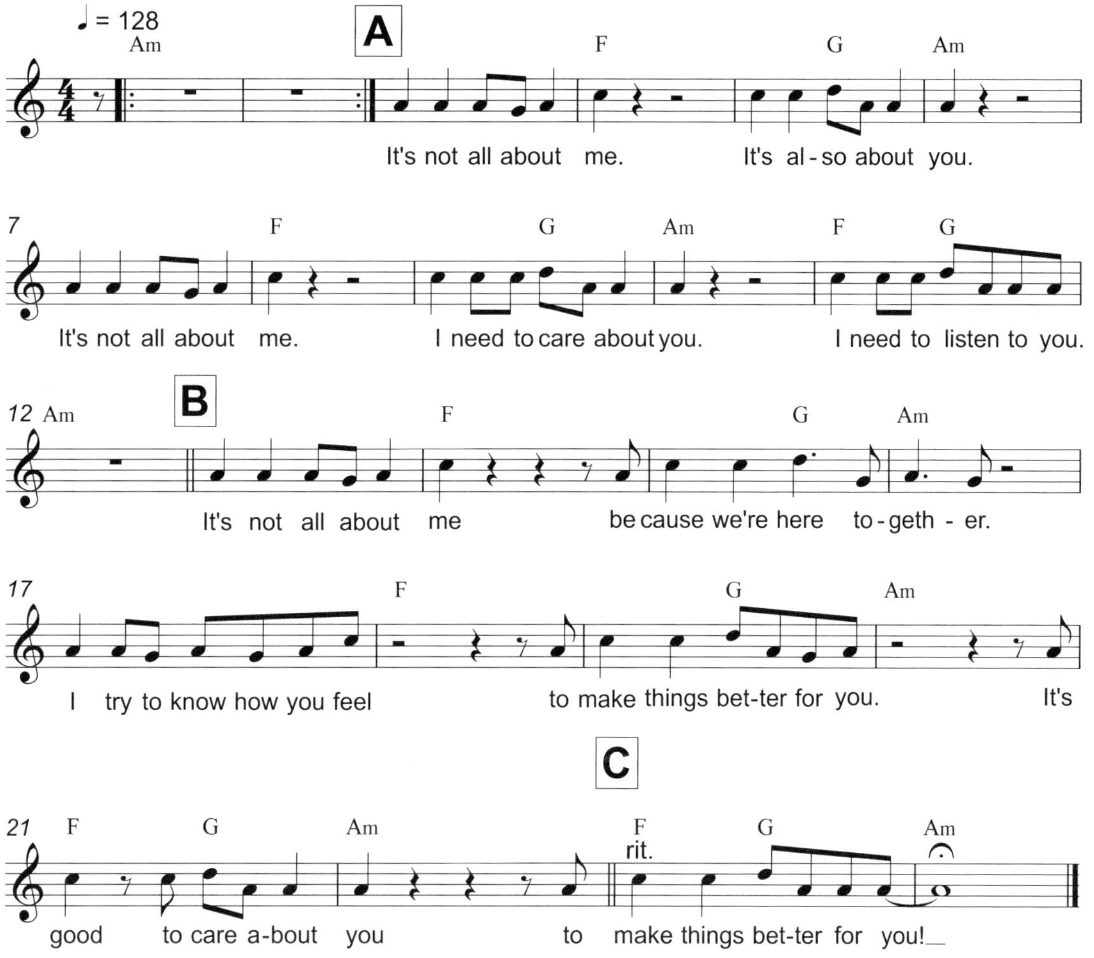

Cooperation's In The Air

Herb Hein

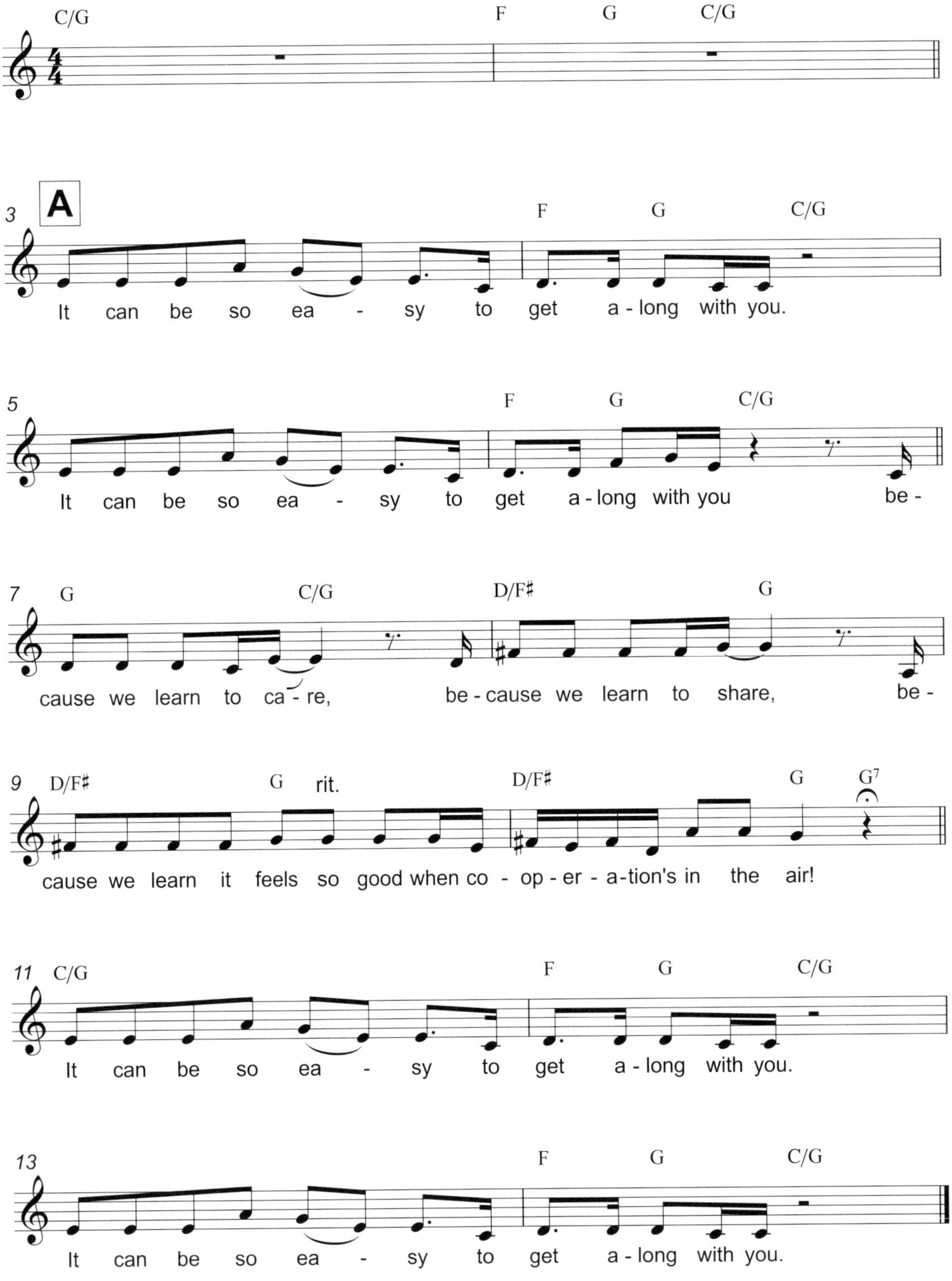

You Are A Friend of Mine

Herb Hein

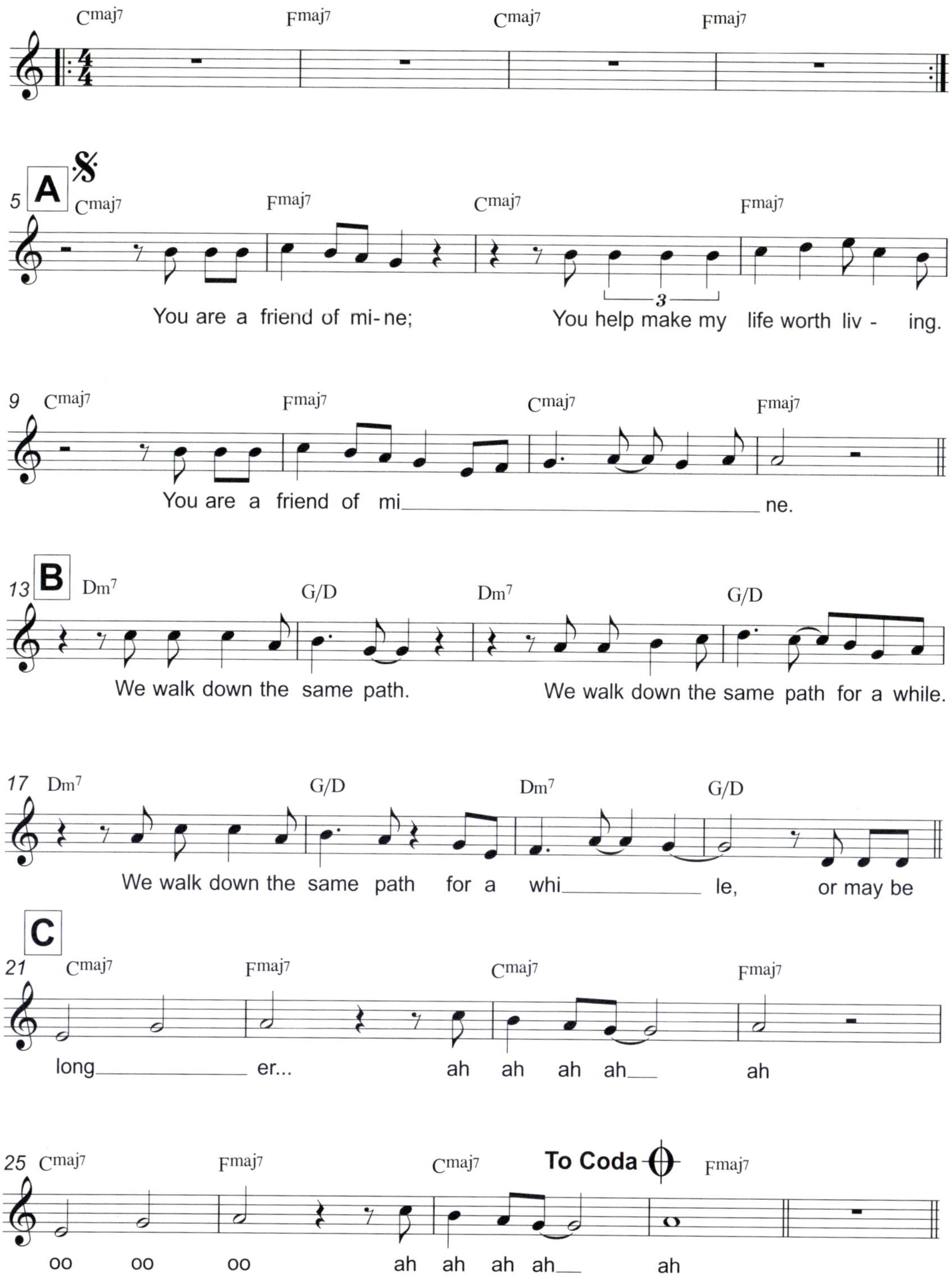

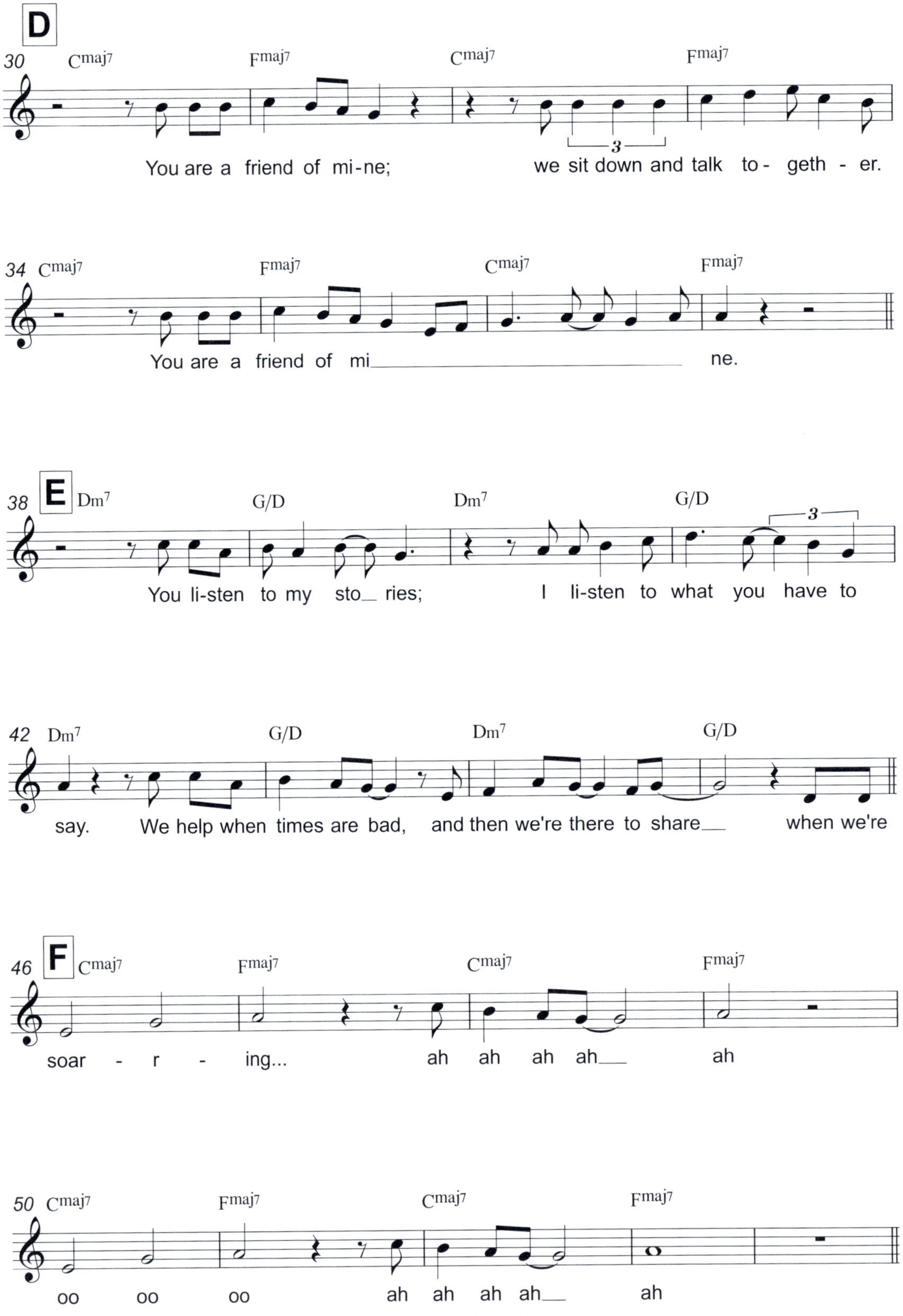
D
30 Cmaj7 Fmaj7 Cmaj7 Fmaj7
You are a friend of mi-ne; we sit down and talk to- geth - er.
34 Cmaj7 Fmaj7 Cmaj7 Fmaj7
You are a friend of mi ne.
38 E Dm7 G/D Dm7 G/D
You li-sten to my sto ries; I li-sten to what you have to
42 Dm7 G/D Dm7 G/D
say. We help when times are bad, and then we're there to share when we're
46 F Cmaj7 Fmaj7 Cmaj7 Fmaj7
soar - r - ing... ah ah ah ah ah
50 Cmaj7 Fmaj7 Cmaj7 Fmaj7
oo oo oo ah ah ah ah ah

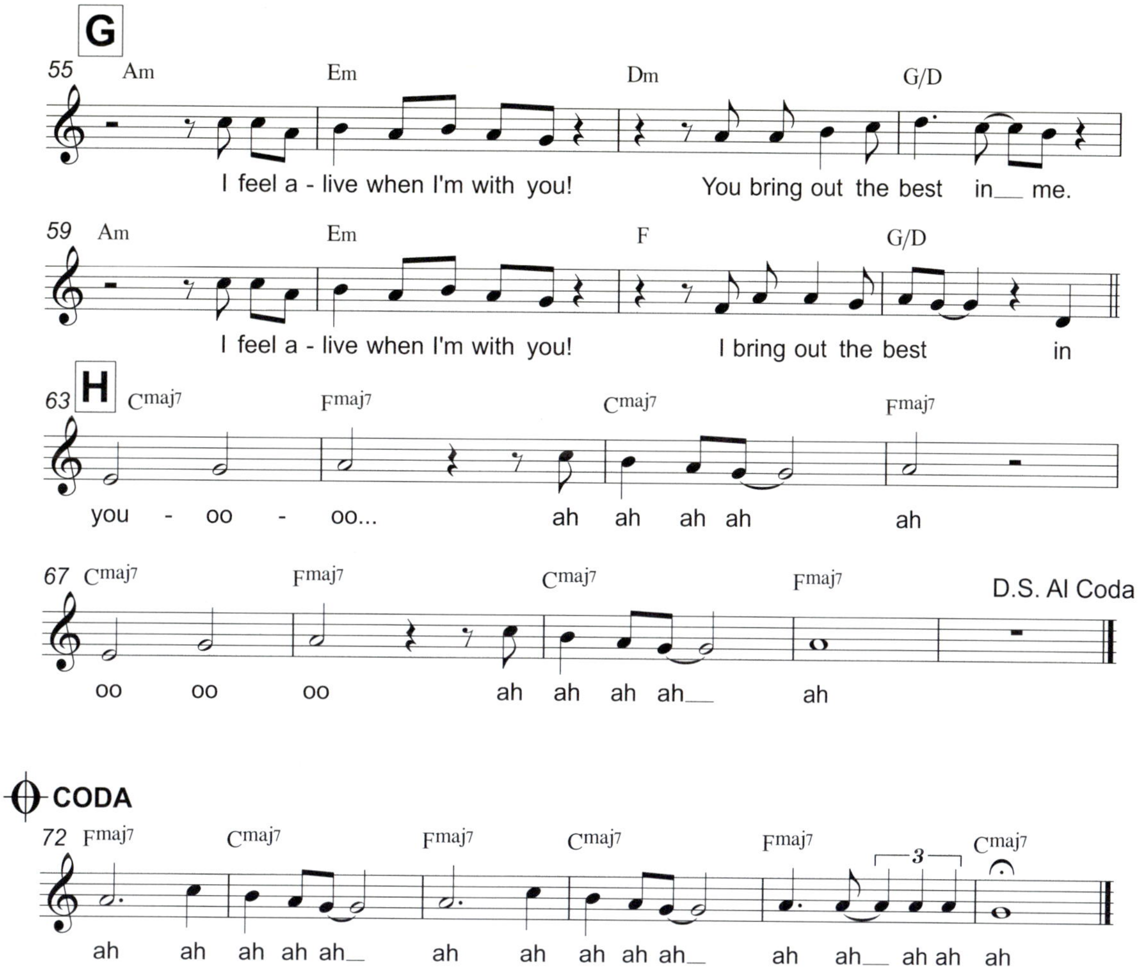
G
55 Am Em Dm G/D
I feel a - live when I'm with you! You bring out the best in__ me.
59 Am Em F G/D
I feel a - live when I'm with you! I bring out the best in
63 H Cmaj7 Fmaj7 Cmaj7 Fmaj7
you - oo - oo... ah ah ah ah ah
67 Cmaj7 Fmaj7 Cmaj7 Fmaj7
D.S. Al Coda
oo oo oo ah ah ah ah__ ah
CODA
72 Fmaj7 Cmaj7 Fmaj7 Cmaj7 Fmaj7 Cmaj7
3
ah ah ah ah ah__ ah ah ah ah ah__ ah ah__ ah ah ah

Made in the USA
Las Vegas, NV
03 November 2026

57424116R00295